HEALTH CARE ISSUES, COSTS AND ACCESS

MEDICAID AND TREATMENT FOR PEOPLE WITH SUBSTANCE ABUSE PROBLEMS

HEALTH CARE ISSUES, COSTS AND ACCESS

Additional books in this series can be found on Nova's website under the Series tab.

Additional E-books in this series can be found on Nova's website under the E-books tab.

HEALTH CARE ISSUES, COSTS AND ACCESS

MEDICAID AND TREATMENT FOR PEOPLE WITH SUBSTANCE ABUSE PROBLEMS

BENTSON H. MCFARLAND
DENNIS MCCARTY
AND
ANNE E. KOVAS
EDITORS

Nova Science Publishers, Inc.
New York

For permission to use material from this book please contact us:
Telephone 631-231-7269; Fax 631-231-8175
Web Site: http://www.novapublishers.com

Library of Congress Cataloging-in-Publication Data

Medicaid and treatment for people with substance abuse problems / [edited by] Bentson H. McFarland, Dennis McCarty, and Anne E. Kovas.
p. ; cm.
Includes bibliographical references and index.
ISBN 978-1-61470-742-4 (softcover)
1. Substance abuse--Treatment--Economic aspects--United States. 2. Medicaid. I. McFarland, Bentson H. II. McCarty, Dennis, Ph.D. III. Kovas, Anne E.
[DNLM: 1. Medicaid--economics. 2. Health Services Accessibility--United States. 3. Managed Care Programs--economics--United States. 4. Mental Health Services--economics--United States. 5. Substance-Related Disorders--therapy--United States. W 250 AA1 M377 2010]
HV4998.M47 2010
362.29'182--dc22
2010015617

Published by Nova Science Publishers, Inc. † New York

CONTENTS

PREFACE

People with substance abuse problems often depend on Medicaid to pay for treatment. Health Care Reform, as specified in the Patient Protection and Affordable Care Act of 2010, will increase the importance of Medicaid as a payment system for chemical dependency care. Now entering its second 50 years, Medicaid is a unique partnership of federal and state agencies financing health care services for low income people. This book is an invaluable resource for patients, family members, clinicians, administrators, and policy-makers concerned about ways to pay for addiction treatment. Written by national experts, the book summarizes the provisions of Medicaid of most relevance to substance abuse treatment, reviews the pertinent history of this complex and ever changing program, and describes key findings from numerous "natural experiments" such as the implementation of Medicaid managed behavioral health care as well as cutbacks in Medicaid coverage. The book is a convenient resource for students in health care professions learning about Medicaid as well as for administrators interested in optimizing provision of care for people with substance abuse problems. Legislators, too, will find that the book documents numerous lessons learned over the last two decades of rapid change in Medicaid.

Chapter 1- Substance abuse is a major public health problem. For example, Kessler et al. (2005) reported that some 15 percent of adults in the United States satisfied lifetime diagnostic criteria for substance use disorder. Medicaid clients are more likely than people with other types of insurance to have chemical dependency problems (Adelmann, 2003). Fortunately, numerous effective treatments are available (see, *e.g.,* Center for Substance Abuse Treatment, 2007; Hester and Miller, 2003). Of course, someone must pay for treatment to be provided.

As it happens, Medicaid is now a major payer for substance abuse treatment services. Mark et al. (2007) found that Medicaid paid for some 18 percent of substance abuse treatment in 2003. Medicaid's share of substance abuse treatment payments nearly doubled from ten percent in 1986 (Mark et al., 2007). At the moment, Medicaid exceeds the Federal substance abuse block grant program in funding for chemical dependency treatment and is itself exceeded only by state and local payments (Mark et al., 2007). Interestingly, Medicaid's share of substance abuse spending now slightly exceeds its 17 percent share of total health care expenditures (Mark et al., 2007). Levit et al. (2008) projected that by 2014 Medicaid will account for some 20 percent of spending on substance abuse treatment. Doubtless the role of Medicaid will become even greater than anticipated thanks to the Patient Protection and Affordable Care Act of 2010.

Chapter 2- Now in its fifth decade, Medicaid is a joint federal-state program with numerous variations and complications. This flexibility allows states to develop programs and funding streams that may be of particular benefit to Medicaid clients with substance abuse problems. This chapter reviews prominent features of Medicaid in the context of chemical dependency treatment program development and financing. The chapter summarizes options available to states within the Medicaid program that can be used to finance addiction treatment. Especially pertinent are the Rehabilitation and Clinic Options; the Early and Periodic Screening, Detection and Treatment program; and the several types of Medicaid waivers. Also relevant are provisions within the Temporary Assistance to Needy Families program. States are encouraged to explore these options with a view to provision of substance abuse treatment services for Medicaid clients.

Chapter 3- Maintenance of insurance coverage is a key concern for Medicaid clients. As discussed in this and later chapters, changes in Medicaid programs have often increased the "churn" of clients into and out of health insurance. Concerns have arisen that loss of coverage may impede utilization of substance abuse treatment by Medicaid clients with chemical dependency problems. This chapter makes the point that substance abuse treatment is delivered in several venues. Service settings include both "specialty" (substance abuse care only) and "non-specialty" (such as medical or mental health care) programs. Impact of Medicaid loss on addiction care utilization appears to differ depending on the setting. The chapter suggests that loss of Medicaid need not decrease use of specialty chemical dependency treatment – perhaps because federal block grant funds make addiction care services available to those who have lost coverage. On the other hand, this work also indicates that loss of Medicaid may substantially decrease use of non-specialty addiction care services. Because non-specialty chemical dependency treatment is notably important, policy-makers would do well to ensure continuous insurance coverage for Medicaid clients with substance abuse problems.

Chapter 4- This chapter summarizes years of substantial change as Medicaid moved largely from fee for service to a managed care environment. Numerous questions have arisen regarding this momentous shift. In particular, it has been suggested that managed care provided incentives for providers to "cherry pick" clients with low substance abuse severity. Beginning with definitions of substance abuse treatment and managed care, the chapter provides detailed historical information on a state-by-state and year-by-year basis regarding the movement away from Medicaid fee for service and towards assorted managed care programs. States adopted numerous Medicaid innovations chiefly via various waiver mechanisms. The chapter provides comprehensive listings in text and tables showing these transitions with emphasis on changes pertinent to chemical dependency care. Building on this carefully assembled (and unlikely to be found elsewhere) record, the chapter examines impact of managed care transition on severity of Medicaid clients in treatment for substance abuse. Using hierarchical linear models, it is concluded that Medicaid managed care led, if anything, to slight increase in severity of substance abuse treatment clients.

Chapter 5- Adolescents are substantially over-represented in Medicaid but little is known about substance abuse treatment for this population. In 1997, the federal Substance Abuse and Mental Health Services Administration (SAMHSA) funded the Human Services Research Institute to conduct a multi-site study examining the impact of managed care on the services received and outcomes achieved for adolescents with substance abuse disorders in managed care and fee for service environments. Study sites included Massachusetts, New York,

Oregon, Pennsylvania, Puerto Rico, Tennessee, and Washington state. Interviews were completed for 1,568 youth at treatment entry. Follow-up interviews were conducted after six months. Administrative data on treatment utilization also were analyzed. This chapter summarizes the methods and results of this large study. Implementation of managed care varied substantially by site with numerous mechanisms involved. There were few if any differences by managed care versus fee for service on the self-report measures. Administrative data showed complex patterns of utilization changes during the study period. While not obviously detrimental to young Medicaid clients in treatment for substance abuse problems, managed care apparently did little if anything to improve outcomes for this population.

Chapter 6- Medicaid managed care and drug courts both grew dramatically during the 1990s. Yet heretofore there has been little or no evaluation of potential impact of Medicaid managed care on drug court participants. This chapter defines drug court, briefly reviews the history of this innovation, and describes one of earliest of such programs. The chapter reviews development of Medicaid managed care in Oregon and shows how there might be impact of Medicaid managed care on substance abuse treatment services for drug court participants. Using before versus after (Medicaid managed care) analyses the project described here tested hypotheses about possible managed care influences on drug court participants. Study subjects included individuals eligible for (but not necessarily participants in) drug court before versus after Medicaid managed care. Under managed care, less time was invested in treatment, especially for participants who chose but did not complete the drug court program. However, there were no more drug court program failures in the managed care period. Moreover, managed care had no effect on measures of recidivism, such as survival time to first arrest and days in the community for drug court participants. Analyses focused on Medicaid eligible drug court participants suggested, overall, that managed care had no impact on this group's numbers of arrests during follow-up, time to first follow-up arrest, or days in the community during follow-up. In summary, implementation of Medicaid managed care appeared not to be detrimental for drug court participants.

Chapter 7- Medicaid clients (and especially clients with substance abuse problems) are often served by multiple agencies. Research and evaluation can be challenged by the need to link data generated by numerous administrative systems. Medicaid clients involved with the criminal justice system may be especially difficult for data linkage owing to numerous identities. This chapter describes methods used to verify matches pertaining to individuals eligible for drug court. Subjects were identified for the drug court and Medicaid managed care research project described in a previous chapter. Especially helpful were flow charts showing (a) the routes of individuals as they made contact with several agencies and (b) the creation of data elements describing those individuals by the numerous organizations. Building on this background, the chapter discusses matching problems as well as the several uncertainties that can arise. Case examples are provided showing results of assorted decisions made about possible linkages. Of some 2,153 potential cases, automated matching software would have retained only about 1,500 matched cases and many of those retained would have lacked demographic and-or service utilization data. Conversely, using manual methods, 214 potential cases were deleted chiefly due to the research project's inclusion and exclusion criteria. Only about 30 potential cases were deleted because of irresolvable data problems. Ultimately, some 1,939 subjects were deemed valid unique cases along with much of their identifying, demographic, and service utilization data. The manual linkage procedures decreased sampling error substantially which increased precision of the research project's data analyses.

Chapter 8- This chapter describes a series of studies examining three facets of methadone maintenance treatment (MMT): access to care, retention in treatment, and outcomes. The work takes advantage of similarities and differences in MMT for the adjoining states of Oregon and Washington. Regarding access, much of the attention in prior research has focused on demonstrating the efficacy of methadone for treating opiate dependence. Very little, if any, research has been conducted on factors that influence access to care. This chapter addresses both systemic influences and client characteristics that predispose to use of services, reflect the need for services, or enable access to care. While MMT is usually considered a long-term form of substance abuse treatment, state systems differ in the typical duration of treatment. Although many previous studies have measured retention, few have examined the impact of Medicaid managed care. This chapter compares retention in a Medicaid managed care state with that in a fee for service state. Turning to outcomes, studies have shown a link between opiate use and crime and suggested that treatment for opiate addiction can reduce criminal activity. However, past studies have generally been short term. The project reported in this chapter followed the arrest history of clients for three years from an initial admission to MMT to take a unique look at the impact of treatment. In general, MMT access was strongly influenced by systemic factors such as geographic proximity to a treatment program as well as capacity. Medicaid coverage also predicted MMT access whereas Medicaid managed care *per se* had little or no impact. Retention in MMT was also strongly influenced by Medicaid coverage. Treatment duration (retention) was longer in Oregon (Medicaid managed care) than in Washington state (fee for service Medicaid). Provider practices (such as administrative discharges which were much less likely in Oregon versus Washington) also appeared to influence retention. Arrests were strongly related to time in MMT but especially so for clients with stable treatment patterns. Multi-level models suggested that long term (over 12 months) MMT retention led to greater than expected reduction in arrests.

Chapter 9- Medicaid clients with co-occurring mental health and substance abuse problems comprise substantial portions of the clienteles served by public sector mental health and chemical dependency treatment systems. However, little is known about implications of managed care for "dual diagnosis" Medicaid clients. This prospective study conducted in eight states used interviews to examine managed care impact on use of mental health services by adult Medicaid clients in treatment for substance abuse (N = 2,424) and on use of chemical dependency services by Medicaid clients with severe mental illness (N = 2,318). Compared with fee for service, managed care had no impact on use of mental health services by clients entering substance abuse treatment. Conversely, there was an apparent 26% reduction in substance abuse treatment ($p < .02$) among managed care (versus fee for service) Medicaid clients with severe mental illness. Managed care impact may vary among Medicaid sub-groups.

Chapter 10- During the early 1990s Oregon dramatically expanded its Medicaid population through a series of federal waivers under a program known as the Oregon Health Plan (OHP). In 2002, the state split the Medicaid population into OHP Plus (traditional mandatory Medicaid-eligible persons), and OHP Standard (the expansion clients). Late in 2002 in response to a substantial budget shortfall, the Oregon legislature eliminated substance abuse, mental health, and dental benefits from OHP Standard coverage effective March 2003,

Coverage for these services remained for the OHP Plus population. This chapter examines the impact of these Medicaid cutbacks. In brief, the benefit cutbacks led to dramatic reduction in the number of OHP Standard clients enrolled in Medicaid. Moreover, of those who remained enrolled, relatively few accessed substance abuse or mental health outpatient treatment while those services were not covered. Enrollment as well as use of mental health and substance abuse services by traditional Medicaid (OHP Plus) clients showed little change. Providers also felt the impact of cutbacks as agencies closed or dramatically reduced services. Medicaid cutbacks for substance abuse and mental health treatment can have substantial impact.

Chapter 11- Cutbacks may differentially affect sub-groups within the Medicaid population. This chapter summarizes 2005 survey data from Oregon Health Plan members including both traditional Medicaid and expansion population clients. The statewide sample was augmented by clients currently in substance abuse treatment who had been Medicaid beneficiaries prior to the 2003 benefit cuts. Among those who had experienced or expressed need for substance abuse or mental health treatment there was no apparent decline in access to behavioral health care for either expansion or traditional Medicaid clients following benefit elimination in 2003. There was also no increase in access following restoration of the benefit in 2004. Clients who were receiving substance abuse or mental health treatment prior to the elimination of these benefits were significantly more likely to maintain access to care following the policy changes than were those who were in need but were not already in treatment prior to the policy change. These results are in marked contrast to the overall declines in behavioral health treatment shown by Oregon Medicaid population data as well as the decreases for Oregon methadone maintenance clients reported in previous chapters. On the other hand, the Oregon data reported here echo findings from California in an early chapter suggesting that at least some Medicaid clients in substance abuse treatment are able to continue care even in the absence of insurance coverage. An important message is that Medicaid policy changes can have assorted and widespread impacts.

Chapter 12- This chapter describes cutbacks in the Oregon Health Plan and the effects of those Medicaid reductions at three distinct levels: individuals' access to substance abuse treatment, the substance abuse delivery system in Oregon, and Oregon's emergency departments. Data from several studies are examined to describe the impacts of major changes to the Oregon Health Plan's Standard (Medicaid expansion) program in early 2003 – particularly the increased cost sharing measures and coverage reduction including outpatient mental health and chemical dependency benefit cutbacks. The preponderance of evidence from these studies suggests that the impacts of program changes were felt profoundly by the individuals enrolled in OHP, by the clinics and treatment centers that form Oregon's substance abuse care delivery system, and in Oregon's emergency departments.

Chapter 13- States often use capitated payment systems when purchasing health and behavioral health care for Medicaid clients. In capitated (prospective) payment programs, the payer sets payment rates for a future time period. A central problem in the development of Medicaid payment systems is that health plans may attempt to avoid enrolling people who are expected to be costly. In particular, because people with substance abuse may be high utilizers of services, health plans paid through capitation may try to avoid such enrollees — either by not enrolling such persons or by not providing access to high-quality substance abuse care. Risk-adjusted payments may improve this situation by reimbursing health plans based on the expected medical need of actual enrolled populations, rather than on the average community risk. However, risk-adjustment systems that only account for demographics and diagnoses are limited in their ability to reduce health plans' incentives to avoid covering people with substance abuse problems under capitation. Another challenge for risk-adjustment is the transient nature of Medicaid enrollment. Most of the literature on risk adjustment for persons with substance abuse problems includes only people who maintain continuous enrollment over the study period. This chapter reports on several risk-adjustment models focused on Oregon Medicaid clients involved with substance abuse treatment in a large health maintenance organization. Models were designed to predict substance abuse treatment expenditures or total health plan costs. Risk-adjustment models that incorporated new variables such as social, clinical, and Medicaid eligibility indicators predicted substance abuse and total health plan expenditures somewhat better than simpler models typical of current risk-adjustment systems. However, models predicting substance abuse expenditures still performed very poorly and explained no more than 11% of the variation in expenditures. On the other hand, models for total health plan expenditures performed better, explaining as much as 35% of variation in expenditures. Although addition of new variables improved prediction modestly, payments would likely be quite inaccurate in some cases. Risk adjustment for capitated Medicaid substance abuse care remains challenging.

Chapter 14- States often use Medicaid as part of innovative strategies to finance publicly funded services for treatment of alcohol and drug dependence. Interviews with officials from eleven states provide case studies and examples of financing innovations. Four management tools (memoranda of understanding, cost-savings analysis, utilization management, and coordinated purchase) and four management strategies (delegated management, dedicated funding, optimization of federal funds, and blended/braided funding) are identified and discussed. Examples from the interviewed states provide concrete illustrations of how these tools and strategies were combined to improve access to alcohol and drug abuse treatment.

Chapter 15- Medicaid has changed continuously since its inception nearly 50 years ago. Major developments of the past two decades include the conversion from Aid to Families with Dependent Children to Temporary Assistance for Needy Families (which affected all states), the switch from fee for service to assorted varieties of Medicaid managed care (which affected most states), expansion and contraction cycles in Medicaid eligibility (which affected many if not most states), and increase in Medicaid as a payer for substance abuse treatment services (which also affected many if not most states). Evaluations of these numerous alterations have, not surprisingly, shown assorted results of interest to people with substance abuse problems, to providers, and to policy makers.

As several chapters in this volume indicate, at least some individuals engaged in specialty sector substance abuse treatment manage to remain in care despite vicissitudes of Medicaid eligibility. But other chapters show that shrinkage of Medicaid eligibility criteria may preclude individuals from entering specialty substance abuse treatment and may adversely affect chemical dependency services delivered in general health care or in mental health care settings. Moreover, sub-groups of Medicaid clients such as persons involved with methadone maintenance treatment may be especially vulnerable to loss of Medicaid coverage.

In: Medicaid and Treatment for People… ISBN 978-1-61470-742-4
Editors: B. H. McFarland, D. McCarty, et al., pp. 1-5

Chapter 1

Introduction: Medicaid and Medicaid Coverage for Treatment of Alcohol and Drug Disorders

Bentson H. McFarland[1] and Dennis McCarty[2]
[1] Departments of Psychiatry and Public Health and Preventive Medicine, Oregon Health and Science University, Portland, OR, USA
[2] Department of Public Health and Preventive Medicine, Oregon Health and Science University, Portland, OR, USA

Substance abuse is a major public health problem. For example, Kessler et al. (2005) reported that some 15 percent of adults in the United States satisfied lifetime diagnostic criteria for substance use disorder. Medicaid clients are more likely than people with other types of insurance to have chemical dependency problems (Adelmann, 2003). Fortunately, numerous effective treatments are available (see, *e.g.,* Center for Substance Abuse Treatment, 2007; Hester and Miller, 2003). Of course, someone must pay for treatment to be provided.

As it happens, Medicaid is now a major payer for substance abuse treatment services. Mark et al. (2007) found that Medicaid paid for some 18 percent of substance abuse treatment in 2003. Medicaid's share of substance abuse treatment payments nearly doubled from ten percent in 1986 (Mark et al., 2007). At the moment, Medicaid exceeds the Federal substance abuse block grant program in funding for chemical dependency treatment and is itself exceeded only by state and local payments (Mark et al., 2007). Interestingly, Medicaid's share of substance abuse spending now slightly exceeds its 17 percent share of total health care expenditures (Mark et al., 2007). Levit et al. (2008) projected that by 2014 Medicaid will account for some 20 percent of spending on substance abuse treatment. Doubtless the role of Medicaid will become even greater than anticipated thanks to the Patient Protection and Affordable Care Act of 2010.

Consequently, it is important to understand substance abuse issues experienced by Medicaid clients. It is equally important to understand the complexities of Medicaid itself. The chapter by Lanahan et al. reviews the origins of Medicaid and addresses the numerous variations in this joint-federal state program pertinent to the provision of services for clients with substance abuse problems.

A major change for this population occurred in conjunction with the conversion from the former Aid to Families with Dependent Children (AFDC) to the current Temporary Assistance for Needy Families (TANF) system during the 1990s (Morgenstern et al., 2009). The chapter by Schmidt et al. describes substance use by Medicaid clients and the use of services by this population (with and without continuous Medicaid coverage) during that time.

Medicaid itself has also changed markedly from its beginnings some 50 years ago as a joint federal-state program intended to fund medical care for the poor. The chapter by Penner et al. reviews Medicaid's conversion from fee to service to managed care with regard to coverage for substance abuse treatment programs and addresses implications for the populations served by chemical dependency care systems.

In fact, Medicaid now serves numerous populations. The chapter by Hughes et al. addresses adolescent Medicaid substance abuse treatment clients, while Bigelow et al. focus on Medicaid and offenders eligible for drug court. Deck examines Medicaid and methadone maintenance programs. A common factor is use of multiple service systems by Medicaid clients with substance abuse problems. Cox and Bigelow show the complexities involved in data linkage procedures designed to give a comprehensive picture of such service utilization. Gabriel et al. address Medicaid services for people with co-occurring mental health and substance abuse problems.

The current financial crisis raises numerous questions about Medicaid retrenchment. As it happens, Oregon has already experienced substantial cutbacks in Medicaid. The chapters by Deck et al., Gabriel et al., and Carlson et al. address several impacts of Medicaid cutbacks on people with substance abuse problems and on the health care and behavioral health care treatment systems.

Looking to the future, it is highly likely that many if not most Medicaid programs providing substance abuse treatment will operate via capitated payment systems (Mangione and Ridgely, 2006). Therefore, Lynch et al. address the challenges in setting capitated payment rates for this population. McCarty et al. summarize administrative and financing strategies that states can employ to enhance substance abuse services via the Medicaid program.

What might be expected of Medicaid in the future and how might this program improve services for clients with substance abuse problems? While forecasting is always perilous, for good or ill some trends seem clear.

First, Medicaid is likely to remain a substantial part of the so-called health care "system" in the United States (Rosenbaum, 2009). The Patient Protection and Affordable Care Act of 2010 notwithstanding, the chaotic, confusing, costly, and perhaps counter-productive collections of "programs" that constitute health care in the United States are unlikely to experience notable change any time soon. While there will doubtless be tinkering and tweaking, this peculiar institution can be expected to persist. This prediction is unsurprising as the federal government in the United States was designed explicitly to resist change. Lacking political leadership of sufficient stature to overcome this structural impediment, Medicaid will continue for decades.

Second, Medicaid's heterogeneity is also likely to persist indefinitely. As noted by Penner et al., Medicaid now varies markedly from state to state and even within states.

Moreover, states (and entities within states) have devised, implemented, and then discontinued numerous Medicaid programs (including those focused on clients with substance abuse problems). Over the last several years, states have obtained considerable authority to shape their Medicaid systems. It is unlikely that states will give up this power. Consequently, Medicaid can be expected to vary substantially in both space and time. In 1932, Justice Louis Brandeis referred to the states as "laboratories of democracy" in the *New State Ice Company versus Liebmann* case (285 U.S. 262, 311). As they manipulate their Medicaid programs, state legislators are conducting complex experiments that, in an academic context, would be unlikely to receive Institutional Review Board approval. This variation will likely continue.

Third, Medicaid programs (and especially those for people with substance abuse problems) will often find themselves under pressure with regard to finances. As in much of health care in the United States, Medicaid financing is irrational. During difficult economic times, Medicaid enrollment rises along with unemployment while state revenues decline (Smith et al., 2009). Not infrequently, Medicaid may be the largest item in state budgets. Legislators find themselves forced to choose between Medicaid and other state services such as education. Not surprisingly, Medicaid programs for clients with substance abuse may well be imperiled.

Given these likely trends, what can be recommended for the next 50 years of Medicaid in relation to treatment for people with substance abuse problems? Hopefully, more than minimal attention will be paid to the numerous chemical dependency prevention programs believed to be effective (Robertson et al., 2003). Nonetheless, addiction will presumably persist in the Medicaid population. What improvements in Medicaid might be both feasible and worthwhile for people with substance abuse? While large scale change is unlikely, incremental enhancement is not impossible.

Indeed, some changes might be implemented relatively easily. For one example, Medicaid could support provision of substance abuse treatment services via the Internet. For another example, Medicaid financing and organization could be structured so as to facilitate connections among substance abuse treatment, mental health treatment, and primary care perhaps via electronic health record systems.

It would also be straightforward to enhance Medicaid program evaluation. For example, state reports to federal agencies on Medicaid programs could be standardized so that interventions are described. In addition, data collection could be improved. The National Survey on Drug Use and Health (NSDUH) could be enhanced to over-sample Medicaid clients whose state of residence would be made known to researchers. Medicaid coverage could become a required Treatment Episode Data Set (TEDS) reporting item. Medicaid client counts could be included in the National Survey of Substance Abuse Treatment Services (N-SSATS).

As science and technology develop, substance abuse treatment may become influenced by genetics (especially pharmaco-genetics), epigenetics, proteomics, and imaging (especially for prediction of relapse). Substance abuse treatment may thereby become tailored to the individual. Medicaid might well be called upon to finance such presumably expensive but hopefully useful approaches. This book provides numerous models for the evaluation of new programs designed to benefit Medicaid clients with substance abuse problems.

Acknowledgment

This book was made possible by generous support from several agencies including the National Institute on Alcohol Abuse and Alcoholism (grants K02 AA000281 and R21 AA014050) and the National Institute on Drug Abuse (grant R01 DA013091) at the National Institutes of Health as well as the Robert Wood Johnson Foundation Substance Abuse Policy Research Program and the Substance Abuse and Mental Health Services Administration.

References

Adelmann, P. (2003). Mental and substance abuse disorders among Medicaid recipients: Prevalence estimates from two national surveys. *Administration and Policy in Mental Health,* 31, 111-129.

Center for Substance Abuse Treatment (2007). *Understanding Evidence-Based Practices for Co-occurring Disorders. Co-occurring Center of Excellence Overview Paper 5.* DHHS Publication Number (SMA) 07-4278. Rockville, MD: Substance Abuse and Mental Health Services Administration.

Hester, R. K., and Miller, W.R. (2003). *Handbook of Alcoholism Treatment Approaches: Effective Alternatives*, third edition. Boston, MA: Allyn and Bacon.

Kessler, R. C., Chiu, W. T., Demler, O., Merikangas, K. R., and Walters, E. E. (2005). Prevalence, severity, and comorbidity of 12-month DSM-IV disorders in the National Comorbidity Survey Replication. *Archives of General Psychiatry, 62,* 617-627.

Levit, K. R., Kassed, C. A., Coffey, R. M., Mark, T. L., Stranges, E. M., Buck, J. A., and Vandivort-Warren, R. (2008). Future funding for mental health and substance abuse: Increasing burdens for the public sector. *Health Affairs (Millwood)* web exclusive, w513-w522 (7 October 2008).

Mangione, M., and Ridgely, M. S. (2006). Is conventional wisdom wrong? Coverage for substance abuse treatment under Medicaid managed care. *Journal of Substance Abuse Treatment*, 30, 285-290.

Mark, T. L., Levit, K. R., Vandivort-Warren, R., Coffey, R. M., Buck, J. A., and SAMHSA Spending Estimates Team. (2007). Trends in spending for substance abuse treatment, 1986-2003. *Health Affairs (Millwood), 26,* 1118-1128.

Morgenstern, J., Neighbors, C.J., Kuerbis, A., Riordan, A., Blanchard, K.A., McVeigh, K.H., Morgan, T.J., and McCrady, B. (2009). Improving 24-month abstinence and employment outcomes for substance-dependent women receiving Temporary Assistance for Needy Families with intensive case management. *American Journal of Public Health*, 99, 328-333.

Robertson, E.B., David, S.L., and Rao, S.A. (2003). *Preventing Drug Use among Children and Adolescents: A Research-Based Guide for Parents, Educators, and Community Leaders, second edition.* National Institutes of Health Publication Number 04-4212(A). Bethesda, MD: National Institute on Drug Abuse, National Institutes of Health.

Rosenbaum, S. (2009). Medicaid and national health care reform. *New England Journal of Medicine,* 361, 2009-2012.

Smith, V.K., Gifford, K., Ellis, E., Rudowitz, R., O'Malley-Watts, M., and Marks, C. (2009). *The crunch continues: Medicaid spending, coverage and policy in the midst of a recession. Results from a 50-state Medicaid budget survey for state fiscal years 2009 and 2010.* Washington, DC: Kaiser Commission on Medicaid and the Uninsured.

In: Medicaid and Treatment for People… ISBN 978-1-61470-742-4
Editors: B. H. McFarland, D. McCarty, et al., pp.7-16

Chapter 2

Overview of Medicaid and Substance Abuse Treatment

***Patrick M. Lanahan*[1], *Alicia D. Smith*[2], *John O'Brien*[3], and *Dennis McCarty*[4]**

[1] Ohio Department of Mental Retardation and Developmental Disabilities, Columbus, OH, USA
[2] Alicia Smith and Associates, LLC, Washington, DC, USA
[3] The Technical Assistance Collaborative, Boston, MA, USA
[4] Department of Public Health and Preventive Medicine, Oregon Health and Science University, Portland, OR, USA

Abstract

Now in its fifth decade, Medicaid is a joint federal-state program with numerous variations and complications. This flexibility allows states to develop programs and funding streams that may be of particular benefit to Medicaid clients with substance abuse problems. This chapter reviews prominent features of Medicaid in the context of chemical dependency treatment program development and financing. The chapter summarizes options available to states within the Medicaid program that can be used to finance addiction treatment. Especially pertinent are the Rehabilitation and Clinic Options; the Early and Periodic Screening, Detection and Treatment program; and the several types of Medicaid waivers. Also relevant are provisions within the Temporary Assistance to Needy Families program. States are encouraged to explore these options with a view to provision of substance abuse treatment services for Medicaid clients.

Introduction

Medicaid is the primary program providing health care and long-term care coverage for low income children, women and men in the United States. For example, during Federal Fiscal Year 2003, almost 52 million individuals received more than $233 billion in health care services (Centers for Medicare and Medicaid Services, 2003). Medicaid was authorized in 1965 under Title XIX of the Social Security Act (Public Law 89-98); certain groups of individuals (women with children, the blind and other disabled, and the elderly) with incomes below the Federal Poverty Level were categorically eligible for Medicaid and, when enrolled, were entitled to coverage for medically necessary services (U.S. General Accounting Office, 1991). States choosing to participate in the Medicaid program are required to provide federally specified benefits and may elect to provide additional optional benefits. State and federal governments share costs. State "matching" requirements vary depending on the poverty level in the state — richer states pay about 50% of the total costs while the share for the poorest states can be as low as 18%.

Initially the federal regulations that implemented the Medicaid program attempted to limit total costs and discouraged states from shifting health care expenses to the federal government. Program design, therefore, limited required benefits to medically necessary services provided by a hospital, physician, rural health clinic, or a federally qualified health center. Outpatient services, in non-hospital settings, were optional benefits and many states did not exercise the options. Moreover, because there was concern that states would use the program to shift long-term costs for psychiatric illnesses to the federal government, Medicaid payments were prohibited for individuals aged 22 to 64 years if they were residents of institutions for mental diseases (IMDs). That is, states were not allowed to bill Medicaid for any medical costs for individuals being treated in state psychiatric institutions and in facilities with more than 16 beds if more than one-half of the residents had a mental health disorder. Subsequently, the IMD prohibition was interpreted to include residential services for the treatment of alcohol and drug dependence. As a result, required Medicaid coverage for alcohol and drug disorders is limited to hospital-based services (*i.e.,* inpatient detoxification and outpatient services provided in a hospital clinic) and services in federally qualified health centers.

Medicaid laws and regulations do not explicitly include coverage for treatment of alcohol and drug disorders but also do not prohibit coverage (U.S. General Accounting Office, 1991). Publicly funded systems of care for alcohol and drug dependent individuals, however, tend to rely on free-standing residential and outpatient clinics (*i.e.,* programs not affiliated with a hospital or health center). Moreover, services in these programs may be considered social services rather than medical care. As a result, Medicaid initially had relatively little role in supporting treatments for alcohol and drug disorders.

States, however, may elect to expand Medicaid coverage and include benefits for alcohol and drug treatments. With a general understanding of Medicaid regulations and a specific knowledge of Medicaid policies related to payment for services, eligible matching funds as well as other applicable federal regulations and state Medicaid operational policy, states can enhance benefits for alcohol and drug use disorders, increase the number of individuals served and grow the overall capacity of the addiction treatment system.

States typically use three general strategies to provide Medicaid coverage for alcohol and drug treatment:

- Optional Medicaid Rehabilitative Services (Medicaid Rehabilitation Option);
- Optional Medicaid Clinic Services (Medicaid Clinic Option); and
- Early and Periodic Screening, Diagnosis and Treatment (EPSDT).

MEDICAID REHABILITATION OPTION

The Medicaid Rehabilitation Option (42 Code of Federal Regulations 440.130(d)) is the most flexible Medicaid category for coverage of substance abuse treatment services and "includes any medical or remedial services recommended by a physician or other licensed practitioner of the healing arts, within the scope of his practice under State law, for maximum reduction of physical or mental disability and restoration of a recipient to his best possible functional level." Licensed practitioners may include (depending on state licensure regulations) physicians, physician assistants, registered nurses, licensed psychologists, licensed clinical social workers and certified addiction counselors, among others.

Under the Rehabilitation Option, covered services are those that restore basic life skills necessary to function independently in the community, redevelopment of communication and socialization skills, and family education and other family services exclusively related to the treatment or rehabilitation of other covered individuals. Medical necessity for rehabilitative services is based on functional criteria, not just diagnosis (O'Brien and Lanahan, 2001).

The tools needed for implementation of the Rehabilitation Option relate to policy and program development, benefit design, coverage limitations and other activities more commonly associated with defining health benefit package. This particular strategy also requires an analysis of current service utilization and reimbursement data in order to set reimbursement rates, establish service limits, define service authorization requirements, and identify sources of matching funds.

Policy Development - Policy development is an all-inclusive term referring to specifying the program's purpose, eligible consumers, covered services and limitations, reimbursement methodologies and claims processing structures and relationships with corollary services in separate, but similar programs. These are the building blocks for a systems approach to financing.

Service Definitions/Provider Qualifications – Because of the flexibility offered under the Rehabilitation Option, states can specify in service definitions: (1) the community resource(s) used to provide the service (*e.g.,* community based treatment program, school settings or outpatient hospital settings); (2) services delivered by type of practitioner, both licensed and unlicensed; (3) allowable settings in which services can be delivered and (4) the service activities and components in ways to reflect the unique nature of community-based services. Service descriptions can also focus on abstinence, recovery, peer support and clearly differentiate substance abuse treatment from mental health services. States that are seeking to optimize Medicaid reimbursement strive to design their service definitions so that they are the same for Medicaid and non-Medicaid funding sources, to the greatest extent practicable (and taking into account Medicaid non-allowable populations and services).

Development of Medical Necessity Criteria – Medical necessity is generally determined by eligibility for treatment in terms of the American Psychiatric Association Diagnostic and Statistical Manual (*e.g.,* the fourth edition or DSM-IV) or the International Classification of Diseases (*e.g.,* the ninth edition clinical modification or ICD-9 CM) diagnosis categories or specifically defined to include levels of functional impairment. Individualized service plans are also used to establish and document medical necessity as well as authorize actual service units for the consumer. A number of states are using standardized utilization management criteria, such as the American Society of Addiction Medicine (ASAM) levels of care.

Identifying Need and Sources of Matching Funds - Once a benefit package is defined, a state must ensure that its Medicaid and substance abuse public purchasers have sufficient matching funds to enable the federal draw-downs. Identifying the annualized amount of matching funds needed involves examining current patterns of utilization around the same or similar services, for populations likely to meet Medicaid eligibility requirements. Where the state substance abuse authority already has client-level data regarding Medicaid eligibility, this analysis can proceed by looking at the utilization patterns of those consumers. Some states, however, either do not have this data, or are just beginning the process of integrating Medicaid funding into their substance abuse systems. These states can arrive at proxies for Medicaid eligibility by looking at common characteristics in the client database which indicate some likelihood that an individual might qualify for Medicaid. For example, a state could look at women with dependent children under the federal poverty level. The state can also apply epidemiological and incidence and prevalence figures to its client database to estimate potential Medicaid eligibility. Once the potential pool of Medicaid eligibility is established, the state can then model various utilization and price expectations to arrive at an annual figure needed for Medicaid match.

A significant issue for state substance abuse authorities is to retain some control over Medicaid matching funds being used for substance abuse services. Some states indicate that they would be very interested in pursuing Medicaid financing strategies, but fear that they will lose their funds to state Medicaid budgets. Arrangements such as delegated management where the state substance abuse authority retains control over Medicaid matching funds for substance abuse services can mitigate these concerns.

Technical Assistance for Providers and Purchasing Partners - States that have successfully optimized use of the Medicaid Rehabilitation Option for substance abuse services use a variety of technical assistance strategies to enable providers to bill appropriately (and to remove disincentives for billing Medicaid) and to prompt local (county or regional) authorities, where applicable, to plan for and purchase the appropriate amounts of Medicaid eligible services. State staff serve as provider relations staff to interact with specialty system providers by answering their questions about billing, eligibility, rates, electronic claims formats, etc. For example, one state provided specialty addiction providers with simple, easy to use claims software to enable them to submit electronic claims for Medicaid services. It also conducted "mock capitation" studies based on converting current levels of local area Medicaid expenditures to "per member per month" allocations, stratifying these results by county, and used the results to identify low-billing areas of the state. This type of "profiling" encouraged the state's local partners to close some of these Medicaid utilization gaps, which resulted in additional federal revenue system-wide. States also conduct frequent statewide or regional meetings with providers and local purchasing partners in order to keep Medicaid reimbursability "on the radar screen." These states have learned that using Medicaid to increase resources to the public substance abuse system is accomplished one recipient, one provider, one service, and one claim at a time. It is the cumulative effect of these Medicaid expenditures that then result in funding growth for the whole system.

Medicaid Clinic Option

Medicaid clinic option services are described in 42 Code of Federal Regulations 440.90: "Clinic services means preventive, diagnostic, therapeutic, rehabilitative, or palliative services that are furnished by a facility that is not part of a hospital but is organized and operated to provide medical care to outpatients. The term includes the following services furnished to outpatients: (a) Services furnished at the clinic by or under the direction of a physician or dentist (b) Services furnished outside the clinic, by clinic personnel under the direction of a physician, to an eligible individual who does not reside in a permanent dwelling or does not have a fixed home or mailing address."

While the clinic option permits the provision of non-hospital based community services, the services arranged under the Medicaid clinic option must be rendered on-site "in the clinic" and must be under the direction of a physician (except for homeless individuals). Many public substance abuse treatment services are provided without the involvement of a physician, and may be provided in the client's natural setting. Some substance abuse treatment programs (*e.g.*, a Mobile Crisis/Emergency Service) must be available "outside of the clinic" to ensure their overall effectiveness. One of the benefits of clinic services is that they can assist in identification screening for substance abuse problems, brief intervention and referral to the specialty system, and coordination with physical health programs for treatment of health complications (*e.g.*, a person with diabetes who is drinking alcohol). Tools related to the management of substance abuse treatment services are rather limited under the clinic option, but can include utilization management (to ensure appropriate utilization of services among programs) and care coordination.

Case Management - Some states also include some form of case management services, within their approved Medicaid State Plan. Case management is an activity that assists individuals eligible for Medicaid in gaining access and coordinating access to necessary care and services appropriate to an individual. While case management services have not been further defined in regulations, activities commonly understood to be allowable include:

- Assessment of an eligible individual to determine service needs;
- Development of a specific care plan;
- Referral activities to help the individual obtain needed services; and
- Monitoring and follow-up.

Because some individuals receiving treatment for alcoholism or substance use/abuse are involved with other systems (*e.g.*, criminal justice, school, juvenile justice, child welfare), the linkage and coordination between systems is essential to increase the likelihood of successful outcomes for all systems involved.

Medicaid has five options for reimbursement of case management services:

1. Case management services under Section 1915(g) of the Social Security Act (targeted case management);
2. Case management as an administrative activity;
3. Case management under the EPSDT program;
4. Coordination of Section 1915(c) Home and Community Based Services Waivers; and
5. Case management of another Medicaid covered service.

Due to case management coverage options, each with unique possibilities and limitations, states devote considerable thought to the design of case management services.

Early and Periodic Screening, Diagnosis and Treatment (EPSDT)

Early and Periodic Screening, Diagnostic, and Treatment (EPSDT) is Medicaid's comprehensive and preventive child health program for individuals under the age of 21. EPSDT was defined in the Omnibus Budget Reconciliation Act of 1989 (OBRA 89) legislation and includes periodic screening, vision, dental, and hearing services. In addition, section 1905(r)(5) of the Social Security Act (the Act) requires that any medically necessary health care service listed at section 1905(a) of the Act be provided to an EPSDT recipient even if the service is not available under the State's Medicaid plan to the rest of the Medicaid population.

The EPSDT program consists of two mutually supportive, operational components: (1) assuring the availability and accessibility of required health care resources; and (2) helping Medicaid recipients and their parents or guardians effectively use these resources. These components enable Medicaid agencies to manage a comprehensive child health program of prevention and treatment, to seek out eligible individuals and inform them of the benefits of prevention and the health services and assistance available, and to help them and their families use health resources, including their own talents and knowledge, effectively and efficiently. It also enables Medicaid agencies to assess the child's health needs through initial and periodic examinations and evaluations, and to assure that the health problems found are diagnosed and treated early, before they become more complex and their treatment more costly.

Some states choose to define a set of substance abuse treatment benefit for adults through the Rehabilitation Option, but not define a set of discrete services for children due, in part, to the state's ability to rely on the EPSDT provision to ensure that the child receives needed services. Tools related to expanding services to children and adolescents utilizing EPSDT include (Legal Action Center, 2002):

- *Identifying Current Gaps in Coverage* – Using tools related to the identification of substance abuse treatment services purchasers and funding streams, states can identify treatment gaps and consider utilizing EPSDT provisions to fill those gaps for children and adolescents.
- *Adopt a Uniform Screening Tool* – By developing and implementing a uniform screening tool, states may be able to increase the number of children and adolescents screened and identified to ensure that they get the treatment or prevention services needed and funded under EPSDT. Many states have yet to implement this approach.
- *Conducting Provider Training* – Physician training to identify and screen for children's health needs early; promotes appropriate referrals to treatment, including referrals to specialty systems.
- *Data Analysis* – States evaluate EPSDT services through analysis of paid claims for services identified through EPSDT screening, and macro and micro comparisons of the needs identified to the services received.

EPSDT based strategies are an excellent opportunity for strong collaboration between the Medicaid agency and the state substance abuse authority.

Blended/Braided Funding

Blended and braided funding is another strategy to leverage funds and improve access, and builds on delegated management, dedicated funding, and optimization of funds. Braided funding maintains separate funding streams but integrates delivery of care seamlessly. Blended funding integrates funding and fosters interchangeable use of resources (Pires, 2002).

Blended/braided funding strategies predominately involve the use of the following, in various combinations:

- State Children's Health Insurance Program (SCHIP);
- Medicaid (whether Rehabilitation Option, Clinic Option, EPSDT);
- Managed Care Waivers and Other Performance Management Strategies (*e.g.,* Section 1915(b) Waivers, 1115 Research and Demonstration Project Waivers);
- Temporary Assistance to Needy Families (TANF);
- Health Insurance Flexibility and Accountability (HIFA) Demonstration;
- Title IV-E Child Welfare funds;
- Criminal Justice Funds;
- Mental Health funds;
- Substance Abuse Treatment and Prevention Block Grant;
- Local tax revenues; and
- Juvenile Justice funds.

More detail follows for some of these resources that relate most directly to the strategies discussed in this chapter.

Temporary Assistance to Needy Families (TANF)

With the de-linking of public cash assistance from medical assistance, states – under TANF provisions – have been increasingly able to provide a set of benefits more suitable to individual client needs. Among the types of services available for funding under TANF is funding for substance abuse treatment services. TANF can fund services including case management, transportation, vocational rehabilitation, and drug treatment, primarily duc to a specific federal provision that permits TANF funds to be spent on substance abuse treatment services.

Medicaid Waivers Under Social Security Act Section 1115 and Section 1915(B)

Section 1115 of the Social Security Act provides the Secretary of Health and Human Services with broad authority to authorize experimental, pilot, or demonstration project(s) which, in the judgment of the Secretary, (are) likely to assist in promoting the objectives of (the Medicaid statute).

As will be seen in subsequent chapters, under Health Care Reform Demonstrations states can expand managed care to include Health Maintenance Organizations (HMOs), partially capitated systems, primary care case managers, or other variations. Savings achieved from managed care arrangements can be used to finance coverage to individuals previously ineligible for Medicaid.

Section 1915(b) Freedom of Choice Waivers permit a waiver of the federal requirements of "statewideness", comparability of services, and freedom of choice. The 1915(b) waivers are limited in that they apply to existing Medicaid eligible beneficiaries; authority under this waiver can not be used for eligibility expansions. There are four 1915(b) Freedom of Choice Waivers: 1) mandate Medicaid Enrollment into managed care, 2) utilize a "central broker", 3) use cost savings to provide additional services, and 4) limit numbers of providers for services

Waivers are used to:

- Require Medicaid recipients to enroll in managed care programs. (States now also have the option, through the Balanced Budget Act of 1997, to enroll certain beneficiaries into mandatory managed care via a State Plan Amendment and can bypass the waiver mechanism).
- Create a "carve out" delivery system for specialty care such as a Managed Behavioral Health Care Plan.
- Create programs that are not available statewide.
- Develop an enhanced service package allowing the State to provide additional services to Medicaid beneficiaries via savings from managed care product. Changes in federal rules (see Federal Register June 4, 2002, Volume 67, Number 115, p 41003), however, limit this opportunity in significant ways.

Health Insurance Flexibility and Accountability (HIFA) Demonstration Waiver

HIFA waivers are a Medicaid waiver (State Children's Health Insurance Program Section 1115 demonstration waiver) designed to encourage new comprehensive state approaches that increase the number of individuals with health insurance coverage within current-level Medicaid and State Children's Health Insurance Program (SCHIP) resources. The Center for Medicare and Medicaid Services hopes that states will utilize the project to:

- Encourage innovation to improve how Medicaid and SCHIP funds are used to increase health insurance coverage for low-income individuals.
- Give States the programmatic flexibility required to support approaches that increase private health insurance coverage options.
- Simplify the waiver application process by providing clear guidance and data templates.
- Increase accountability in the State and federal partnership by ensuring that Medicaid and SCHIP funds are effectively being used to increase health insurance coverage, including substantially more private health insurance coverage options.
- Give priority review to State proposals that meet the general guidelines of the HIFA demonstration project outlined below.

States are encouraged to utilize the waiver to identify ways that the demonstration project can assist them in increasing populations receiving substance abuse treatment services.

The Substance Abuse and Mental Health Services Administration has released technical reports that may provide additional guidance on Medicaid coverage for the treatment of alcohol and drug disorders (Fox et al., 1993; Rosenbaum et al., 1997). A report from the National Institute on Drug Abuse may also be helpful (Horgan et al., 1994).

Conclusion

Medicaid is a complicated but potentially flexible financing mechanism that can assist states in paying for substance abuse treatment. Numerous options are available for directing federal Medicaid dollars toward the care of people with chemical dependency. Of course, key considerations are enrollment in and maintenance of coverage by Medicaid. The following chapter addresses continuity of Medicaid coverage in the context of substance abuse and its treatment. Subsequent chapters address Medicaid waivers pertinent to clients with substance abuse problems.

Acknowledgments

An award from the Robert Wood Johnson Foundation (Resources for Recovery: State Practices that Expand Treatment Opportunities) supported the preparation of the manuscript.

References

Centers for Medicare and Medicaid Services. (2003). Medicaid Statistical Information System State Summary FY2003. U.S. Department of Health and Human Services. http://www.cms.hhs.gov/MedicaidDataSourcesGenInfo/Downloads/MSISTables2003.pdf

Fox, H. B., Wicks, L. N., McManus, M. A., and Kelly, R. W. (1993). *Medicaid financing for mental health and substance abuse services for children and adolescents* (Rep. No. SMA 93-1743). Rockville, MD: Substance Abuse and Mental Health Services Administration.

Horgan, C., Larson, M. J., and Simon, L. (1994). Medicaid funding for drug abuse treatment: A national perspective. In G. Denmead and B. A. Rouse (Eds.), *Financing drug treatment through state programs.* Rockville, MD: National Institute on Drug Abuse.

Legal Action Center (2002). *Resources for recovery: State policy options for increasing access to alcohol and drug treatment through Medicaid and TANF.* New York: Legal Action Center.

O'Brien, J. and Lanahan, P. (2001). *Recovery in the community: Funding mental health rehabilitative approaches under Medicaid.* Washington, DC: Bazelon Center for Mental Health Law.

Pires, S. A. (2002). *Promising approaches for behavioral health services to children and adolescents and their families in managed care systems* (Rep. No. FMHI Publication

#211-1). Tampa, FL: Louis de la Parte Florida Mental Health Institute, University of South Florida.

Rosenbaum, S., Silver, K., and Wehr, E. (1997). *An evaluation of contracts between state Medicaid agencies and managed care organizations for the prevention and treatment of mental illness and substance abuse disorders* (Rep. No. Managed Care Technical Assistance Series: Volume Two). Rockville, MD: Substance Abuse and Mental Health Services Administration.

U.S. General Accounting Office (1991). *Substance abuse treatment: Medicaid allows some services but generally limits coverage.* (GAO/HRD-91-92 ed.) Washington, DC: U.S. General Accounting Office.

In: Medicaid and Treatment for People... ISBN 978-1-61470-742-4
Editor: B. H. McFarland, D. McCarty, et al., pp.17-46

Chapter 3

INSURANCE INSTABILITY: REPLACEMENT OF AID TO FAMILIES WITH DEPENDENT CHILDREN BY TEMPORARY ASSISTANCE FOR NEEDY FAMILIES AND IMPACT ON MEDICAID CLIENTS WITH SUBSTANCE ABUSE PROBLEMS

Laura A. Schmidt[1], Tammy Tam[2], James Wiley[3], and Constance M. Weisner[4]

[1] Philip R. Lee Institute for Health Policy Studies, Department of Anthropology, History and Social Medicine, University of California, San Francisco, CA, USA
[2] Alcohol Research Group, Public Health Institute, Emeryville, CA, USA
[3] Biobehavioral Research Center, San Francisco State University, CA, USA
[4] Department of Psychiatry, University of California, San Francisco, CA, USA

ABSTRACT

Maintenance of insurance coverage is a key concern for Medicaid clients. As discussed in this and later chapters, changes in Medicaid programs have often increased the "churn" of clients into and out of health insurance. Concerns have arisen that loss of coverage may impede utilization of substance abuse treatment by Medicaid clients with chemical dependency problems. This chapter makes the point that substance abuse treatment is delivered in several venues. Service settings include both "specialty" (substance abuse care only) and "non-specialty" (such as medical or mental health care) programs. Impact of Medicaid loss on addiction care utilization appears to differ depending on the setting. The chapter suggests that loss of Medicaid need not decrease use of specialty chemical dependency treatment – perhaps because federal block grant funds make addiction care services available to those who have lost coverage. On the other hand, this work also indicates that loss of Medicaid may substantially decrease use of non-specialty addiction care services. Because non-specialty chemical dependency treatment is notably important, policy-makers would do well to ensure continuous insurance coverage for Medicaid clients with substance abuse problems.

INTRODUCTION

Medicaid, the government insurance plan for low-income Americans, makes an important contribution to the overall financing of treatment for alcohol and drug problems. Reimbursements by Medicaid provide for one-fifth of national treatment expenditures annually (U.S. Department of Health and Human Services, 1999; Coffey et al., 2000). Some, but not all, studies suggest that the Medicaid population has both a greater need for, and better access to, chemical dependency treatment than other groups of insured Americans (Substance Abuse and Mental Health Services Administration, 2001). Given the importance of Medicaid funding for alcohol and drug treatment, declines in the program's enrollment and benefits are a major concern (Ku and Bruen, 1999). Most state governments, in the face of worsening fiscal crises, have revamped their Medicaid programs to reduce costs, sometimes leading to reductions in benefits traditionally used to fund chemical dependency treatment (Smith et al., 2004). Other policy developments, such as welfare reform and the spread of behavioral managed care, have increased the complexity and uncertainty of Medicaid enrollment and claims payment. These changes have often made it more difficult for beneficiaries to navigate the Medicaid system, *i.e.,* to enroll in the plan and maintain stable coverage year-to-year (Ellwood, 1999).

Studies have also shown that low-income adults, such as those eligible for Medicaid, experience the greatest instability in health insurance coverage over time (Doty and Holmgren, 2004). Other studies have shown that instability in Medicaid coverage, in turn, leads to substantial reductions in access to medical care (*e.g.,* Lurie et al., 1986; Brown and Cousineau, 1991). But researchers have not, as yet, examined these effects for chemical dependency treatment. This chapter investigates how patterns of variation in insurance coverage over time influence access to services for chemical dependency, comparing the experiences of Medicaid beneficiaries with other, less economically disadvantaged, populations of people with health coverage. Our work is based on a secondary analysis of the National Institute on Alcohol Abuse and Alcoholism-funded *Drinking Trajectories Study* (R01 AA-19231) that followed large samples of people with alcohol and drug problems in California over a five-year period, from 1995 to 2000.

BACKGROUND

Instability in Medicaid

Changes in Medicaid enrollment and benefits have heightened concerns about the unmet need for alcohol and drug treatment in America (Felland et al., 2004; Kessler et al., 1996; SAMHSA, 2002; Wang et al., 2000; Woodward et al., 1997). During the mid-1990s, Medicaid spending on behavioral health care slowed dramatically (Coffey et al., 2000), and many states reduced Medicaid benefits in efforts to control costs (Holahan et al., 1998; Mann et al., 2002; Pear and Toner, 2002b). Moreover, on a national basis, Medicaid enrollment steadily declined between 1995 and 2000 (Chavkin et al., 2000; U.S. Census Bureau, 2003), although more recently, enrollment has begun to creep back up, in part, due to a worsening economy (Strunk and Reschovsky, 2004). Studies show that the growing complexity of eligibility rules, as well as new state requirements for paperwork and in-person eligibility interviews, accounted for declining Medicaid enrollment (Chavkin et al., 2000; Garrett and Holahan, 2000a; Post, 2001).

A careful study of enrollment processes in five states found that confusion and complexity in eligibility rules contributed to problems with premature drop-out from the plan as well (Ellwood, 1999; for general discussions of changing Medicaid eligibility, enrollment and spending, see: Berk and Schur, 2001; Smith, Ramesh et al., 2004; U. S. Department of Health and Human Services, 2003).

Several forces conspired to produce these changes in Medicaid. The first has been a fiscal crisis in state government occasioned by what some have called a "perfect storm" (Johnson et al., 2003). Next to education, Medicaid is typically the largest line item in a state's budget. As the business cycle took a downturn in the late 1990s, higher unemployment rates drove up demand for Medicaid coverage. At the same time, the souring economy meant a drop in state tax revenues just as the costs of health insurance premiums had begun to climb (Ku et al., 2002). In the face of these budget pressures, many state legislatures were forced to revamp their Medicaid programs (Pear and Toner, 2002a). By 2003, 46 states had enacted legislation to alter Medicaid eligibility, benefits and reimbursement rates. Half of these states reduced or eliminated optional benefits, including those benefits traditionally used to fund alcohol and drug treatment (Johnson et al., 2003). In California, the Governor's 2002 budget proposed to reduce Medicaid spending by a monumental $1.1 billion through a myriad of small cuts to be made with "scalpels rather than battle axes" (Broder, 2004).

The spread of managed care to Medicaid also contributed to the program's instability. Between 1996 and 1999, the number of states experimenting with public sector managed care tripled so that, by the decade's end, over half of all Medicaid beneficiaries were in a managed care plan (Fox et al, 1999; Rowland and Hanson, 1996; U.S. Department of Health and Human Services, 1999; U.S. Center for Health Statistics, 1999). While managed care helped some Medicaid plans to control costs, it also added a new layer of complexity to enrollment and claims-payment systems. Many state plans now operate through additional layers of administration set up under contracts with private sector managed behavioral health care firms. Medicaid contracts are regularly put out for competitive bidding, which can mean frequent changes year-to-year in plan administration. Case studies from some states, such as Massachusetts and Oregon, suggested that the movement to managed care in Medicaid can have a positive impact on access to care (Callahan et al., 1995; Cavanaugh, 1999; Deck et al., 2000; Huskamp, 1999; Sabin and Daniels, 1997). In other states, however, such as Tennessee, experiments at reform dramatically failed, leaving many beneficiaries without health coverage (Chang et al. 1998; Holahan et al. 1998).

The advent of federal welfare reform in 1996 is another force that contributed to instability in Medicaid. Numerous studies show that the implementation of welfare reform contributed to an overall decline in Medicaid enrollment nationally (Andrulis and Hopkins, 2001; Chavkin et al., 2000; DeChiara and Wolff, 1998; Klein and Fish-Parcham, 1999; Ku and Coughlin, 1997; Maloy et al., 1999; Mann et al., 2002; U.S. General Accounting Office, 1998b). Prior to welfare reform, welfare recipients were automatically enrolled in Medicaid. But when Congress passed the 1996 welfare reform package, it decoupled enrollment procedures so that recipients would not lose their Medicaid coverage when they left welfare due to new federal time limits (Ku and Bruen, 1999; Mann et al., 2002). In the aftermath of reform, this system encountered significant implementation problems due to growing complexity of the rules and to ongoing difficulties with educating clients about new administrative procedures (Mann et al., 2002). Despite efforts to the contrary, it appears that nearly half of welfare recipients are uninsured within one year of leaving welfare. Only 22 percent remain on Medicaid after one year despite the fact that most remain eligible (Garrett and Holahan, 2000a, 2000b). In some states, including California, governments have mitigated this problem by setting up special state supplemental funds. These programs automatically re-enroll individuals in Medicaid when they transition from welfare to work thus preserving continuity in Medicaid coverage (Cox et al., 2001; Gresenz and Klerman, 2002; Mauldon et al., 2002).

Since the mid-1990s, Medicaid, therefore, underwent several key changes. Policy developments in state fiscal affairs, including welfare reform and Medicaid managed care, reshaped state plans, often making it more difficult for beneficiaries to maintain stable coverage over time. Medicaid contributes one-fifth of the funding for chemical dependency treatment nationally. Instability in Medicaid, therefore, added to concerns about making chemical dependency treatment available and affordable to low-income people in America.

Chapter Questions

Our analysis of Medicaid coverage and access to care is motivated by two questions. First, *how did the insurance coverage of people with chemical dependencies – particularly Medicaid coverage – change given policy developments since the mid-1990s?* Here, we are interested in the kinds of insurance coverage that people with chemical dependencies possess, and how stable Medicaid coverage is in relation to other forms of insurance. We are also interested in what happens when individuals lose their Medicaid coverage: Are they more likely to become uninsured or to shift to some other form of coverage, such a private plan or Medicare?

Second, *how does instability in insurance coverage — particularly in Medicaid coverage — influence access to chemical dependency treatment?* Some cross-sectional studies suggest that the Medicaid population has a greater need for, and better access to, chemical dependency treatment than other groups of insured people (SAMHSA, 2001). But growing instability in access to Medicaid coverage could threaten access to care. In considering access to care, it is important to include encounters with specialty treatment providers in chemical dependency programs, as well as mainstream medical and mental health providers who often provide care for alcohol and drug problems in the context of non-specialty settings. It has been shown that individuals with alcohol and drug problems obtain help from mutual aid and non-specialty service settings more readily than from specialty chemical dependency programs (Kessler et al., 1996; Regier et al., 1993; Weisner et al., 1995). Moreover, benefits and insurance policies surrounding coverage for services provided by specialty and non-specialty providers are likely to differ.

Insurance and Access to Care

Our approach to answering these questions is informed by Aday and Andersen's model of medical care seeking (Aday and Andersen, 1974; Andersen, 1995; Andersen and Newman, 1973). Some studies have examined the medical care utilization model and its adaptations to treatment seeking for alcohol and drug problems (Booth et al., 1996, 1997; Grant, 1996; Padgett et al., 1990; Weisner, 1990a, 1990b, 1993; Weisner et al., 2002; Weisner and Schmidt, 2001). As Figure 1 illustrates, this approach argues that demographic and background characteristics *predispose* help seeking for alcohol and drug problems by shaping the propensity to seek care before the onset of illness symptoms. For example, men are more likely to seek treatment than women after controlling for differences in need, and prior treatment experiences predispose people to enter treatment again. Illness factors reflect the *need* for treatment. Thus, higher-severity alcohol and drug problems and comorbidities are strong predictors of chemical dependency treatment utilization. Finally there are factors that *enable* treatment by increasing the individual's ability to secure services. Disposable income to pay for services and insurance coverage are examples of enabling factors.

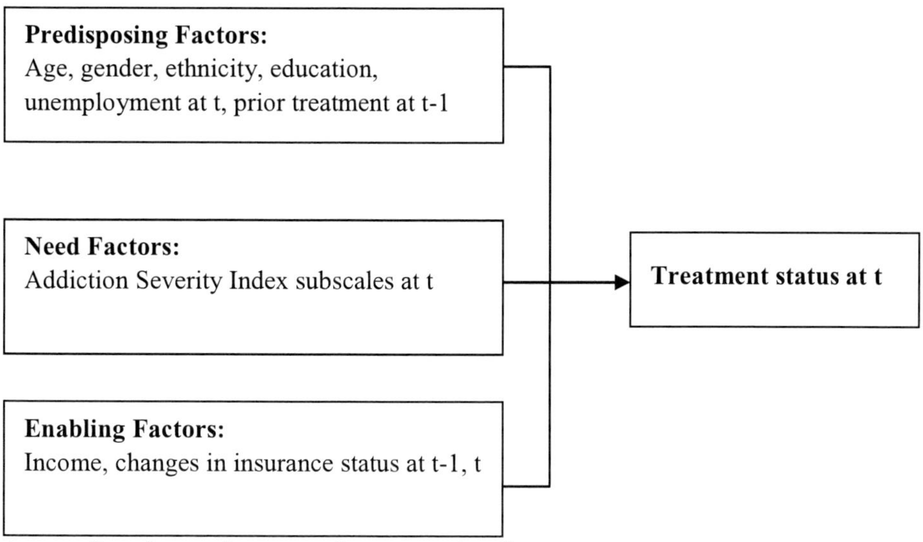

Note: t ranges from 1-year, 3-years, to 5-years post baseline.

Figure 1. Longitudinal model of treatment utilization.

As Figure 1 suggests, we are interested in how access to care at one time point (represented by "t" which, in this study, can be 1, 3 or 5 years after baseline) is affected by changes in insurance coverage at a time point prior to that (represented by "t-1"). Prior work suggests that various aspects of insurance coverage may enable treatment entry for alcohol and drug problems. Researchers have examined whether having any insurance coverage at all affects the utilization of substance abuse treatment using a cross-sectional approach (*e.g.*, Booth et al., 2000; Booth and McLaughlin, 2000; Grant, 1996; Weisner et al., 2002). Notably, researchers have rarely found that having health coverage has a strong impact on the likelihood of receiving treatment for a chemical dependency problem. They have interpreted this finding to mean that public sector funding through Medicaid, Medicare and block grants provides an effective public safety net that allows even the uninsured to enter care more readily than is typically the case (Rogowski, 1993; Weisner et al., 2002).

Some studies have examined whether different types of insurance coverage influence access to care. Analyses suggest that people with public insurance — including Medicaid – are as or more likely than those with private coverage to obtain treatment for an alcohol or drug problem, perhaps due to more extensive coverage of specialty and inpatient care (Harwood et al., 2001; Schmidt and Weisner, 2005; SAMHSA, 2001; Wu, Kouzis and Schlenger 2003). Again, the argument is that, because the public sector heavily subsidizes chemical dependency treatment, having public insurance or access to treatment slots subsidized by federal block grants may promote treatment entry.

METHODS

Overview

We conducted a secondary analysis of the *Drinking Trajectories Study*, which includes representative samples of adults in chemical dependency treatment programs and dependent and problem drinkers in the general population of the same county in California. Both portions of the sample were followed and re-interviewed three times over a 5-year period. The sample drawn from treatment programs includes consecutive admissions of individuals entering public and private alcohol and drug programs throughout the study site. Our analysis uses this group to examine how insurance influences subsequent episodes of care following the baseline episode, that is, we are interested in episodes of "re-treatment". The general population sample involved screening over 13,000 adults in the county's household population to obtain a representative sample of problem drinkers who had not obtained treatment in the past year. Our analysis uses this group to examine how insurance influences initial treatment encounters. While the sampling strategy focused on selecting problem drinkers, the study ultimately included large numbers of individuals with illicit drug problems as well. Over one-third of all study participants reported the use of any type of illicit drugs on a weekly basis or more often, and 29 percent met psychiatric criteria for American Psychiatric Association Diagnostic and Statistical Manual fourth edition (*DSM-IV)* drug dependence diagnosis. The most prevalent drugs used were marijuana and stimulants, such as methamphetamine.

Our analysis develops a generalized linear transition model to examine chemical dependency treatment entry as a function of predisposing, need and enabling factors. The key factor of interest is instability in insurance coverage, which is measured by observing transitions from one insurance status to another between time points. To perform this analysis, we created a stacked data set that converted survey data on individuals into a sample of person-years and treatment events (see Figure 2). Each individual in the study was interviewed at four time points over the 5-year study period, thus contributing three data points to the new sample of person-years. Some variables in the data set are fixed or time-invariant, such as gender. Other variables are time varying, such as the stability of insurance, which is defined by experiencing a shift in insurance status from one time point to the next.

Case ID	Year (t)	Treatment status at t	Baseline age	Change in insurance status t-1, t	Treatment status at t-1
001	1	Yes	37	Continuously uninsured	No
001	3	Yes	37	Got insurance	Yes
001	5	No	37	Lost insurance	Yes

Note: Unit of analysis is the person-year.

Figure 2. Illustration of "stacked" data structure for longitudinal analysis of treatment utilization.

Study Site

Data were collected in a northern California county whose population is over one million people. A county was chosen as the universe for the *Drinking Trajectories Study* because, in many states, including California, services are organized at that level. This particular county was chosen because of its mix of urban and rural areas, the range of economic and ethnic characteristics in its population, as well as its treatment system characteristics. The county offers a full range of public and private treatment services for chemical dependency problems at all levels of care.

At the time of the baseline data collection, in 1995, private insurance plans operating in the county were mostly marketing managed care products, although some traditional indemnity coverage was also still available. The vast majority of private plans at this time provided coverage for alcohol and drug detoxification and most also covered alcohol and drug rehabilitation. Medicare covered these services, as well as residential care, and the majority of beneficiaries remained in the traditional, non-managed Medicare plan. Medicaid provided coverage for outpatient rehabilitation and detoxification exclusively through contracted health maintenance organizations (HMOs). County residents on Medicaid had the choice of four separate HMO options, although the specific plans could change yearly as contracts were renegotiated.

Sample

Baseline Sample

Two sampling procedures were used: in-person interviews were conducted with individuals entering the county's public and private chemical dependency programs and with dependent and problem drinkers from the county general population (for a combined N=1598). Signed informed consent was obtained from both samples.

The treatment program sample (n=926) included consecutive admissions to all ten public and private programs in the county that met the following inclusion criteria (Kaskutas et al., 1997): (1) at least one new intake per week, (2) detoxification and treatment for drugs other than alcohol were not the primary focus (*e.g.,* methadone maintenance programs were not included), and (3) first line treatment entry (*i.e.,* programs limited to aftercare were excluded). Although the study excluded treatment programs that confined their focus to illicit drug problems, as noted above, a majority of the sample used illicit drugs and many met diagnostic criteria for drug abuse or dependence.

Trained survey interviewers, who were independent of participating agencies, collected data from the *treatment program sample*. All new intakes to treatment programs were included in the sampling frame. The interviewers administered structured in-person questionnaires to all participants by the end of their third day of residential treatment or third outpatient visit, which often occurred within one month's time. Participation was independent of receiving agency services. The overall recruitment rate for individuals in all programs in this portion of the study was 80 percent. In order for the sample to reflect the true population attending treatment programs, statistical weights were created. These weights took into account differences in fieldwork duration (the length of time spent interviewing in each agency in order to equally represent across agencies the number of individuals who would have entered during the same given time period) and differences in sampling fractions across agencies (*i.e.,* variation in every "nth" client sampled). Sampling weights also adjusted for non-response by gender and ethnicity using post-stratification. For example, non-white women were over-represented in one public program and were therefore down-weighted (.39) and non-white men were under-represented in one public program and were thus weighted up (3.0) (Humphreys and Weisner, 2000; Tam, 1997; Weisner et al., 2002).

The same interviewers collected data from a *general population sample* (N=672) of dependent and problem drinkers in the same county. Telephone interviews using random digit dialing methods were conducted with a probability sample of 13,394 adults. Individuals were recruited for an in-person interview if they met specific criteria for problem drinking (described below in *Measures*) and reported that they had not received chemical dependency treatment during the previous 12 months. Only 22 percent of problem drinkers in the general population reported a treatment episode in the past twelve months, with a mean of 1.5 episodes per lifetime.

Participants in the general population portion of the study were interviewed in person, in a private location at home, using a survey instrument that contained identical items to those used with the treatment program sample. The recruitment rate in the general population sample was 70 percent of eligible respondents. This rate was calculated using a standard designed for random-digit-dialing telephone surveys (American Association for Public Opinion Research, 2000). It takes into account the percent of eligible unknowns who would have been problem drinkers and loss at the point of telephone screening, as well as refusals of the in-person interview. There were no significant differences between those who did and did not agree to the in-person interview in age, gender, ethnicity, or problem severity characteristics. Moreover, prevalence rates and characteristics of the general population sample are similar to those obtained by other household population studies conducted in this study site (Weisner et al., 1995; Weisner and Schmidt 1995).

Follow-Up Procedures

One-, three- and five-year follow-up interviews were conducted with all study participants using Computer Assisted Telephone Interviewing (CATI). Respondents were tracked every three months using postcard mailings and telephone check-ins; once located, an interviewer called the respondent, asked questions and entered the respondent's answers into the computer system. Those who could not be reached by telephone were referred to a fieldwork agency for further searching. Seven percent of respondents who could not be located through telephone contacts were successfully found and interviewed in person at the 1-year follow-up. Eight percent were found and interviewed in person at the 3-year follow-up, and 5 percent at the 5-year follow-up. Follow-up response rates were 84 percent at Year 1, 82 percent at Year 3, and 79 percent at Year 5 (75 percent, 78 percent, and 72 percent, respectively, for the treatment program sample, and 93 percent, 91 percent, and 88 percent, respectively, for the general population sample).

Sample Characteristics

It is notable that the overall distribution of insurance in the pooled sample of participants in the *Drinking Trajectories Study* is not that different from the nation as a whole (see: U.S. Census Bureau 2003). As the bottom row of Table 1 shows, despite high levels of unemployment, 62 percent of study participants had a private policy as their main source of insurance coverage at baseline, as compared to 69 percent of the nation's general population. In most cases, the coverage was provided through the employer(s) and labor union of the respondent. Eight percent were on Medicaid, 12 percent on Medicare, and 4 percent on other public plans (*e.g.*, Veterans Affairs coverage, Civilian Health and Medical Program of the Uniformed Services (CHAMPUS), or locally-sponsored coverage for medical indigents). Fourteen percent reported being uninsured at baseline, which is roughly consistent with the national average.

Table 1. Pooled sample characteristics by baseline insurance status (percents and means)

Characteristic	Private Coverage	Medicare	Medicaid	Other Public Coverage	Uninsured	Total
Female, %	40	23	49	25	28	36
Ethnic Minority, %	28	48	65	46	50	39
Age, M (SD)	37 (11.9)	45 (13.5)	36 (9.4)	40 (9.7)	35 (8.6)	37 (11.6)
Unemployed, %	31	81	83	76	68	52
High school dropout, %	10	25	37	18	28	18
Income < 20K, %	17	74	86	70	65	42
ASI alcohol severity, *M* (SD)	0.29 (0.01)	0.38 (0.04)	0.28 (0.02)	0.35 (0.03)	0.28 (0.02)	0.30 (0.01)
ASI drug severity, *M* (SD)	0.60 (0.003)	0.13 (0.01)	0.14 (0.10)	0.14 (0.01)	0.10 (0.07)	0.09 (0.003)
ASI psychiatric severity, *M* (SD)	0.25 (0.01)	0.40 (0.02)	0.39 (0.02)	0.33 (0.03)	0.28 (0.01)	0.29 (0.003)
Unweighted N	(973)	(183)	(125)	(66)	(224)	(1571)
Percent of Sample	62	12	8	4	14	100

Notes:
ASI = Addiction Severity Index
M = mean
SD = standard deviation
All differences are statistically significant at $p<0.001$ level based on chi-square or F test.
Data are weighted for non-response and sample design.

Table 1 also compares demographic and severity characteristics by baseline insurance status within the pooled sample. Large differences in demographic and severity characteristics across insurance groups underscore the need for multivariate analyses that allow one to observe the effects of insurance on treatment entry independent of other factors. There were some differences between Medicaid recipients and others on public plans. While the severity of drug problems was roughly the same, Medicaid beneficiaries experienced lower average alcohol severity than others who were publicly insured. Those on Medicaid were somewhat more likely to be ethnic minorities and lower income, as compared with Medicare and other public plan beneficiaries. Note that many Medicare beneficiaries in this sample were on the plan in connection with their receipt of disability benefits. This explains why so many Medicare beneficiaries in this study were male and under age 65. Compared to the privately insured, those on Medicaid were much more disadvantaged. As would be expected based on eligibility criteria, significantly larger proportions of Medicaid beneficiaries were unemployed, poorly educated, low income and unmarried. There were more women and ethnic minorities on Medicaid, and alcohol, drug and psychiatric severity were higher than among the privately insured.

Measures

Individuals in the general population were screened in order to produce a sample of individuals with current alcohol problems. General population cases met criteria for *problem drinking* by reporting at least two of the following during the 12 months prior to the baseline interview: (1) drinking five or more drinks in a day at least once a month for men (three drinks in a day weekly for women), (2) one or more alcohol-related social consequences (from a list of eight), and (3) one or more alcohol dependence symptoms (from a list of nine). This measure is consistent with the predominant approach taken in research on alcohol epidemiology and similar measures have been used in a wide variety of published studies (Institute of Medicine, 1990; Schmidt, 1998; Weisner, 1992; Wilsnack, 1991). Alcohol-related social consequences covered a range of ways that individuals with substance abuse problems come to the attention of others in the community (Hilton, 1987; Weisner, 1990, 1992, 1995). This measure pertained to the 12 months prior to each interview and included drinking-driving arrests, public drunkenness arrests, other alcohol-related criminal arrests, traffic crashes when drinking, other (non-traffic) alcohol-related accidents, and/or confrontations about an alcohol-related health problem by a medical practitioner, serious alcohol-related family problems caused by respondents' drinking, or confrontations about an alcohol-related job problem by a supervisor or employer. Dependence symptoms included assessment of nine criteria commonly used in clinical and general population research (American Psychiatric Association, 2000; Caetano, 1995).

Our analyses focus on two dependent variables reflecting chemical dependency treatment encounters at each wave of follow-up. The first is *specialty treatment encounters*, which includes professional services provided in alcohol and drug treatment programs, including inpatient and outpatient substance abuse settings that provide detoxification, rehabilitation or both. This measure does not include treatment provided in mental health programs, and our analysis does not distinguish between detoxification and rehabilitation services. Also, our measure of specialty treatment is confined to professional services rendered at some cost and therefore excludes help provided through mutual aid or self-help groups, such as Alcoholics Anonymous and Narcotics Anonymous. Membership in the treatment program versus general population sample defines specialty treatment use at the baseline observation. At each follow-up interview, treatment experiences 12 months prior to the interview are included. Lifetime treatment history prior to baseline is also evaluated. In all cases, we created dichotomous variables to indicate treatment received during each referenced time period.

Non-specialty medical and mental health treatment encounters is the second outcome variable of interest. Respondents were asked whether they had contact with the medical system (through a physician visit, emergency room visit or overnight hospital stay) and the mental health system (through inpatient or outpatient visits). For each type of care, they were asked whether an alcohol problem had been addressed during the encounter. We created dichotomous variables to indicate one or more non-specialty treatment encounters with any medical or mental health provider for each referenced time frame. It is notable that the majority of chemical dependency encounters took place in the non-specialty sector, which included treatment encounters for substance abuse problems in medical and mental health treatment settings. At the first year follow-up interview, 22 percent of the pooled sample reported a mental health treatment encounter that addressed a chemical dependency problem, while 15 percent reported a medical encounter. In contrast, only 22 percent of the pooled sample had a specialty treatment encounter at the first year follow-up. Notable differences were also found between the treated and general population samples. While 44 percent of the treated sample received substance abuse services from a medical or mental health setting, only 12 percent of the general population sample reported similar encounters.

In keeping with the medical care utilization model, independent variables represent three clusters of factors in treatment use: predisposing, need and enabling factors. *Predisposing factors* include gender, age (categorized as 17-29 years, 30-44 years, and 45+ years), ethnicity, education, employment, and prior treatment use. Ethnicity is represented by two dichotomous variables indicating blacks (=1) and Hispanics and others (=1), respectively, with whites (=0) as the reference group for each. Education is represented by a dichotomous variable indicating high school and greater than high school education (=1) versus others (=0). Unemployed individuals are coded as 1 versus others who are coded as 0. Prior specialty and non-specialty treatment are represented by dichotomous variables indicating whether individuals had received each type of care at least once prior to the referenced time frame at each follow-up interview (within 12 months prior to the interview).

The *need* for treatment is represented by alcohol, drug, psychiatric, and legal problem severity. Severity in each problem area was assessed using an abbreviated form of the *Addiction Severity Index* (*ASI*). The *ASI* is a valid and reliable instrument that assesses the severity of alcohol, drug, employment, medical, psychiatric, family/social relations, and legal problems (McLellan et al., 1992). In each domain, questions measure the number, frequency and duration of these problems in the patient's lifetime and in the past 30 days. The resulting score is a continuous measure from 0 (no problems) to 1.0 (high severity) within each area of problem severity. Initial descriptive statistics indicated skewed distributions for all of the *ASI* measures. We therefore use logarithmic transformations that allow these distributions to more closely approximate the normal distribution. Scores range from 0 to 1 with higher values suggesting more severe problems within each domain.

Enabling factors include household income and insurance status. We use a dichotomous measure of family income. Insurance status is assessed at baseline and at each follow-up interview. The survey instruments contained a set of standard questions on insurers, type of coverage and number of policies that have been used in prior published studies (Schmidt and Weisner, 2005; Weisner et al., 2002). To increase reliability, the study team also independently researched the community's insurance market to cross check the coverage in cases where respondents were uncertain. Our measures of insurance reflect the first payer if an individual had multiple insurance policies, although only 11 percent of the pooled sample at baseline reported multiple coverage.

To evaluate the stability of insurance coverage over time, we created a variable to capture transitions in insurance status, including any form of coverage, from one time point to the next. This procedure resulted in a four-category variable that measures the full range of possible transitions in insurance status between each data point: continuously insured, lost insurance, gained insurance and continuously uninsured. Thus, respondents who switched types of health plans (*e.g.,* moved from Medicaid to a private plan, or vice versa) were coded as "continuously insured," and only those who transitioned from some form of coverage to no coverage were coded as "lost insurance." In cases where an individual shifted plans but did not shift types of plans – *e.g.,* moved from one type of private coverage to another – we considered the coverage stable. It was only when individuals shifted from one type of insurance status to another (*e.g.*, from private coverage to being uninsured, or from Medicaid to a private plan) that we coded a transition in insurance coverage. We further developed dummy codes that compared the effects of losing or gaining insurance or being continuously insured versus being continuously uninsured. Thus, we created three dichotomous variables indicating losing insurance (=1) versus continuously uninsured (=0); gaining insurance (=1) versus continuously uninsured (=0); and continuously insured (=1) versus continuously uninsured (=0). Below, under *Methodological limitations* we describe the potential for reporting bias and efforts to mitigate this problem.

Data Analysis

The analysis began by examining the stability of insurance coverage for all individuals in the study using the pooled sample of cases from treatment programs and the general population. These bivariate comparisons used Pearson's chi-square test to assess significant differences between categorical variables, and t-tests and analysis of variance to examine differences for continuous variables, with Bonferroni adjustments to address multiple comparisons. The weighted sample size of the pooled sample was normalized to the observed sample size to maintain correct proportions of treated and untreated problem drinkers in the county. The analysis then moved to a multivariate regression approach that examined the impact of insurance on treatment encounters after controlling for other factors. Here, we estimated regression models for substance abuse-related service encounters in specialty (*i.e.,* substance abuse) and non-specialty (*i.e.,* medical or mental health) settings separately, and conducted our analyses in the samples of general population and treatment program cases separately, to show differences between initial treatment (or those occurring after at least one year without treatment) and re-treatment encounters. In a small number of cases, general population respondents experienced more than one treatment episode during the study period and all encounters were included in the analysis.

For the regression analyses, we used a generalized linear transition model that estimated the probability of a treatment encounter at any given time point as a function of predisposing, need, and enabling factors (Diggle et al., 1994; Neuhaus, 1992). The transition model explicitly specified correlations among outcome variables measured at different time points. Here, we used a first order autoregressive model where treatment use at any given time of follow-up had a direct dependence on treatment use at the previous interview (Bonney, 1987; Neuhaus, 1992). This approach is particularly relevant to the analysis of treatment utilization because there is abundant evidence that prior use is an important predictor of current treatment. Because we used treatment at the prior time point as an independent variable, only data from the Year 1, Year 3, and Year 5 follow-up interviews were candidates for dependent variables in this analysis.

As noted above, we used a data stacking approach where, for each individual case, data from each of the three follow-up interviews were arranged in a single record assigned with the same case identifier but different time indicators. Each person-year record contained both time invariant and time varying variables. Gender, age, and ethnicity, as measured at baseline, were modeled as time invariant variables in our analysis. Income and education were also treated as time invariant because a preliminary survey of the data found no major changes from baseline status over the five-year period. *ASI* scores, employment status and changes in insurance status were allowed to vary over time. Treatment use at the prior time point was an additional independent variable. Note that our analyses controlled for year-to-year changes in employment status. This control is important because insurance coverage may be linked to employment status, as well as possibly changes in alcohol and drug problem severity, and our interest was in examining the independent role of insurance instability.

We estimated the models using maximum likelihood estimation, specifically, the *xtgee* commands in Stata Version 8.0 (Stata Corp., 2003). One concern is that in stacked data, observations of the same individual at different time points are not independent and therefore, the data do not meet statistical assumptions for regression analysis. We accounted for the non-independence of observations using standard autoregression techniques. This approach meant first estimating within-individual correlations with an unrestricted structure for each model. Here, the estimated correlation matrix consistently showed a lagged structure, where the serial correlation of residuals diminished as the lag increased. The within-individual correlation was therefore specified as a first order lag structure for subsequent analyses. The resulting first order autoregressive transition models included data from at least two consecutive interviews regardless of the number of interviews successfully completed for each respondent. Maximum likelihood estimation allowed the use of all non-missing data for each individual case.

Our strategy for adjusting for autocorrelation was a conservative one and sample sizes were sometimes too small to detect effects of the expected size. Therefore, while we adhered to the standard threshold for statistical significance of $p < .05$, we also interpreted trends in the data where results appeared robust across analyses and where $p < .10$.

Methodological Limitations

One set of limitations in this analysis involved the generalizability of results, given our focus on a single California county. The selection of a confined geographic area facilitated an intensive data collection effort that allowed the study team to capture comparable samples of people in need of treatment, some in treatment and some not. However, this approach meant potentially limiting the relevance of results to other regions of the country. To maximize generalizability, the study site was selected carefully on the basis of its treatment system characteristics, ethnic and socioeconomic diversity in its population, as well as similarities to national patterns of alcohol and drug use, health and social problems (Greenfield and Weisner, 1995; Weisner et al., 1995; Weisner and Schmidt, 1992). We provide detail above under *Study site* on the county's insurance market and coverage for chemical dependency.

This information can be useful in assessing the degree to which the results of this analysis are applicable to other places within the U.S.

Another set of limitations involves sample coverage. First, the sample drawn from treatment programs did not include people receiving care in non-specialty treatment settings, such as private psychiatric settings, doctor's offices and hospital wards. The logistical challenges and costs of locating and representatively sampling individuals from such settings were prohibitive. As noted above, however, many individuals in this portion of the sample reported contact with these non-specialty providers for help with alcohol and drug problems. Second, the general population portion of the sample used a random-digit dial survey to screen individuals for eligibility in the study. This method excluded individuals who did not have telephones and who did not reside in the household population. Prior studies suggest that the omission of these individuals could produce conservative estimates of alcohol and drug problems (U.S. General Accounting Office, 1998a; U.S. National Institute on Drug Abuse, 1992, Weisner et al., 1995).

This analysis was also limited by the range of independent variables incorporated into our models of treatment utilization. In particular, this analysis did not incorporate coercion into treatment, which may involve pressuring from the courts, family or employer to obtain treatment. Such factors have been shown to be important predictors of treatment utilization, but were beyond the scope of this analysis, which focuses on insurance and financial predictors receiving care. For separate analyses of coercion in these data, see: Schmidt and Weisner, 2005; Weisner et al, 2001.

Finally, there are limitations in the data on insurance coverage. Ideally, our measures of insurance coverage would include information on whether the respondent's insurance policy included a specific chemical dependency treatment benefit. However, self-report survey data on insurance coverage are unreliable due to the fact that many beneficiaries lack detailed knowledge about what their policies do or do not cover in the way of services for chemical dependency. While the study team did not attempt to collect these data from respondents, the majority of private benefits plans covered inpatient detoxification (97 percent), inpatient rehabilitation (76 percent) and outpatient rehabilitation (80 percent) in 1995 (Bureau of Labor Statistics, 1998), and Medicaid mainly provided coverage for outpatient rehabilitation and detoxification. A final limitation is that our measures of instability in insurance coverage only captured changes between survey time points. Turnover in insurance may occur more rapidly and therefore, our estimates of change are likely to be conservative. Also, it is possible that in some cases, treatment providers assisted uninsured respondents in obtaining insurance during a treatment episode, and thus the time-ordering of insurance and treatment admission would have been reversed. Because we were confined to yearly measurements of insurance coverage, it was not possible to identify specific cases in which this reversal occurred.

RESULTS

Instability in Insurance Coverage

We began by examining instability in insurance coverage, particularly Medicaid coverage, among dependent and problem drinkers. Figure 3 shows the cumulative proportion of people in the study who changed from their baseline insurance status at each wave of follow-up. Notably, those who started the study with Medicaid coverage were among the most likely to have transitioned off the plan at subsequent time points. This pattern was contrasted by those with a private insurance plan, who had a far greater chance of staying with that form of coverage over the course of the study. Thus, within the first year of the study, over half of Medicaid recipients had changed coverage, as contrasted by the privately insured, among whom only 15 percent had shifted status by Year 1. By Year 5 of the study, over three-quarters of those who began on Medicaid had changed coverage, as contrasted by only one third of the privately insured. Only the uninsured surpassed Medicaid recipients in the degree to which their insurance status was unstable by Year 5, when slightly more of those who began uninsured had changed status. Note that in 1997, changes in the Supplemental Security Income (SSI) program categorically denied eligibility to individuals who qualified for SSI on the sole basis of an alcohol or drug disorder. Consequently, this shift led to changes in Medicare coverage which had been automatically conferred with SSI eligibility for these individuals (Baumohl, Speiglman et al., 2003; Hanrahan, Luchins et al., 2004). This SSI change could account for some of the instability we observed in Medicare within this sample of problem drinkers. However, controlling for SSI eligibility in our analyses did not significantly change the findings.

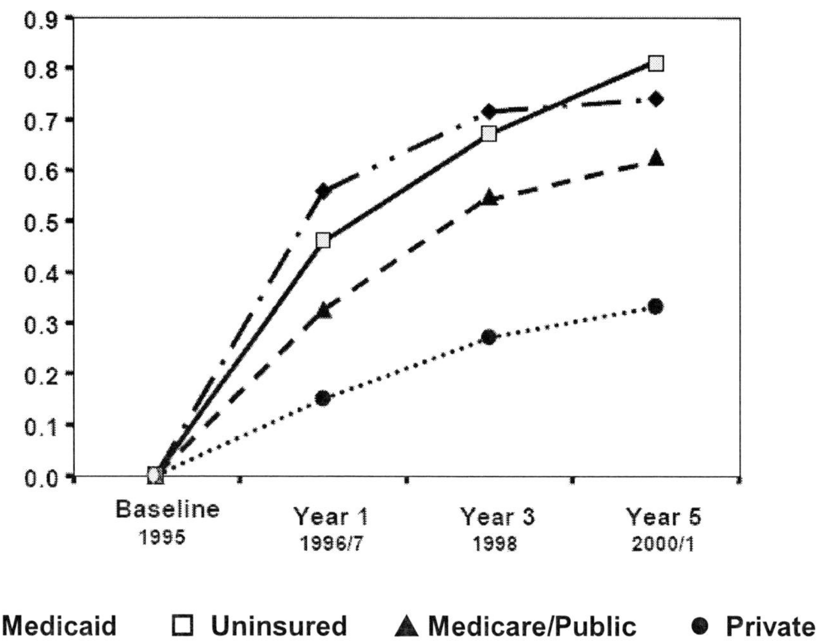

Figure 3. Cumulative proportion of pooled sample who changed from baseline insurance status.

To understand the nature of the instability in Medicaid coverage, we characterized the predominant patterns of variation over time among those who were on the plan at baseline (see Figure 4). The most common pattern, experienced by one third of the people in this group, was cycling on and off Medicaid into other statuses over the course of time. The second most common was to stay on Medicaid continuously for all five years; about one quarter experienced this pattern. Other patterns were less common. Thirteen percent shifted from Medicaid to a private plan, while 10 percent were in a different status at each wave, and another nine percent became stably insured on a different public plan, such as Medicare. It is notable that nine percent of those who began the study on Medicaid lost their coverage and became uninsured for the remainder of the study. While this course was not the predominant pattern among former Medicaid recipients, moving from Medicaid to a state of being continuously uninsured is of great significance from the perspective of public policy. These uninsured and low-income individuals are likely to face significant economic barriers to obtaining needed health and addiction services.

As noted, research has linked changes in enrollment procedures under welfare reform to growing instability in Medicaid coverage. In California, welfare reform began implementation in 1997, or during the Year 1 follow-up wave of the *Drinking Trajectories Study*, thus allowing us to examine this question. We compared the proportion of welfare recipients and non-welfare recipients who remained on Medicaid at each transition point during the study. While some in the comparison group of non-welfare recipients received other forms of aid, such as SSI or local General Assistance, many did not. As Figure 5 illustrates, the Medicaid retention rate among welfare participants in this study was consistently better – not worse – than the retention rate among non-welfare participants. Retention rates for welfare recipients ranged from 64 to 75 percent depending on the year of transition, whereas they ranged from 20 to 45 percent among non-welfare recipients. Equally noteworthy is the fact that Medicaid retention rates did not decline among welfare recipients following the implementation of welfare reform at the Year 1 follow-up wave. These results, while contrary to expectation, are interpretable. This finding is likely the result of a special transitional Medicaid fund set up for the purpose of keeping California welfare recipients covered by Medicaid as they transitioned from welfare to work.

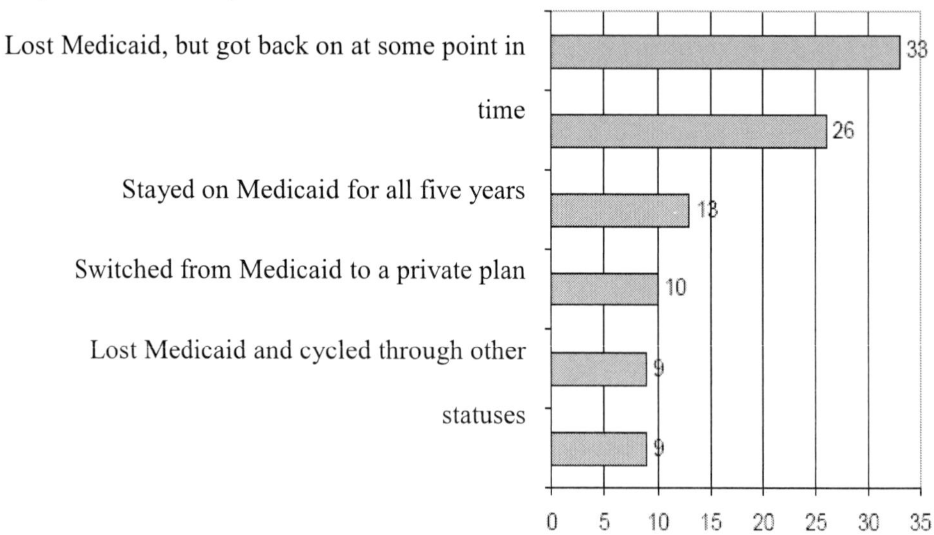

Figure 4. Insurance patterns over five years for those who began study on Medicaid .

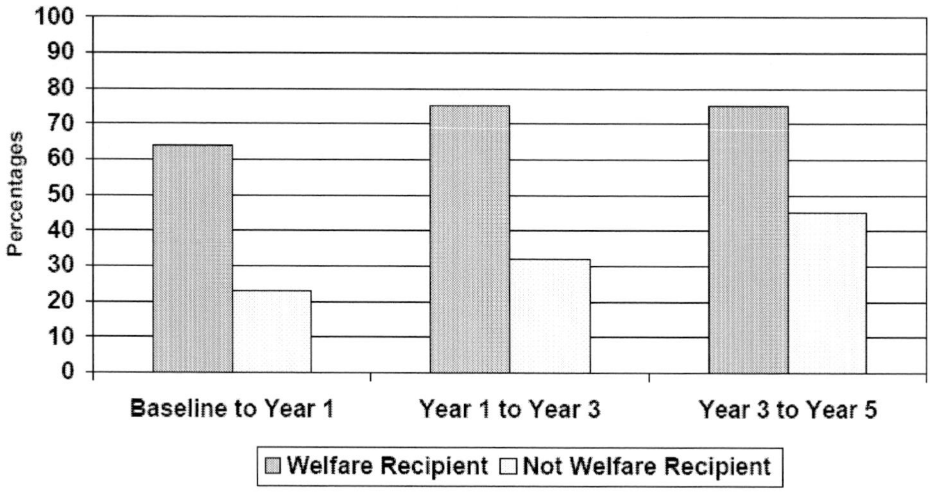

Figure 5. Medicaid enrollees who remained covered over time .

Instability of Insurance Coverage and Access to Treatment

We next turned to the question of how instability in insurance coverage influences access to chemical dependency treatment. As a first step, we examined the associations between baseline characteristics and different patterns in insurance coverage over the course of this five-year study. Over three-quarters of the pooled sample (76 percent) remained continuously insured at each time point over the course of all five years (see Table 2, bottom row). Equal proportions of others (eight percent in each case) experienced more unstable patterns involving transitions from being insured to uninsured or vice versa. Another eight percent remained continuously uninsured at each time point over the course of all five years.

There were significant differences in the characteristics of groups experiencing each of these patterns in insurance coverage, as shown in Table 2. Those who were continuously insured were, on the whole, more socioeconomically advantaged. As would be expected, they were more likely to be white, employed, higher income, married, to have never relied on welfare, and as a group, they were slightly older than other groups. In contrast, the most disadvantaged were the continuously uninsured, who notably were also disproportionately male, twice as likely to be African-American and had higher drug and psychiatric severity scores. These individuals were unlikely to have private coverage due to being unemployed and may not have met eligibility criteria for SSI-linked Medicare coverage after the 1997 policy change that rendered those disabled solely by virtue of a substance abuse disorder ineligible for assistance. The characteristics of those who lost or obtained insurance were roughly similar, and generally ranged somewhere between the two other groups on most indicators of socioeconomic deprivation and problem severity.

Table 2. Insurance status change by baseline characteristics in pooled sample (percents and means)

Characteristic	Continuously Insured	Lost Insurance	Got Insurance	Continuously Uninsured	Total
Female, %	42	33	39	24	40
Ethnicity					
White	69	59	60	50	66
Black	16	25	23	30	19
Other	15	16	17	20	16
Age, *M* (SD)	38 (12.2)	34 (9.8)	34 (9.0)	34 (9.2)	37 (11.7)
Unemployed, %	14	32	35	46	20
High school dropout, %	56	67	67	73	59
Income < 20K, %	29	47	53	63	35
Marital status (unmarried), %	57	77	76	81	62
Prior welfare use, %	9	21	24	33	13
ASI alcohol severity, *M* (SD)	0.27 (0.25)	0.30 (0.28)	0.27 (0.27)	0.25 (0.25)	0.27 (0.26)
ASI drug severity, *M* (SD)	0.06 (0.10)	0.10 (0.13)	0.09 (0.12)	0.10 (0.12)	0.07 (0.11)
ASI psychiatric severity, *M* (SD)	0.25 (0.24)	0.31 (0.24)	0.29 (0.25)	0.30 (0.23)	0.27 (0.24)
Unweighted N	(2852)	(312)	(285)	(296)	(3745)
Percent of Sample	76	8	8	8	100

Notes:

ASI = Addiction Severity Index

M = mean

SD = standard deviation

All differences by insurance stability, except for *ASI* alcohol severity, are statistically significant at $p<0.001$ level based on chi-square or F tests.

Data are weighted for non-response and sample design.

We next examined the role that variation in the stability of insurance coverage over time played in shaping the chances that an individual would obtain treatment for an alcohol or drug problem. Here, we used logistic autoregressive models to predict the odds of entering treatment at any given point in time as a function of shifts in insurance status at the prior time point and other factors. Table 3 shows the results of this analysis for episodes of specialty chemical dependency treatment, comparing initial treatment episodes in the general population sample with episodes of re-treatment in the sample drawn from alcohol and drug programs (odds ratios that achieve statistical significance at $p < .05$ are bolded). With respects to many factors in treatment entry, findings from the two models run in parallel. In both cases, having a specialty treatment encounter at one time point more than quadruples the chances of another encounter at the next point in time. Need factors are also significant predictors of treatment utilization in both models, although there is some minor variation in which kinds of problems play a greater role. In both samples, high psychiatric scores stand out as strong predictors of specialty treatment entry. After controlling for these factors, some patterns of insurance coverage are significantly associated with the receipt of specialty treatment over time. In the general population sample, losing one's insurance at one point in

Table 3. Logistic autoregressive model results for specialty substance abuse treatment

Factors in Treatment Entry	Initial Treatment General Population Sample of Problem Drinkers Odds Ratio	P-value	Repeat Treatment Treatment Program Sample Odds Ratio	P-value
Predisposing Factors				
Male	1.92	0.088	1.14	0.393
Age (vs. under 30)				
30-44	0.86	0.691	1.01	0.950
45 and above	0.76	0.507	1.10	0.694
Ethnicity (vs. White)				
Black	0.69	0.437	**1.58**	**0.011**
Other	0.54	0.203	1.46	0.109
More than high school education	0.47	0.065	1.07	0.682
Unemployed	1.29	0.610	1.30	0.113
Treatment at t-1	**4.85**	**0.000**	**4.41**	**0.000**
Need Factors				
ASI alcohol severity	1.39	0.078	1.35	0.001
ASI drug severity	**1.48**	**0.034**	1.12	0.156
ASI psychiatric severity	**1.89**	**0.029**	1.59	0.000
ASI legal severity	1.43	0.268	1.41	0.040
Enabling Factors				
Income < $35K	1.89	0.060	1.08	0.629
Insurance (vs. Continuously insured)				
Lost insurance	2.34	0.075	1.42	0.179
Got insurance	1.22	0.754	1.50	0.143
Continuously uninsured	0.94	0.914	**1.79**	**0.036**
Wald chi-squared	110.39		196.05	
Degrees of freedom	16		16	
p-value	0.000		0.000	
N of transitions	1580		1618	
N of persons	536		548	

time (as compared to being continuously insured) more than doubles the chances of receiving treatment at the next point. In the sample drawn from treatment programs, being continuously uninsured increases the chances of treatment by 79 percent at the next time point.

Table 4 shows a similar analysis of non-specialty chemical dependency treatment encounters, which include treatment in medical and mental health settings. Again, most results run parallel for initial treatment episodes and re-treatment episodes. In both cases, having a health or mental health treatment encounter for a chemical dependency problem at one time point increases the likelihood of another at the next point in time. Higher levels of psychiatric severity are also strong predictors of non-specialty care, while drug severity drops out as a predictor of treatment in non-specialty settings. What is particularly notable, however, is that the role of insurance in obtaining non-specialty care differs markedly from its role in specialty treatment entry, as was shown above. In both samples, losing insurance at one point in time reduces the chance of obtaining treatment in a non-specialty setting by more

Table 4. Logistic autoregressive model results for non-specialty treatment

	Initial Treatment		**Repeat Treatment**	
	General Population Sample of Problem Drinkers		Treatment Program Sample	
Factors in Treatment Entry	Odds Ratio	P-value	Odds Ratio	P-value
Predisposing Factors				
Male	1.20	0.334	0.88	0.373
Age (vs. under 30)				
30-44	1.06	0.762	0.99	0.937
45 and above	1.23	.0384	1.14	0.551
Ethnicity (vs. White)				
Black	0.71	0.366	0.85	0.340
Other	0.72	0.186	0.83	0.389
More than high school education	1.13	0.509	1.24	0.142
Unemployed	1.05	0.862	1.11	0.495
Non-specialty treatment at t-1	**4.84**	**0.000**	**1.79**	**0.000**
Need Factors				
ASI alcohol severity	**1.46**	**0.002**	**1.63**	**0.000**
ASI drug severity	0.99	0.993	1.11	0.124
ASI psychiatric severity	**1.85**	**0.000**	**2.39**	**0.000**
ASI legal severity	**1.73**	**0.009**	1.10	0.537
Enabling Factors				
Income < $35K	1.39	0.079	1.07	0.638
Insurance (vs. Continuously insured)				
Lost insurance	**0.43**	**0.034**	**0.37**	**0.001**
Got insurance	1.23	0.505	1.10	0.686
Continuously uninsured	0.54	0.135	0.67	0.117
Wald chi-squared	146.78		191.43	
Degrees of freedom	7		17	
p-value	0.000		0.000	
N of transitions	1583		1628	
N of persons	537		551	

than half, as compared to being continuously insured. Recall that in our models of specialty treatment, losing insurance had the opposite effect – the effect of increasing the chances of receiving specialty care.

Treatment Access among Medicaid Recipients

As noted above, individuals in this study with Medicaid coverage experienced some of the greatest instability in insurance coverage over time. Our final analyses, therefore, examined how such instability in Medicaid coverage influenced access to care over time. Here, we conducted our transitional regression analyses on the subset of participants who were on Medicaid at the beginning of the study, in 1995 (see Table 5). To achieve sufficient sample size for this analysis, we pooled Medicaid recipients from the general population and treatment program samples.

Findings from this sub-analysis of Medicaid recipients run in parallel to our findings for the whole sample. As in our earlier regression analyses, prior treatment and need factors prove to be important predictors of obtaining both specialty and non-specialty treatment for alcohol and drug problems. While this result does not meet the standard for statistical significance of $p < .05$, we do see a trend in the data that would likely reach this threshold if not for our conservative approach to autocorrelation and small sample size of Medicaid recipients. The data suggest that instability in Medicaid coverage may be more likely to reduce the likelihood of receiving care in a non-specialty treatment setting than in a specialty setting. When individuals lost their Medicaid to become continuously uninsured, the odds of receiving non-specialty care at the next time point was three times lower than those who were continuously insured. There is also a trend in the data suggesting that obtaining insurance may be positively associated with obtaining specialty care.

Table 5. Logistic autoregressive model results for specialty and non-specialty treatment (pooled Medicaid recipient sample)

Factors in Treatment Entry	Initial Treatment General Population Sample of Problem Drinkers Odds Ratio	P-value	Repeat Treatment Treatment Program Sample Odds Ratio	P-value
Predisposing Factors				
Male	0.87	0.762	1.09	0.848
Age (vs. under 30)				
30-44	1.19	0.742	0.88	0.789
45 and above	2.90	0.226	0.87	0.842
Ethnicity (vs. White)				
Black	2.27	0.115	1.34	0.539
Other	2.41	0.303	**2.82**	**0.058**
More than high school education	0.93	0.920	0.82	0.752
Unemployed	0.54	0.151	0.47	0.076
Treatment at t-1	**28.48**	**0.000**	**3.90**	**0.002**
Need Factors				
ASI alcohol severity	1.15	0.553	**1.79**	**0.003**
ASI drug severity	1.39	0.145	1.02	0.904
ASI psychiatric severity	1.45	0.239	**2.61**	**0.001**
ASI legal severity	1.20	0.663	0.50	0.146
Enabling Factors				
Income < $35K	0.46	0.13	1.77	0.660
Insurance (vs. Continuously insured)				
Lost insurance	0.99	0.994	0.31	0.188
Got insurance	3.44	0.97	0.33	0.280
Continuously uninsured	2.45	0.387	0.30	0.066
Wald chi-squared	77.02		58.69	
Degrees of freedom	16		17	
p-value	0.000		0.000	
N of transitions	208		214	
N of persons	70		72	

Conclusion

Medicaid beneficiaries in this study experienced some of the greatest instability in insurance coverage over time. By the end of a five-year period, more than three quarters of individuals on Medicaid had switched insurance plans or had become uninsured at least once, as compared to only one-third of those who began the study with private insurance. Once individuals left the Medicaid program, the most common result was a pattern of cycling back on and off the plan over subsequent years. However, nine percent of those who lost their Medicaid coverage became continuously uninsured over subsequent time points. Further analyses found that those individuals who left Medicaid to become uninsured would ultimately face significant difficulties with accessing treatment services from mainstream medical and mental health providers. Those who left Medicaid to become continuously uninsured were three times less likely than those with stable Medicaid coverage to obtain services for chemical dependency in a medical or mental health setting.

Some have pointed to changes in the Medicaid enrollment process following welfare reform as a major source of the kind of instability in coverage we observed. Prior to welfare reform, welfare recipients were automatically enrolled in Medicaid. But following reform, legislators decoupled the welfare and Medicaid application processes and gave states more flexibility in how they administered their plans. While national studies show that welfare recipients have experienced much more instability in Medicaid coverage in the aftermath of reform, we found the opposite to be the case. Following welfare reform implementation, welfare recipients in this study were, in fact, *more* likely to keep their Medicaid coverage than others on the plan. This is likely due to the fact that, in California, legislators sought to mitigate the problem by providing supplemental funds that preserved continuity in Medicaid coverage for former welfare recipients. What is remarkable, however, is that even in the absence of enrollment gaps generated by welfare reform, Medicaid recipients in this study still experienced the greatest instability in coverage. And that instability in coverage had significant consequences for their access to care.

Some of the most interesting findings from this analysis emerged from our comparisons of access to specialty and non-specialty chemical dependency treatment. Here, we found that most factors other than insurance coverage played similar roles in predicting the odds of accessing specialty and non-specialty care. Thus, factors that predispose one to seek substance abuse treatment, such as having had a prior treatment experience, had similar effects on access to services from specialty and non-specialty treatment providers. Results across measures of the severity of need for treatment were also relatively uniform. Regardless of whether the treatment was in a specialty or non-specialty setting, indicators of need had a roughly similar magnitude of effect in predicting service use, with psychiatric severity proving to be one of the strongest factors.

Our results concerning insurance coverage, however, differed markedly in analyses of specialty and non-specialty treatment. Indicators of insurance instability – losing insurance and being continuously uninsured – significantly increased the chances of receiving care in a specialty chemical dependency treatment program, but significantly decreased the chances of receiving care from a medical or mental health provider. Moreover, the magnitude of these effects was, at times, quite large. For example, controlling for other factors, losing one's health coverage reduced the chances of obtaining care from a medical or mental health provider by more than half.

These results should, of course, be interpreted within the confines of this study's analytic limitations. As detailed above, there were limitations in sample coverage and in variables included in the analysis. In particular, our models of treatment entry do not include independent variables reflecting coercion into treatment, and our measures of insurance are imprecise in that they only capture year-to-year changes in health coverage.

Policy Implications

Since the mid-1990s, we have seen declines in the numbers of eligible people enrolled in the Medicaid plan, reductions in Medicaid spending on behavioral health care, and changes in plan administration that make it more difficult for Medicaid beneficiaries to stay covered year-to-year. These policy developments have fueled concerns about meeting the need for chemical dependency treatment among low-income Americans. On the whole, the results of our analysis justify these concerns and underscore the need for policy changes that reduce instability in Medicaid coverage. In this study, Medicaid beneficiaries who experienced some of the greatest degree of instability in insurance coverage over time. And this instability in coverage, in turn, had pronounced effects on access to care for a chemical dependency problem in mainstream health and mental health settings, where most care for these problems is delivered.

While our analysis supports the conclusion that instability in Medicaid since the mid-1990s is a growing problem with real consequences, we also found evidence that the problem can be remedied through deliberate policy changes. This evidence came in the form of unexpected findings concerning the impact of welfare reform. Numerous studies have found that welfare recipients are particularly susceptible to losing Medicaid coverage as a consequence of special provisions under welfare reform. However, our analysis of a sample drawn from California found precisely the opposite (see also: Cox et al., 2001; Gresenz and Klerman, 2002; Mauldon et al., 2002). We believe this is because California legislators earmarked supplemental funds to preserve continuity in Medicaid coverage for welfare recipients. The case of California's supplemental plan thus suggests that policy interventions can offset the problems with Medicaid retention if states, as under welfare reform, are given the flexibility to design specialized solutions. It further suggests that the model of targeted transitional coverage to groups at high risk for losing Medicaid may be a useful one to replicate more broadly.

Our findings on insurance and access to different types of chemical dependency services point to some larger policy issues concerning the design and implementation of insurance benefits. Here we found that losing health coverage and being continuously uninsured increased the chances of receiving care from specialty chemical dependency treatment providers, but that it decreased the chances of receiving care from mainstream medical and mental health providers. This result may be attributable to the fact that the federal government provides block grant funds to states that help to cover specialty chemical dependency treatment for individuals with limited means to pay. Block grants provide a unique source of funding that subsidizes addiction care provided in specialty treatment programs. Our results suggest that this funding has an impact where it is most needed. The fact that those who lose their health coverage have a greater likelihood of receiving specialty care than those who are stably insured is testimony to the important role played by block grant funds in providing care to individuals who might otherwise not be served. At a time of fiscal crisis in many state Medicaid programs, findings such as this underscore the importance of preserving other sources of public funding for addiction treatment, namely, block grant funding.

We also found that, in the absence of public subsidies for specialty care, individuals with alcohol and drug problems who lose their insurance coverage will have limited treatment alternatives. In this study, those with stable insurance coverage were twice more likely than those who lost their coverage to receive care from a medical or mental health provider. Our analysis also showed that individuals with a propensity to lose health coverage or to become continuously uninsured had higher-severity alcohol and drug problems than those who were consistently insured. Given the crises in many Medicaid programs, policymakers should be most concerned about the adverse consequences of Medicaid cutbacks on access to care in non-specialty settings, such as medical and psychiatric settings. Encounters in these settings account for the majority of services provided to people in this study as well as others. Non-specialty services, therefore, make a very important contribution to the overall supply of treatment services. However, in mental health and medical settings, there is no block grant-funded alternative for the uninsured seeking care for substance abuse problems.

Our findings around specialty and non-specialty care point to the role played by insurance coverage in sorting individuals across different types of care. In an ideal world, we would rather find that characteristics of need – namely, higher-severity alcohol and drug problems – factor into this sorting process more than they did here. However, in this analysis, need factors played rather similar roles in predicting the odds of obtaining specialty and non-specialty treatment. Meanwhile, stability in insurance coverage made a significant difference in predicting which type of care one received.

These findings may ultimately reflect the broader fragmentation in coverage for treatment within our mixed system of public and private insurance plans in the United States. Some public sector funding streams, such as block grants, flow into specialty facilities but not mainstream facilities such as general hospitals. Meanwhile, the Medicaid and private funding streams more readily flow into mainstream health care and mental health settings. Within this broad division of responsibility, one payer may fill the gaps left open by another. But this arrangement may also mean that choices about where one receives care are driven less by the severity of need and more by the types of benefits provided under one's particular insurance plan. What would ultimately be needed to produce a more need-driven system for delivering care is a more uniform insurance benefits policy that promotes the blending of financing streams, for example, through centralized purchasing collaboratives. Such a system is not just possible, based on the growing body of evidence on treatment effectiveness, but essential if access to care is to be provided on the basis of clinical need. As discussed in the next chapter, managed care may (at least in theory) be one strategy that could facilitate blending of financing streams

Acknowledgments

This chapter was developed under a contract from the Substance Abuse and Mental Health Services Administration (SAMHSA), U.S. Department of Health and Human Services

(DHHS) (No. 270-01-7097). Report contributors included Christopher Tompkins, Brandeis University, Mary Jo Larson, New England Research Institutes, and Sharon Reif, Brandeis University. Government Project Officers included Patrice Roth, Center for Substance Abuse Treatment and Joan Dilonardo, Center for Substance Abuse Treatment. Views and opinions expressed are those of the authors and do not necessarily reflect those of SAMHSA or DHHS.

REFERENCES

Aday, L. A, and Andersen, R. A. (1974). A framework for the study of access to medical care. *Health Services Research, 9,* 208-220.

American Association for Public Opinion Research. (2000). *Standard definitions: Final dispositions of case codes and outcome rates for surveys.* Ann Arbor, MI: AAPOR.

Andersen, R. and Newman, J. P. (1973). Societal and individual determinants of medical utilization in the United States. *Milbank Memorial Fund Quarterly, 51,* 95-124.

Andersen, R. (1995). Revisiting the behavioral model and access to medical care: Does it matter? *Journal of Health and Social Behavior, 36,* 1-10.

Andrulis, D., and Hopkins, S. (2001). Public hospitals and substance abuse services for pregnant women and mothers: Implications for managed-care programs and Medicaid. *Journal of Urban Health-Bulletin of the New York Academy of Medicine, 78,* 181-198.

Baumohl, J., Speiglman, R., Swartz, J. A. and Stahl, R. (2003). Substance abuse and welfare policy at the new century. *Contemporary Drug Problems, 30,* 501-537.

Berk, M. L., and Schur, C. L. (2001). Access to care: How much difference does Medicaid make? In C. Harrington and C. L. Estes (Eds.), *Health policy: Crisis and reform in the U.S. health care delivery system* (pp. 276-283). Sudbury, MA: Jones and Bartlett Publishers.

Bonney, G. E. (1987). Logistic regression for dependent observations. *Biometrics, 43,* 951-973.

Booth, B. M., Blow, F. C., Cook, C. A., Bunn, J. Y., and Fortney, J. C. (1997). Relationship between inpatient alcoholism treatment and longitudinal changes in health care utilization. *Journal of Studies on Alcohol, 58,* 625-637.

Booth, B. M., Blow, F. C., Ludke, R. L., and Ross, R. L. (1996). Utilization of acute inpatient services for alcohol detoxification. *The Journal of Mental Health Administration, 23,* 366-374.

Booth, B. M., Kirchner, J., Fortney, J., Ross, R., and Rost, K. (2000). Rural at-risk drinkers: Correlates and one-year use of alcoholism treatment services. *Journal of Studies on Alcohol, 61,* 267.

Booth, B. M., and McLaughlin. Y. S. (2000). Barriers to and need for alcohol services for women in rural populations. *Alcoholism-Clinical and Experimental Research, 24,* 1267--1275.

Broder, J. M. (2004, January 18). Schwarzenegger budget denies some health care. *The New York Times.*

Brown, E. R., and Cousineau, M. R. (1991). Loss of Medicaid and access to health services. *Health Care Financing Review, 12,* 17-26.

Bureau of Labor Statistics. 1998. *Employee benefits in medium and larger private establishments, 1995.* Washington, DC: Bureau of Labor Statistics.

Callahan, J., Shepard, D., Beinecke, R., Larson, M. J., and Cavanaugh, D. (1995). Mental health/ substance abuse treatment in managed care: The Massachusetts Medicaid experience. *Health Affairs, 14,* 174-184.

Cavanaugh, D. A. (1999). Substance abuse and mental health services for children and adolescents: Experience under the Massachusetts Medicaid carve-out. *Dissertation Abstracts International, 59,* 3342-B.

Chang, C. F., Kiser, L. J., Bailey, J. E., Martins, M., Gibson, W. C., Schaberg, K. A., Mirvis, D. M., and Applegate, W. B. (1998). Tennessee's failed managed care program for mental health and substance abuse services. *The Journal of the American Medical Association, 279,* 864-869.

Chavkin, W., Romero, D., and Wise, P. H. (2000). State welfare reform policies and declines in health insurance. *American Journal of Public Health, 90,* 900-908.

Coffey, R.M., Mark, T., King, E., Harwood, H., McKusick, D., Genuardi, J. Dilonardo, J., and Buck, J. (2000). *Health care spending: National expenditures for mental health and substance abuse treatment 1997,* p. 57. Rockville, MD: U.S. Department of Health and Human Services.

Cox, A., Klerman, J. A., and Happoldt, I. A. (2001). *Medi-Cal after welfare reform: Enrollment among former welfare recipients* (p. 16). Oakland, CA: Medi-Cal Policy Institute.

DeChiara, M., and Wolff, T. (1998). Topics for our times: If we have the money, why is it so hard? *American Journal of Public Health, 88,* 1300-1302.

Deck, D. D., McFarland, B. H., Titus, J. M., Laws, K. E., and Gabriel, R. M. (2000). Access to substance abuse treatment services under the Oregon Health Plan. *The Journal of the American Medical Association, 284,* 2093-2099.

Diggle, P. J., Liang, K-Y., and Zeger, S. L. (1994). *Analysis of longitudinal data.* Oxford, UK: Clarendon Press.

Doty, M. M., and Holmgren, A. L. (2004). Unequal access: Insurance instability among low-income workers and minorities. In *Task Force on the Future of Health Insurance: Issue Brief.* New York: The Commonwealth Fund.

Ellwood, M. R. (1999). *The Medicare eligibility maze.* Washington, DC: Urban Institute.

Felland, L. E., Felt-Lisk, S., and McHugh, M. (2004). Health care access for low-income people: Significant safety net gaps remain. In *Issue brief: Findings from HSC* (pp. 1-4). Washington, DC: Center for Studying Health System Change.

Fox, A., Graves, M. C., and Garris, K. (1999). *The yearbook of managed behavioral health market share in the United States, 1999-2000.* Gettysburg, PA: Open Minds.

Garrett, B., and Holahan, J. (2000a). Health insurance coverage after welfare. *Health Affairs, 19,* 175-184.

Garrett, B., and Holahan, J. 2000b. *Welfare leavers, Medicaid coverage, and private health insurance* (pp. 1-5). Washington, DC: The Urban Institute.

Grant, B. (1996). Toward an alcohol treatment model: A comparison of treated and untreated respondents with DSM-IV alcohol use disorders in the general population. *Alcoholism: Clinical and Experimental Research, 20,* 372-378.

Greenfield, T. K., and Weisner, C. M. (1995). Drinking problems and self-reported criminal behavior, arrests and convictions: 1990 U.S. alcohol and 1989 county surveys. *Addiction, 90,* 361-373.

Gresenz, C. R., and Klerman, J. A. (2002). *Beyond Medi-Cal: Health insurance coverage among former welfare recipients* (p. 30). Oakland, CA: RAND.

Hanrahan, P., Luchins, D., Cloninger, L., and Swartz, J. (2004). Medicaid eligibility of former Supplemental Security Income recipients with drug abuse or alcoholism disability. *American Journal of Public Health, 94,* 46-47.

Harwood, H., Sullivan, K., and Malhorta, D. (2001). Data analysis identifies major disparities in alcohol treatment access across various groups. *Front Lines: Linking Alcohol Services Research and Practice, 4,* 7.

Holahan, J., Zuckerman, S., Evans, A., and Rangarajan, S. (1998). Medicaid managed care in thirteen states. *Health Affairs, 17,* 43-63.

Humphreys, K., and Weisner, C. M. (2000). Use of exclusion criteria in selecting research subjects and its effect on the generalizability of alcohol treatment outcome studies. *American Journal of Psychiatry, 157,* 588-594.

Huskamp, A. A. (1999). Episodes of mental health and substance abuse treatment under a managed behavioral health care carve-out. *Inquiry: The Journal of Health Care Organization Provision and Financing, 36,* 147-161.

Johnson, P., Curtigan, S., and Dixon, L. (2003). *FY 2003-2004 NCSL Medicaid budget survey executive summary.* Washington, DC: Health Policy Tracking Service, National Conference of State Legislatures.

Kaskutas, L., Russell, G., and Dinis, M. (1997). *Technical report on the alcohol treatment utilization study in public and private sectors.* Berkeley, CA: Alcohol Research Group.

Kessler, R. C., Nelson, C. B., McGonagle, K. A., Edlund, M. J., Frank, R. G. and Leaf, P. J. (1996). The epidemiology of co-occurring addictive and mental disorders: Implications for prevention and service utilization. *American Journal of Orthopsychiatry, 66,* 17-31.

Klein, R., and Fish-Parcham, C. (1999). *Losing health insurance: The unintended consequences of welfare reform* (p. 45). Washington, DC: Families USA Foundation.

Ku, L., and Bruen, B. (1999). The continuing decline in Medicaid coverage, p. 1-7. Washington, DC: The Urban Institute.

Ku, L., and Coughlin, T. (1997). How the new welfare reform laws affects Medicaid. *The Urban Institute,* Series A (A-5).

Ku, L., Ross, D. C., and Nathanson, M. (2002). *State Medicaid cutbacks and the federal role in providing fiscal relief to states* (p. 5). Washington, DC: Center on Budget and Policy Priorities.

Lurie, N., Ward, N. B., and Shapiro, M. F. 1986. A termination of Medi-Cal benefits: A follow-up study one year later. *New England Journal of Medicine, 314,* 1266-1268.

Maloy, K., Pavetti, L., Darnell, J., and Shin, P. (1999). *Diversion as a work-oriented welfare reform strategy and its effect on access to Medicaid: An examination of the experiences of five local communities* (p. 152). Washington, DC: The George Washington University School of Public Health and Health Services: Center for Health Policy Research.

Mann, C., Hudman, J., Salganicoff, A., and Folsom, A. (2002). Five years later: Poor women's health care coverage after welfare reform. *Journal of the American Medical Women's Association, 57,* 16-22.

Mauldon, J., Nayeri, K., and Dobkin, C. E. (2002). Transitional Medi-Cal for families leaving welfare is underused. In *CPRC Brief.* Berkeley, CA: California Policy Research Center.

McLellan, T. A., Kushner, H., Metzger, D., Peters, R., Smith, I., Grissom, G., Pettinati, H., and Argeriou, M. (1992). The fifth edition of the Addiction Severity Index. *Journal of Substance Abuse Treatment, 9,* 199-213.

Neuhaus, J. M. (1992). Statistical methods for longitudinal and clustered designs with binary responses. *Statistical Methods in Medical Research, 1,* 249-273.

Padgett, D., Struening, E., and Andrews, H. (1990). Factors affecting the use of medical, mental health, alcohol, and drug treatment services by homeless adults. *Medical Care, 28,* 805-821.

Pear, R., and Toner, R. (2002a, January 14). Amid fiscal crisis, Medicaid is facing cuts from states. *New York Times.*

Pear, R., and Toner, R. (2002b, January 14). States face hard choices on Medicaid cuts. *The New York Times.*

Post, P. A. (2001). *Casualties of complexity: Why eligible homeless people are not enrolled in Medicaid* (p. 73). Nashville, TN: National Health Care for the Homeless Council.

Regier, D. A., Narrow, W. E., Rae, D. S., Manderscheid, R. W., Locke, B. Z., and Goodwin, F. K. (1993). The *de facto* U.S. mental and addictive disorders service system: Epidemiologic catchment area prospective 1-year prevalence rates of disorders and services. *Archives of General Psychiatry, 50,* 85-94.

Rogowski, J. A. (1993). *Private versus public sector insurance coverage for drug abuse* (p. 53). Santa Monica, CA: RAND.

Rowland, D., and Hanson, K. (1996). Medicaid: Moving to managed care. *Health Affairs, 15,* 150-152.

Sabin, J. E., and Daniels, N. (1997). Setting behavioral health priorities: Good news and crucial lessons from the Oregon Health Plan. *Psychiatric Services, 48,* 883-884.

Schmidt, L. (2001). *Technical report: Coding scheme for insurance variables, study of treated and untreated problem drinkers, baseline and wave 1 of follow-up.* Berkeley, CA: Alcohol Research Group.

Schmidt, L. A., and Weisner, C. M. (2005). Private insurance and the utilization of chemical dependency treatment. *Journal of Substance Abuse Treatment*, *28,* 67-76.

Smith, V., Ramesh, R., Gifford, K., Ellis, E., Wachino, V., and O'Malley, M. (2004). States respond to fiscal pressure: A 50-state update of state Medicaid spending growth and cost containment actions, p. 20. In *Kaiser Commission on Medicaid and the Uninsured.* Washington, DC: The Henry J. Kaiser Family Foundation.

Stata Corp. (2003). *Stata statistical software: Release 8.0.* College Station, TX: Stata Corporation.

Strunk, B. C., and Reschovsky, J. D. (2004). Trends in U. S. health insurance coverage, 2001 - 2003. In *Tracking Report: Results from the Community Tracking Study No. 9* (pp. 1-5). Washington, DC: Center for Studying Health System Change.

Substance Abuse and Mental Health Services Administration. (2001). *Prevalence of and access to substance abuse and mental health treatment by type of insurance coverage.* Fairfax, VA: The Lewin Group, Inc.

Substance Abuse and Mental Health Services Administration. (2002). *National and state estimates of the drug abuse treatment gap: 2000 National Household Survey on Drug Abuse,* p. 73. Rockville, MD: SAMHSA, Office of Applied Studies.

Tam, T. (1997). *Technical report on the alcohol treatment utilization study in public and private sectors: Within and across sector weights.* Berkeley, CA: Alcohol Research Group.

United States Census Bureau. (2003). Income, poverty, and health insurance coverage in the United States: 2003. In C. DeNavas-Walt, B. D. Proctor, and R. J. Mills (Eds.), *Current Population Reports: Consumer Income*. Washington, DC: U.S. Bureau of the Census.

United States Department of Health and Human Services. (1999). *Lewin Group state profiles, 1999, on public sector managed behavioral health care,* p. 345. Falls Church, VA: U.S. Department of Health and Human Services (SAMHSA).

United States Department of Health and Human Services (2003). *The application process for TANF, Food Stamps, Medicaid, and SCHIP: Issues for agencies and applicants, including immigrants and limited English speakers.* Washington, DC: U. S. Department of Health and Human Services.

United States Center for Health Statistics. (1999). *Health United States, 1999.* Hyattsville, MD: United States Department of Health and Human Services.

United States General Accounting Office. (1998a). *Drug abuse treatment: Data limitations affect the accuracy of national and state estimates of need* (p. 24). Washington, DC: United States General Accounting Office.

United States General Accounting Office. (1998b). *Welfare reform: States are restructuring programs to reduce welfare dependence.* Washington, DC: United States General Accounting Office.

United States National Institute on Drug Abuse (1992). *The Washington DC Metropolitan Area Drug Study: Prevalence of drug use in the DC metropolitan area household population: 1990.* Rockville, MD, United States Department of Health and Human Services, National Institute on Drug Abuse, Division of Epidemiology and Prevention Research.

Wang, P. S., Berglund, P., and Kessler, R. C. (2000). Recent care of common mental disorders in the United States. *Journal of General Internal Medicine, 15,* 284-292.

Weisner, C. (1990a). Coercion in alcohol treatment. In Institute of Medicine, *Broadening the base of treatment for alcohol problems. Report of a study by a committee of the Institute of Medicine* (pp. 579-609). Washington, DC: National Academy of Sciences Press.

Weisner, C. (1990b). The role of alcohol-related problematic events in treatment entry. Berkeley, CA: Alcohol Research Group.

Weisner, C. M. (1993). Toward an alcohol treatment entry model: A comparison of problem drinkers in the general population and in treatment. *Alcoholism: Clinical and Experimental Research, 17,* 746-752.

Weisner, C. M., Greenfield, T. K., and Room, R. (1995). Trends in the treatment of alcohol problems in the U.S. general population, 1979 through 1990. *American Journal of Public Health, 85,* 55-60.

Weisner, C. M., Matzger, H., Tam, T, and Schmidt, L. A. (2002). Who goes to alcohol and drug treatment? Understanding utilization within the context of insurance. *Journal of Studies on Alcohol, 63,* 673-682.

Weisner, C. M., and Schmidt L. A. (1992). Gender disparities in treatment for alcohol problems. *The Journal of the American Medical Association, 268,* 1872-1876.

Weisner, C. M., and Schmidt L. A. (1995). The community epidemiology laboratory: Studying alcohol problems in community and agency-based populations. *Addiction, 90,* 329-342.

Weisner, C. M., and Schmidt L. A. (2001). Rethinking access to alcohol treatment. In M. Galanter, *Recent Developments in Alcoholism* (pp. 107-136). New York, NY: Plenum Press.

Weisner, C. M., and Schmidt L. A., and Tam, T. (1995). Assessing bias in community-based prevalence estimates: Toward an unduplicated count of problem drinkers and drug users. *Addiction 90,* 391-406.

Woodward, A., Epstein, J., Gfroerer, J., Melnick, D., Thoreson, R., and Wilson, D. (1997). The drug abuse treatment gap: Recent estimates. *Health Care Financing Review, 18,* 1-13.

Wu, L.-T., Kouzis, A. C., and Schlenger, W. E. (2003). Substance use, dependence, and service utilization among the U.S. uninsured non-elderly population. *American Journal of Public Health, 93,* 2079-2085.

In: Medicaid and Treatment for People... ISBN 978-1-61470-742-4
Editors: B.H. McFarland, D. McCarty et al., pp.47-109 © 2011 Nova Science Publishers, Inc.

Chapter 4

History of Medicaid Managed Care and Substance Abuse Treatment

Norman Penner*[1]*, Bentson H. McFarland*[2]*,
***and Anne E. Kovas*[1]**

[1] Department of Psychiatry, Oregon Health and Science University, Portland, OR, USA
[2] Departments of Psychiatry and Public Health and Preventive Medicine, Oregon Health and Science University, Portland, OR, USA

Abstract

This chapter summarizes years of substantial change as Medicaid moved largely from fee for service to a managed care environment. Numerous questions have arisen regarding this momentous shift. In particular, it has been suggested that managed care provided incentives for providers to "cherry pick" clients with low substance abuse severity. Beginning with definitions of substance abuse treatment and managed care, the chapter provides detailed historical information on a state-by-state and year-by-year basis regarding the movement away from Medicaid fee for service and towards assorted managed care programs. States adopted numerous Medicaid innovations chiefly via various waiver mechanisms. The chapter provides comprehensive listings in text and tables showing these transitions with emphasis on changes pertinent to chemical dependency care. Building on this carefully assembled (and unlikely to be found elsewhere) record, the chapter examines impact of managed care transition on severity of Medicaid clients in treatment for substance abuse. Using hierarchical linear models, it is concluded that Medicaid managed care led, if anything, to slight increase in severity of substance abuse treatment clients.

Introduction

Medicaid changed substantially during the 1990s with both marked growth in its role as a payer for substance abuse treatment and replacement in many states of fee for service payment systems by managed care programs. These Medicaid alterations comprise a nation-wide "natural experiment" regarding the impact of organizational and financing arrangements on provision of services for people with substance abuse problems. Results of this experiment are important both for Medicaid clients and for decision-makers.

This chapter documents on a state-by-state and year-by-year basis the implementation, adaptation, and (in some cases) discontinuation of various so-called "managed care" alternatives to traditional Medicaid fee for service payments for chemical dependency treatments. Building on this history, the chapter then examines the impact of Medicaid managed care on a key measure of substance abuse treatment delivery. These analyses are of considerable interest to Medicaid clients with substance abuse problems and also to policy makers concerned about provision of health care services. To put this work in context, the nature of substance abuse treatment is summarized, managed care definitions are provided, and single state studies on Medicaid managed care for chemical dependency services are reviewed.

SERVICES AND THEIR VALUE FOR PEOPLE WITH SUBSTANCE ABUSE PROBLEMS

Services for people with substance use disorders are usually divided into the acute detoxification stage, the rehabilitation phase of treatment, and the maintenance phase or recovery (Institute of Medicine, 1990; McLellan et al., 1996). There are many types of treatment available including, to cite just a few examples, self-help programs such as Alcoholics Anonymous (Humphreys and Moos, 1996; Tonigan et al., 1996), brief interventions delivered by primary health care providers (Bien et al., 1993; Fleming et al., 1997; Parish, 1997; Sullivan and Fleming, 1997), and the treatments provided by professionals working in the behavioral health specialty sector (Institute of Medicine, 1990). This chapter is concerned chiefly with rehabilitation phase services delivered by behavioral health professionals.

While the evidence is not unequivocal (Finney, 1995; Finney and Monahan, 1996), it is generally believed that professional rehabilitation services for people with substance abuse problems are efficacious (Institute of Medicine, 1990; McLellan et al., 1996; Moos and Finney, 1995; O'Brien and McLellan, 1996). By and large, the literature suggests that people with substance abuse problems who receive treatment have better outcomes than their untreated counter-parts (McLellan et al., 1996; Moos and Finney, 1995; Timko et al., 1995).

There are several types of professional rehabilitation phase treatments (Zwick and Berman, 1992) for clients with substance abuse problems. One important aspect of treatment is the modality (*e.g.,* outpatient, residential, hospital inpatient, etc.). In a frequently cited review, Miller and Hester (1986) found little evidence for superiority of one treatment modality over another. However, randomized trials by Walsh et al. (1991) and Pettinati et al. (1993) at least raised the possibility that for some clients there may be advantages to residential over outpatient care.

Key issues regarding substance abuse treatment include the extent of use (which may reflect availability of services and ease of access thereto), the characteristics of people who obtain treatment (which may reflect both self-selection and programmatic selection of clients), and the outcomes of care. Regarding managed care, Weisner et al. (1999) pointed out that "concerns have been raised by providers and consumers that these changes (*i.e.,* managed care implementation) may affect the availability of services, access to them, and the results of treatment".

Managed Care and its Impact on Substance Abuse Treatment

Managed care may be defined as the provision of services in accordance with "medical necessity" which, in turn, is the "health care service that will effectively and efficiently address the patient's medical condition" (McFarland and George, 1995). Numerous managed care mechanisms have evolved that seek to limit treatment services to those deemed medically necessary (Alexander and Lemak, 1997, 1997; McFarland and Minkoff, 1996). Approaches including capitation (also known as pre-payment), discounted fee for service, prior authorization, utilization review, and case rate payments have been adopted by states and counties (Alexander and Lemak, 1997). Some states, such as Oregon, assigned responsibility for chemical dependency services to capitated health maintenance organizations serving Medicaid clients so as to link alcohol and drug abuse treatment with general medical care (Laws et al., 2002). At one time or another, some 20 states adopted "integrated" models that attempted to combine behavioral health care with physical health care in managed (typically capitated) Medicaid programs (McFarland, 1994; Policy Resource Center and George Washington University Center for Health Policy Research, 1996). Conversely, states such as Massachusetts adopted a carve-out approach in which a statewide vendor managed the Medicaid substance abuse treatment benefit (Callahan, 1995). Egnew (1996) pointed out that states have not necessarily created (or purchased services from) new entities. Rather, at least in the 20 "strong county" states where services are delivered by local government agencies, state authorities often switched reimbursement away from fee for service and towards capitation or other payment systems operated by county programs (McFarland, 1996).

There has also been variation over time within state Medicaid programs for clients with chemical dependency problems. For example, Montana and New Mexico switched back from managed care to fee for service. Yet another variation has been to devise special programs for distinct sub-populations of Medicaid clients (such as people with disabilities) in what might be called a "population carve-out". Adoption and adaptation of these and other managed care approaches created considerable ferment among agencies that provided substance abuse treatment.

Indeed, speaking of the 1990s, Horgan (2001) noted that "there has been dramatic growth in managed care for substance abuse treatment". At least in the private sector, managed care implementation was usually accompanied by a shift from inpatient or residential to outpatient treatment (Goldman et al., 1998). The replacement of fee for service with other payment mechanisms in the private sector also led to consolidation of provider programs in a process termed "horizontal integration" (McFarland, 2000).

Impact of managed care on privately funded substance abuse treatment was substantial. In the commercial sector, a survey of 1,043 large employers showed that from 1988 to 1997 the value of general health care (*i.e.,* medical-surgical) benefits declined by seven percent whereas the value of addiction treatment benefits dropped by 71 percent (Galanter et al., 2000). This change may well have been related to the poor opinions about alcohol and drug treatment held by private sector payers (McFarland et al., 2003). Other work in the private sector by Stein et al. (1999) suggested that access to substance abuse treatment declined when a large employer implemented a "carve-out" managed behavioral health care program. In their review, Steenrod et al. (2001) concluded that "substance abuse services may be especially vulnerable to reductions in utilization (due to managed care)". However, some studies in the private sector found that managed behavioral health care led to an increase in numbers of enrollees served but decreases in intensity of treatment (Goldman et al., 1998).

Public Sector Managed Care for Substance Abuse Treatment

Managed care also arrived in the public behavioral health sector during the 1990s (Alexander and Lemak, 1997; Alexander et al., 1998; Gustafson et al., 1999; McFarland and Minkoff, 1996; Maglione and Ridgely, 2006). The Substance Abuse and Mental Health Services Administration found that the fraction of substance abuse treatment agencies holding managed care contracts increased dramatically from 32 percent in 1995 to 54 percent in 1999 (Office of Applied Studies, 2001). This increase was especially noteworthy among the non-profit programs (Alexander and Lemak, 1997). In addition, Alexander et al. (1998) reported that managed care had substantial impact on the internal operations of substance abuse treatment agencies. In its survey of state alcohol and drug abuse agencies, the National Association of State Alcohol and Drug Abuse Directors found that "managed care and its consequences" was the most frequently mentioned policy concern (Gustafson et al., 1999). Alexander et al. (2003) noted that in the 1990s public sector managed care arrangements for substance abuse treatment increased whereas those in the private sector decreased.

Medicaid Managed Care and Public Sector Substance Abuse Treatment

Also during the 1990s, Medicaid grew markedly as a payer for chemical dependency services and now finances considerable public sector substance abuse treatment (Coffey et al., 2000). Coffey et al. (2000) estimated that Medicaid accounted for 12 percent of chemical dependency treatment expenditures in 1987 whereas by 1997 the comparable figure had nearly doubled to 20 percent. Similarly, Mark et al. (2007) found that Medicaid accounted for 10 percent of substance abuse treatment expenditures in 1986, accounted for 18 percent by 1998, and remained at about 18 percent through 2003. These percentages are especially important because people with substance abuse problems depend heavily on the public sector for treatment (Coffey et al., 1997; (Mark et al., 2003; Mark et al., 2007; McKusick et al., 1998). Mark et al. (2007) found that the percentage of chemical dependency treatment funding provided by the public sector rose from 50 percent in 1986 to 77 percent in 2003.

Conversely, during that time period public sector funding for all health care only rose from 41 percent to 45 percent (Mark et al., 2007).

Medicaid overall (*i.e.,* physical health care plus behavioral health) changed dramatically during the 1990s as assorted managed care programs replaced the previous fee for service system (McFarland, 2000). The fraction of Medicaid clients enrolled in managed care rose from 10 percent in 1991 to 48 percent in 1997 (Iglehart, 1999) with the majority in managed care by 1998. Several authors noted that state Medicaid agencies increasingly embraced managed care approaches such as health maintenance organizations and-or financial risk sharing even as the private sector moved away from these programs (Draper and Gold, 2003; Draper, Hurley, and Short, 2004; Hurley and Somers, 2003).

Similarly, Medicaid behavioral health systems underwent marked change in the 1990s (McKusick et al., 1998) as programs shifted away from fee for service and towards managed care approaches such as case rates or capitation (Maglione and Ridgely, 2006; Mark et al., 2003; McCarty et al., 2003; McFarland, 2000). A report from the Substance Abuse and Mental Health Services Administration (Bergman, 1999; SAMHSA, 1998) showed that most states either implemented or considered some form of managed care in their Medicaid behavioral health programs. In particular, many states adopted Medicaid managed care systems pertaining to substance abuse treatment (Bergman, 1999; SAMHSA, 1998). The Substance Abuse and Mental Health Services Administration's Managed Care Tracking System reported that most states implemented Medicaid managed care for substance abuse during the middle 1990s. In some states, block grant funded substance abuse treatment programs were also converted to managed care (American Managed Behavioral Healthcare Association and the National Association of State Alcohol and Drug Abuse Directors, 1999; Bergman, 1999; SAMHSA, 1998).

Medicaid Managed Care for Substance Abuse Treatment and Concerns About Provision of Care

Concerns have been expressed about the impact of these changes on treatment outcomes and access to services (Chang et al., 1998). Whereas the fee for service system rewards treatment delivery, managed care financing mechanisms such as capitation may motivate providers to reduce services (McFarland, 2000; Sosin and D'Aunno, 2001; Steenrod et al., 2001). Mechanic pointed out that providers operating under managed care arrangements have "a disincentive to offer a level of comprehensiveness and quality of care that will attract particularly needy and expensive clients" (Mechanic, 1999).

Critics of managed care suggested that clients may be given services that are less intense or of shorter duration than clinically indicated (Galanter et al., 2001). The implication here is that client outcomes would be worse under managed care than under fee for service. Ettner, Denmead et al. (2003) noted that capitated programs in particular may be tempted to minimize service provision (which might be called "short-changing"). Indeed, Etheridge et al. (1995) found nationwide a significant reduction over time in the number and range of services that substance abuse clients received. Moreover, studies in Iowa (Ettner, Argeriou et al., 2003) and Maryland (Ettner, Denmead et al., 2003) showed a shift from inpatient and residential to outpatient substance abuse treatment programs following introduction of

Medicaid managed care. While it is conceivable that such changes in service provision might lead to poor treatment outcomes, no adverse impact was found in Maryland (Ettner, Denmead et al., 2003). Similarly, a Colorado study found that youth with alcohol problems had reduced contact with juvenile justice authorities after the change from fee for service to capitated Medicaid behavioral health care (Scott et al., 2002). In addition, work in Oregon by McFarland, McCamant et al. (2005) showed no impact of managed care on outcomes for adult Medicaid clients with substance abuse problems.

Another concern has been the impact of managed care and-or state Medicaid enrollment policies on treatment duration for public sector chemical dependency clients. This topic is of interest to policy makers because a large body of literature suggests that there is a minimum duration of treatment for people with substance abuse problems (Finney and Moos, 2002; Simpson and Brown, 1997). Indeed, the National Institute on Drug Abuse states in its Thirteen Principles of Effective Drug Addiction Treatment that "remaining in treatment for an adequate period of time is critical for treatment effectiveness" (NIDA, 1999). While this statement is not entirely without controversy (Manski et al., 2001), the National Institute on Drug Abuse has also suggested that "the threshold of significant improvement is reached at about three months in treatment" (NIDA, 1999). However, work from Maryland suggested that the implementation of managed care led if anything to increased treatment duration for Medicaid clients with substance abuse problems (Ettner, Denmead et al., 2003).

Access to services under Medicaid managed care has also been an area of controversy (Chang et al., 1998). As it happens, increased access to chemical dependency treatment was observed in Oregon when Medicaid alcohol and drug abuse treatment converted from fee for service to capitation in 1995 (Deck et al., 2000). On the other hand, states such as Montana, New Mexico, and Tennessee had unfortunate experiences when their Medicaid systems adopted managed care. For example, it was alleged (but not demonstrated quantitatively) that Medicaid client access to chemical dependency treatment declined in Tennessee when the state adopted Medicaid managed care (Chang et al., 1998). Projects in Oregon (Deck et al., 2000), Iowa (Ettner, Argeriou et al., 2003; McCarty and Argeriou, 2003), and Maryland (Ettner, Denmead et al., 2003) examined the impact of Medicaid managed care on use of substance abuse treatment services. In general, these studies showed that overall access to services apparently increased following the shift to managed care (Deck et al., 2000; McCarty and Argeriou, 2003).

Medicaid Managed Care and Substance Abuse Treatment Client Severity

There have also been concerns that managed care programs such as capitation could motivate providers to ignore more severely impaired clients. Ettner, Denmead et al. (2003) pointed out that capitation may provide incentives for health plans to focus on less severely impaired patients (sometimes referred to as "cream-skimming"). In other words, the issue is the impact of Medicaid managed care on what might be called the "case mix" of substance abuse treatment clients in the public sector. Critics have asserted that managed care programs "cream skim" by selectively serving people with few impairments (Institute of Medicine, 1996; Talbott and Hales, 2001). Interestingly enough, the severity of patients entering publicly funded substance abuse treatment programs was about the same before and after Medicaid managed care in Oregon (Sosin and D'Aunno, 2001) and even increased in Iowa (Ettner, Argeriou et al., 2003). However, there appear to be few if any nation-wide data that address this issue.

A question of some interest, then, is whether or not the implementation of managed care (including financial risk) has had an impact on severity of clients admitted for care in publicly funded substance abuse treatment programs. To address this topic, the present chapter reviews the history of Medicaid and the conversion of this program from a fee for service system into a markedly heterogeneous enterprise characterized by assorted managed care approaches. Both qualitative and quantitative methods are employed to describe this state-by-state and year-by-year transformation. The chapter then addresses the severity of substance abuse treatment clients during the transformation of Medicaid from fee for service to managed care. Information came chiefly from materials provided on-line by the United States Centers for Medicare and Medicaid Services (CMS) and from national databases maintained by the United States Substance Abuse and Mental Health Services Administration (SAMHSA).

Medicaid History

The Medicaid program, Title XIX of the Social Security Act, was authorized by Federal legislation in 1965 to provide medical assistance for certain individuals and families with low incomes and resources (Maglione and Ridgely, 2006). Medicaid eligibility was limited to individuals who fell into specific categories. The program was structured as a jointly-funded cooperative venture between the Federal and state governments. The Federal government, in addition to providing a portion of the funding, also established broad national guidelines regarding eligibility and scope of benefits. For their part, the states were allowed (within the broad national guidelines) to establish their own eligibility standards; determine the type, amount, duration, and scope of services; set the rates of payment for services; and administer their own programs. As a result, the Medicaid program has varied considerably from state to state over time. There have also been significant variations within individual states.

With regard to substance abuse, it is important to note that Medicaid has not had a defined set of reimbursable alcohol and drug treatment services. Initially, Medicaid beneficiaries suffering from medical conditions resulting from the abuse of alcohol were provided treatment under the provisions of the law that stated they were entitled to "Inpatient Hospital Care" or "Outpatient Hospital Care" or "Physician Services" or their treatment was determined to be "Medically Necessary". Beneficiaries were free to seek treatment from any qualified provider in the state under the "freedom of choice" provisions of the law (Section 1902(a)(23). Once the acute medical condition was alleviated, care was terminated. The long-term needs of the addicted patient in dealing with his or her addiction were not specifically addressed in the original Medicaid legislation. Because states had significant latitude in deciding what services -- and the amount, duration, and scope -- to include in their Medicaid plans, not all states chose to cover mental health and-or substance abuse services and those that did cover these services applied a variety of limits to them. One state may have limited the type of service or delivery setting, another the duration of service, a third the dollar amount per year, and in some instances all three limits were applied.

Moreover, Medicaid was not designed to provide medical assistance to all poor people. Under the original provisions of the Federal statute, individuals seeking medical services under Medicaid were required not only to be poor but also to belong to one or more of several specific groups, *e.g.*, recipients of (then) Aid to Families with Dependent Children (AFDC), children under the age of six in a family that was below Federal poverty level, pregnant women below the Federal poverty level, Supplemental Security Income (SSI) recipients, recipients of adoption or foster care assistance, or persons deemed "medically needy". (Medically Needy programs were designed for people who meet the basic eligibility criteria for Medicaid and who have resources and income that are limited, but that exceed the guidelines for Family Independence Programs [FIP] and Supplemental Security Income [SSI]).

The benefits to be provided under the provisions of Title XIX were set forth in terms of basic services a state had to offer in order to receive Federal matching funds. There was no mention of disease, disability types, or diagnoses for which services could be provided. Services were to be inpatient or outpatient hospital care delivered by a physician. Neither physical nor mental diagnoses were specifically cited in the listing of "certain basic services" that states had to offer in order to receive Federal matching funds. As a result, there has been substantial variation in services provided by state Medicaid plans.

Over the intervening years, both the states and the Federal government have changed the qualification rules as well as the scope of covered services. As a result, over the past decades, Medicaid has changed from a narrowly defined program available only to persons eligible for cash assistance into a large and costly enterprise with complex eligibility rules. Today Medicaid is a heterogeneous program reflecting both Federal policy and individual state decisions concerning eligibility as well as the scope and types of services.

Early Medicaid Managed Care

Due to the program's loose construction, Federal legislation, and fluctuations in the nation's economic condition, as well as continual healthcare price increases, Medicaid costs experienced a general upward trend from the outset of the program. From the program's beginnings in the mid-1960s, Medicaid policymakers struggled with financing and coverage, provider participation, and access for covered beneficiaries.

This situation led state Medicaid managers to search for new concepts and models for the financing and delivery of services including managed care. With its focus on utilization of services and restrictions on service providers, managed care seemed to be the best cost-containment solution for Medicaid. However, states could not simply adopt a managed care concept and restrict beneficiaries to specific providers. Such an approach would be in violation of beneficiaries' right to choose their service providers. Federal law prevented states from deviating from the basic procedures set down in Title XIX without review and approval of their plans by the Secretary of Health and Human Services.

There was, however, nothing that prevented a Medicaid beneficiary from voluntarily enrolling in a health maintenance organization (HMO) and several states chose this approach as a way to begin obtaining some benefits from managed care. In the early 1970s, California (1970), Pennsylvania (1972), Michigan (1974) and Illinois (1975) were the first states to allow some of their Medicaid population to enroll voluntarily in commercial HMO plans. California began its Prepaid Health Program on January 1, 1970 involving both HMO as well as Seniors and Persons with Disabilities (SPD) components. The California program covered both mental health and substance abuse. Pennsylvania started a "Vol. HMO Contracts" program on January 1, 1972 with HMO, SPD, mental health and substance abuse aspects. Michigan started its "Health Maint. Org." program on January 1, 1974 including HMO, SPD, mental health and substance abuse components. Illinois started Voluntary Medical Care on July 1, 1975 including Prepaid Health Plan (PHP), HMO, mental health and substance abuse programs. These HMOs were either Federally qualified or were defined by state Medicaid plans.

All the HMOs involved with these early California, Pennsylvania, Michigan, and Illinois Medicaid programs provided coverage for mental conditions and substance abuse. However, commercial HMOs had limits on their mental health and substance abuse benefits. Mental health benefits were generally limited to 30 inpatient days and 20 outpatient visits per calendar year. Substance abuse benefits were limited to 5 inpatient days per calendar year for acute care or detoxification. Outpatient substance abuse treatment was limited to 20 visits per calendar year.

It should be noted too that some early Medicaid managed care programs omitted mental health and substance abuse services. For example, Florida began its Managed Health Care system on October 1, 1981 with both Primary Care Case Management (PCCM) and HMO aspects but with neither mental health nor substance abuse services. Similarly, Nevada began its Vol. PHP/PCCM Program on November 1, 1983 with PHP and PCCM but with neither mental health nor substance abuse.

There were also special programs addressing aspects of behavioral health care. For example, the New York Office of Mental Health began a Partial Capitation program on May 1, 1987 involving a Prepaid Health Plan for mental health (Babigian et al., 1991; Babigian and Marshall, 1989; Cole et al., 1994; Reed and Babigian, 1994; Reed et al., 1994; Reed et al., 1995). In addition, New York began a Voluntary Managed Care program on April 1, 1987 that included HMO, SPD, mental health and substance abuse components. Maryland started a Voluntary HMO Contracts program prior to 1992 (state personnel were unable to provide the implementation date) including PHP, Health Insuring Organization (HIO) plus mental health and substance abuse aspects.

However, during the 1970s HMOs were only operating in a few urban markets so the numbers of Medicaid beneficiaries who chose this option were small. Generally, individuals with disabilities or chronic conditions chose to stay with their providers under the fee-for-service system. To benefit fully from managed care, Medicaid would have to find a way to mandate beneficiaries' participation in managed care. This development did not occur until the early 1980s.

Waivers for Medicaid Managed Care Programs

Federal law already had a provision permitting the introduction of managed care concepts into Medicaid plans. This provision was part of a 1962 amendment to the Social Security Act. This amendment added Section 1115 to that Act and gave the Secretary of Health and Human

Services discretion in waiving compliance with requirements of the Act in order to conduct "any experiment, pilot, or demonstration project which in the judgment of the Secretary, is likely to assist in promoting the objectives of title I, X, XIV, XVI, or XIX...in a State or States…". It is significant that this provision predated the Medicaid legislation by some three years. Initially, Section 1115 waivers were used for research or demonstration pilot projects designed to test new ideas on a small scale.

Section 1115 was the first waiver authority available to state Medicaid program managers to modify their plans. It provided the Secretary of Health and Human Services with broad authority to grant experimental, pilot, or demonstration projects that have the potential to assist in the promotion of the objectives of Medicaid. These demonstration projects required evaluation, should demonstrate a new approach, and produce significant findings. These waivers were generally approved for a five-year period and were to be budget neutral over the term of the project.

Implementation of Medicaid managed care arrangements has not been the only purpose of Section 1115. It has been used to extend financial coverage to individuals previously ineligible for Medicaid or to provide payments directly to beneficiaries to select and/or direct goods and services. It has also been used to establish pharmacy programs to provide prescriptions and over-the-counter drugs to a range of individuals. One use of the 1115 waiver authority is the Health Insurance Flexibility and Accountability (HIFA) Demonstration Initiative.

Additional legislation was passed in 1981 that added Section 1915(b) to the Social Security Act. This section allowed states to waive certain requirements under the original act. The Medicaid Freedom of Choice (FOC) requirement was the requirement most frequently requested to be waived in the coming years. Under the original provisions, Medicaid beneficiaries had freedom to select their health care providers. A Section 1915(b) waiver would allow a state to require Medicaid beneficiaries to enroll in specific managed care programs and receive care from only those providers who were part of these plans.

Section 1915 is a frequently cited authority used by states to make programmatic changes to their Medicaid programs. It has three significant subsections. Section 1915(b) is known as the "freedom of choice" waiver authority. It allows states to waive "state-wideness", comparability of services, and freedom of choice of providers. There are several kinds of 1915(b) waivers but only one pertains to managed care. Section 1915(b)(1) mandates Medicaid enrollment into managed care. There is also Section 1915(c) - Home and Community-Based Services Waivers. Section 1915(b) and (c) are so-called "Combo" Waivers that contain certain elements of managed care for the purpose of controlling provider resources and the cost of care.

In 1995 Congress established Section 1931 of the Social Security Act which also influenced Medicaid. Section 1931 was added by the Personal Responsibility and Work Opportunity Act of 1995, part of a Congressional effort to reform welfare. These efforts continued in 1996 with the passage of the Welfare Reform Law. This law created the Temporary Assistance for Needy Families (TANF) Program. TANF became effective July 1, 1997, and replaced Aid to Families with Dependent Children (AFDC) and the Job Opportunities and Basic Skills Training (JOBS) programs. Temporary Assistance for Needy Families (TANF) provided assistance and work opportunities by granting states the Federal funds and wide flexibility to develop and implement their own welfare programs.

The TANF Program also established a new mandatory eligibility group of low-income families with children. Historically, the majority of Medicaid beneficiaries became categorically eligible for the program as a result of their enrollment in Aid to Families with Dependent Children (AFDC). Welfare reform disconnected Medicaid from cash assistance and created a new eligibility category, which was based on state AFDC eligibility standards in effect on July 16, 1996. As of February 2002, some 13 states and the District of Columbia had made the adjustments to their eligibility requirements allowed by Section 1931.

The Balanced Budget Act of 1997 added yet another section to the Social Security Act, which further altered Medicaid. This addition was Section 1932(a) and it allowed a state to "require an individual who is eligible for medical assistance under the State plan under this title to enroll with a managed care entity as a condition of receiving such assistance". The first state to take advantage of the provisions of Section 1932 was Nevada in 1995. North Carolina followed in 1996 and Wisconsin in 1997. States that opted to use the provisions of Section 1932 would no longer be required to seek a Freedom of Choice waiver (Section 1915[b]). As of June 30, 2002 some 12 states had opted for this provision.

Although Section 1115 was added to the Social Security Act in 1962, twenty years passed before a state would request authority under this provision to modify its Medicaid program. Arizona was the first state to use the provisions of Section 1115 regarding Medicaid which were employed to establish its Medicaid program. Arizona had no Medicaid program before 1982. On October 1, 1982 Arizona became the first state to implement a "managed care" Medicaid program and to mandate HMO enrollment in its Medicaid program. In that year, five states implemented waivers. However four were under the provisions of the newly added section 1915(b) and only one (Arizona) was under Section 1115. Minnesota was the second state to implement a Section 1115 waiver in 1985 but it was not statewide. The next state to seek a statewide 1115 waiver was Oregon. Its 1991 application was the first request since 1982 to modify a statewide Medicaid program to allow it to operate a comprehensive, statewide demonstration project. But after a year of review the first Bush administration rejected it. Oregon revised and resubmitted its waiver application in late 1992 and it was approved.

During the ten years from 1982 through 1992, 19 additional states sought approval for and implemented 24 waivers. All but four waivers were under the authority of 1915(b). Michigan and Utah implemented the first Section 1915(b) waivers on July 1, 1982. The Section 1915(b) waiver was the most frequently used waiver (107) while the Section 1115 waiver was used for only 22 plans. Several states used both types. California, with 17 plans functioning under waivers, used the Section 1915(b) waiver for 15 plans and Section 1115 for only two plans. It appears that the Section 1932(a) waiver had been implemented in only seven plans.

Peak waiver activity occurred in the years 1992 through 1998 when 88 waivers were implemented in 43 states. California implemented the most, a total of 12, during that period. Again, most (67) waivers were implemented under the authority of Section 1915(b).

By 2002 almost every state plus the District of Columbia had implemented at least one waiver. The exceptions were Alaska, Illinois, New Hampshire, South Carolina and Wyoming. Illinois, New Hampshire and South Carolina did have managed health plans but because they were organized as voluntary programs they did not require waivers and individuals with chronic conditions still had freedom to choose their care providers who would in turn be paid under a fee for service system. Some 135 waivers were in force as of June 30, 2002. These waivers fostered numerous approaches to managed care for Medicaid clients.

Medicaid Managed Care Mechanisms

The term "managed care" is generic and does not specify operational procedures or financial arrangements in a given program. Table 1 shows several Medicaid managed care arrangements. There are three basic types of Medicaid managed care systems: 1) Primary care case management systems (PCCMs), 2) partial capitation systems, and 3) comprehensive risk contracting plans. However, many variations are found within each prototype (Lewin-VHI, 1995; Maglone and Ridgely, 2006).

Table 1. Medicaid managed care arrangements

Year	HIO	MCO		PCCM	PHP		PACE	Other	Total
1995	6	250		48	99		--	--	403
1996	7	349		59	89		--	7	511
1997	6	370		60	113		--	19	568
		Commercial	Medicaid Only						
1998	6	283	136	56	--			11	585
1999	6	237	136	60	--			13	581
2000	5	210	127	37	--			20	367
2001	5	202	122	41	152		--	24	546
2002	5	186	117	38	121		--	24	491
					PAHP	PIHP			
2003	5	161	121	41	27	107	22	27	505

HIO = Health Insuring Organization
MCO = Managed Care Organization
PACE = Program of All inclusive Care for the Elderly
PCCM = Primary Care Case Management
PAHP = Prepaid Ambulatory Health Plan
PHP = Prepaid Health Plan
PIHP = Prepaid Inpatient Health Plan

In a primary care case management system the Medicaid agency pays a primary care provider (called a "gatekeeper") a monthly management fee to manage the beneficiary's care but all of the services are paid on a fee-for-service basis. The primary care physician bears no financial risk. Under a partial capitation program the state contracts with a group of providers or clinics to assume the financial risk for some of the recipient's health care needs. These arrangements are sometimes referred to as "prepaid health plans," although the concept of prepaid health plans also includes plans that offer a comprehensive array of services on a non-risk basis. Common forms of partial capitation programs include primary care capitation programs in which the providers assume financial risk for primary care only or special service capitation programs such as mental health "carve-outs (Lewin-VHI, 1995).

Comprehensive risk programs generally fall into two categories: health maintenance organizations (HMOs) and health insuring organizations (HIOs). Both HMOs and HIOs create networks of providers and assume risk for a comprehensive list of services. One of the major differences between HMOs and HIOs is whether risk is passed to the providers (Lewin-VHI, 1995).

As states obtained their waivers they instituted a variety of managed care concepts. Initially the most popular approach was the Managed Care Organization (MCO) model. In 1995, the earliest year for which there is national data, there were 403 Managed Care Entities reported of which 250 were MCOs. The next most frequent model was the Prepaid Health Plan (PHP) of which there were 99. The Primary Care Case Management (PCCM) provider program was the third model used with 48 reported to be in use. The final model was the Health Insuring Organization (HIO) with a total of six in place. Table 1 shows how each model either increased or decreased over time. Definitions and concepts changed as well.

In 1998 the MCO category was further broken down into two categories – commercial and Medicaid only. However, the MCO category increased to a total of 288 by 2003. The PHP category was the other entity to increase significantly during the nine years (from 99 to 134).

There were still Primary Care Case Management providers (PCCM) and Health Insuring Organizations (HIO). The Prepaid Health Plan (PHP) has also been separated into two new types: Prepaid Inpatient Health Plan (PIHP) and Prepaid Ambulatory Health Plan (PAHP). The type of service further defines these two types. For example there are Dental PAHPs and Transportation PAHPs as well as Medical-only PAHPs and Mental Health PAHPS. There is even a Substance Use Disorders PAHP reported in Deschutes County, Oregon. Table 2 shows prevalence of assorted Medicaid managed care approaches by state during 2003.

DOCUMENTING MEDICAID SUBSTANCE ABUSE TREATMENT MANAGED CARE IMPLEMENTATION

Mapping the transition from fee for service to managed care for Medicaid substance abuse treatment services is challenging because alcohol or drug abuse services are not mentioned in the original Federal legislation nor in regulations of states that converted to managed care. The operational definition of managed substance abuse treatment programs included the following: (a) some type of substance abuse care delivered through an entity that was placed at some degree of financial risk and-or used managed care technologies (*e.g.*, administrative services only and managed fee-for-services programs) and (b) the state Medicaid agency, state mental health agency, state substance abuse agency, and-or county mental health and-or substance abuse departments were identified as purchaser(s) of the program.

Table 2. Medicaid managed care program summary for 2003

State	HIO	Commercial MCO	Medicaid MCO	PCCM	PAHP	PIHP	PACE	Other	Totals
AL	0	0	0	2	0	1	0	0	3
AK	0	0	0	0	0	0	0	0	0
AZ	0	2	26	0	0	1	0	0	29
AR	0	0	0	1	1	0	0	0	2
CA	5	24	0	2	11	0	1	3	46
CO	0	0	1	1	0	9	1	0	12
CT	0	2	2	0	0	0	0	0	4
DE	0	1	0	0	0	0	0	0	1
DC	0	0	4	0	0	1	0	0	5
FL	0	9	2	1	0	2	1	1	16
GA	0	0	0	1	2	0	0	0	3
HI	0	2	1	0	0	2	0	1	6
ID	0	0	1	0	0	0	0	0	1
IL	0	4	1	0	0	0	0	0	5
IN	0	0	3	2	0	0	0	0	5
IA	0	3	0	1	0	1	0	0	5
KS	0	0	1	1	0	0	1	0	3
KY	0	0	1	1	1	0	0	0	3
LA	0	0	0	1	0	0	0	0	1
ME	0	0	0	1	0	0	0	0	1
MD	0	0	6	0	0	0	1	0	7
MA	0	2	2	1	0	1	6	0	12
MI	0	9	9	0	0	20	0	0	38
MN	0	6	3	0	0	0	0	1	10
MS	0	0	0	0	0	0	0	0	0
MO	0	3	4	0	0	0	1	0	8
MT	0	0	0	1	0	0	0	0	1
NE	0	1	0	1	0	0	0	1	3
NV	0	2	0	0	0	0	0	0	2
NH	0	1	0	0	0	0	0	0	1
NJ	0	1	4	0	0	0	0	0	5
NM	0	3	0	0	0	0	0	0	3
NV	0	2	0	0	0	0	0	0	2
NY	0	14	15	6	1	0	4	13	53
NC	0	1	0	2	0	0	0	0	3
ND	0	1	0	1	0	0	0	0	2
OH	0	4	2	0	0	0	2	0	8
OK	0	0	3	2	0	0	0	0	5
OR	0	4	9	1	8	10	0	0	32
PA	0	2	9	1	0	28	1	0	41
RI	0	3	0	0	0	0	0	0	3
SC	0	0	1	0	1	0	0	0	2
SD	0	0	0	1	1	0	0	0	2
TN	0	5	3	0	0	2	1	0	11
TX	0	10	2	2	0	1	0	0	15
UT	0	0	0	3	1	12	0	0	16
VA	0	6	1	1	0	0	0	0	8
VT	0	0	0	1	0	0	0	0	1
WA	0	6	2	1	0	14	1	0	24
WI	0	28	3	0	0	2	1	1	35
WV	0	2	0	1	0	0	0	0	3
WY	0	0	0	0	0	0	0	0	0
Total	5	161	121	41	27	107	22	21	505

HIO = Health Insuring Organization

MCO = Managed Care Organization

PACE = Program of All inclusive Care for the Elderly

PCCM = Primary Care Case Management
PAHP = Prepaid Ambulatory Health Plan
PHP = Prepaid Health Plan
PIHP = Prepaid Inpatient Health Plan

Additional criteria were applied to differentiate and define managed substance abuse treatment within broad national guidelines established by Federal statutes, regulations, and policies. These criteria included that each state a) established its own eligibility standards; b) determined the type, amount, duration, and scope of services; c) set the rate of payment for services; and d) administered its own program.

Moreover, Medicaid policies for eligibility, services, and payments are complex and vary considerably even among states of similar size or geographic proximity. Thus, a person who is eligible for Medicaid in one state may not be eligible in another state and the services provided by one state may differ considerably in amount, duration, or scope from services provided in a similar or neighboring state. In addition, state legislatures may change Medicaid eligibility and-or services during the year. Considerable effort was made to establish accurate guidelines to discern when and through what mechanisms each state converted to managed care for substance abuse treatment. Part of this effort included an examination of state waiver programs using information provided either on paper or on-line by the U.S. Centers for Medicare and Medicaid Services.

As was mentioned, states were unable to implement Medicaid managed care programs without some sort of Federal approval. For example, Section 1915(b) of the Social Security Act authorizes the Secretary of Health and Human Services to waive compliance with certain portions of the Medicaid Statute that prevent a state from requiring Medicaid beneficiaries to obtain their care from a single provider or health plan. Examination of these waiver mechanisms using online and paper documents from the Federal Centers for Medicare and Medicaid Services provided data on each state's switch to managed care.

States began requesting 1915(b) freedom of choice waivers that increased the Medicaid enrollment in managed care plans beginning in 1993. Initial waiver requests were for enrollment in managed medical plans. The early managed care plans often excluded psychiatric conditions (such as substance abuse diagnoses). Many waivers had little to do with medical care but rather, such matters as expanding eligibility, housing, transportation, etc. Therefore it was important to determine, on a state-by-state basis, where and when waiver requests specifically addressing alcohol and other substance abuse were first submitted.

Tracking waivers and assessing their impact on beneficiary services was complicated by several factors. Some waivers were originally approved for a specific number of years (as little as two and as long as six years). Some waivers were not renewed when their authority expired while others were renewed with a new name and-or under one of the new authorities (Sections 1931 or 1932).

Although waivers began to be implemented in 1982, a computerized National Summary of State Medicaid Managed Care Programs files was not produced until 1995. These files contain a description of the plans implemented in each state, population covered and services provided, and the date the plan(s) were originally implemented.

Information was obtained on when and by what state the first waiver specifically addressing the behavioral health area was instated. Key words used in the on-line search of the U.S. Centers for Medicare and Medicaid Services web sites included "mental health", "behavioral health", "substance abuse", "alcoholism", and "substance abuse services". The search process included documents through June 30, 2002. Matrices of yes-no indicator variables were constructed showing for each state and each year whether or not the state Medicaid program included a substance abuse treatment managed care component.

A search was also conducted of the National Summaries of State Medicaid Managed Care Programs for five key terms: alcoholism, chemical dependency, mental health, behavioral health, and substance abuse. The data searched were for the years 1995, 1997, 1998, 1999, 2000, 2001 and 2002. Due to a data file defect in the database, data for 1996 was not available. A hard copy was requested and provided by the Office of Managed Care at the (then) Health Care Financing Administration (HCFA). Because the file for 1996 data could not be accessed electronically, the hard copy was visually scanned.

Each state's summary contained the title of the plan, program data and a list of included services. The search for terms was conducted by looking at these lists of included services. The term that appeared most frequently was "mental health". The term "alcoholism" did not appear in any state's files.

Information on implementation dates for Medicaid waivers addressing mental health and-or substance abuse came from the Centers for Medicare and Medicaid Services' National Summary of State Medicaid Managed Care Programs as of June 30, 2002 (revised February 2, 2004 as downloaded from the CMS web site). This approach complemented the survey of state Medicaid agencies conducted in 2000 by Maglione and Ridgely (2006).

Conversion from Fee for Service to Managed Care for Medicaid Substance Abuse Treatment

An Internet search of the Centers for Medicare and Medicaid Services files found no references to "alcoholism". The two terms most frequently found were "substance abuse" and "mental health". The term "chemical dependency" was also found. Quite often these terms were used interchangeably. Also, substance abuse was not cited in the reports on Medicaid Managed Care submitted annually by the states to the (then) Health Care Financing Administration nor to its successor the Centers for Medicare and Medicaid Services. Substance abuse is frequently included in the larger category "mental diseases". In addition, although a search for these terms might find one or more of them, such a finding did not necessarily mean that the waiver plan covered the related services. For example, both mental health and substance abuse were found in the District of Columbia plan, but they were in a statement setting forth excluded services.

In 1982 there were a total of five waiver plans implemented. Three of the five (California, Michigan and Utah) did not contain any of the search terms. Arizona's plan included both mental health and substance abuse. The Colorado plan listed mental health as a service provided but offered no information as to what that term might include. In 1983 there were four waiver plans implemented. One contained the term "mental health" and another included the term "substance abuse". Arizona, the first state to implement an 1115 waiver, specifically listed both mental health services and substance abuse services as included in its Arizona Health Care Cost Containment System (AHCCCS). In Iowa the managed care plan required a primary diagnosis of mental illness before a person could receive substance abuse services. Pennsylvania, West Virginia and Wisconsin allowed Medicaid recipients to "self-refer" for mental health, drug and alcohol services. This approach may put some recipients of those services outside the constraints or review required by managed care.

The use of the key word "substance abuse" in a search of the 1995 files produced 11 hits. Ten were in 1915(b) plans and one was in an 1115 plan. The term "chemical dependency" was found in only one state's plan, the Minnesota Consolidated Chemical Dependency Treatment Fund (CCDTF). This program was a statewide fee-for-service plan created by combining existing state appropriations for chemical dependency (CD) rehabilitative services from the following sources: General Assistance (state funds), General Assistance Medical Care (state funds), Medical Assistance or Medicaid (Federal and state funds), Regional Treatment Centers (state funds), and other state and Federal grants administered by the Department of Human Services. The Minnesota system was a carve-out program in which individuals chose their own provider so there was no case management by a primary care physician.

By 1995 states had implemented 89 waivers. Nineteen of those waivers contained a reference to mental health services, while 33 provided both mental health services and substance abuse services. One listed substance abuse services alone. While many states had implemented multiple waivers, only five states had no waivers: Alaska, Illinois, New Hampshire, South Carolina and Wyoming.

From 1982 through 2002 some 135 waivers were implemented of which 56 (41 percent) were without mental health or substance abuse. Conversely, 79 waivers (59 percent) listed mental health and substance abuse as provided services.

MEDICAID WAIVER IMPLEMENTATION BY YEAR 1982 THROUGH 2002

The Medicaid legislation provided for waivers from the outset but no state requested a waiver until 1982. The first five states were Arizona, California, Colorado, Michigan, and Utah. Four used the 1915(b) authority and only Arizona used 1115. Colorado's waiver included mental health services while Arizona's included both mental health and substance abuse services. Over the following eight years (1983 through 1990) only a few states each year applied for waivers. The number jumped in 1991 to six, followed by seven in 1992 and 11 in 1993. The most waivers implemented in any year was 22 in 1995. The numbers gradually dropped off in the following years to a low of only one in 2002.

Looking at each year to determine the number of waivers that included either mental health, substance abuse, or both showed the following: 1982 (five waivers, three with neither mental health nor substance abuse, one with mental health and substance abuse, and one with mental health only), 1983 (four waivers, two with neither mental health nor substance abuse, one with mental health only, and one with mental health plus substance abuse), 1984 (three waivers, one with neither mental health nor substance abuse, and two with both mental health and substance abuse), 1985 (two waivers, both with mental health plus substance abuse), 1986 (two waivers, one with neither mental health nor substance abuse, and one with both mental health plus substance abuse), 1987 (two waivers, one with neither mental health nor substance abuse, and one with both mental health plus substance abuse), 1988 (two waivers, one with only mental health and the other with only substance abuse), 1989 (one waiver with both mental health and substance abuse), 1990 (one waiver for mental health only), 1991 (six waivers, two with neither mental health nor substance abuse, three with mental health only, and one with both mental health plus substance abuse), 1992 (seven waivers, four with neither mental health nor substance abuse and three with both mental health plus substance abuse), 1993 (11 waivers, six with neither mental health nor substance abuse, two with mental health only, and three with both mental health plus substance abuse), 1994 (21 waivers, eight with neither mental health nor substance abuse, five with mental health only, and eight with both mental health plus substance abuse), 1995 (22 waivers, eight with neither mental health nor substance abuse, five with mental health only, and nine with mental health plus substance abuse), 1996 (15 waivers, nine with neither mental health nor substance abuse, one with mental health only, one with substance abuse only, and four with mental health plus substance abuse), 1997 (ten waivers, two with neither mental health nor substance abuse, two with mental health only, and six with mental health plus substance abuse), 1998 (eight waivers, four with neither mental health nor substance abuse, and four with both mental health plus substance abuse), 1999 (five waivers, one with neither mental health nor substance abuse, one with mental health only, and three with mental health plus substance abuse), 2000 (five waivers, three with neither mental health nor substance abuse, and two with mental health plus substance abuse), 2001 (two waivers, one with neither mental health nor substance abuse, and one with both mental health plus substance abuse), and 2002 (one waiver for both mental health plus substance abuse). Table 3 shows implementation by year of Medicaid waivers as well as inclusion (or not) of mental health and-or substance abuse within the waivers.

Total waivers from 1982 through 2002 were 135. Of those, 56 (41 percent) had neither mental health nor substance abuse whereas 79 (59 percent) included mental health and-or substance abuse. Eighteen states or 35 percent (of the 50 states and the District of Columbia) did not have a waiver to the basic Medicaid law that specifically addressed substance abuse services. This finding could be interpreted as suggesting that services for substance abuse continued to be delivered without any managed care control or restrictions.

Implementation by state occurred as follows. Alabama in 1988 without substance abuse but with mental health, Alaska neither mental health nor substance abuse, Arizona mental health and substance abuse in 1982, Arkansas mental health in 1996 but no substance abuse waiver, California mental health in 1983 and substance abuse in 1994, Colorado mental health in 1982 but no substance abuse, Connecticut mental health and substance abuse in 1995, Delaware mental health and substance abuse in 2000, District of Columbia mental health and substance abuse in 1995, Florida mental health and substance abuse in 1993, Georgia mental health and substance abuse in 1993, Hawaii mental health and substance abuse in 1994, Idaho mental health and substance abuse in 1993, Illinois neither mental health nor substance abuse, Indiana neither mental health nor substance abuse, Iowa mental health in 1990 with substance abuse in 1995, Kansas mental health and substance abuse in 1984, Kentucky neither mental health nor substance abuse, Louisiana neither mental health nor substance abuse, Maine neither mental health nor substance abuse, Maryland mental health in 1991 with substance abuse in 1997, Massachusetts mental health and substance abuse in 1992, Michigan mental health and substance abuse in 1983, Minnesota mental health and substance abuse in 1985,

Table 3. Medicaid waivers

	Waivers and Services				
Year	Neither mental health nor substance abuse	Mental health	Substance abuse	Mental health plus substance abuse	Total
1982	3	1	0	1	5
1983	2	1	0	1	4
1984	1	0	0	2	3
1985	0	0	0	2	2
1986	1	0	0	1	2
1987	1	0	0	1	2
1988	0	1	1	0	2
1989	0	0	0	1	1
1990	0	1	0	0	1
1991	2	3	0	1	6
1992	4	0	0	3	7
1993	6	2	0	3	11
1994	8	5	0	8	21
1995	8	5	0	9	22
1996	9	1	1	4	15
1997	2	2	0	6	10
1998	4	0	0	4	8
1999	1	1	0	3	5
2000	3	0	0	2	5
2001	1	0	0	1	2
2002	0	0	0	1	1
Total	56	23	2	54	135

Data from key word searches of Centers for Medicare and Medicaid Services (CMS) web sites and data bases including the national summary of state Medicaid managed care programs.

Mississippi neither mental health nor substance abuse, Missouri mental health and substance abuse in 1987, Montana mental health and substance abuse in 1995, Nebraska mental health and substance abuse in 1995, Nevada mental health in 1995 but no substance abuse waiver, New Hampshire neither mental health nor substance abuse, New Jersey neither mental health nor substance abuse, New Mexico mental health and substance abuse in 1997, New York mental health and substance abuse in 1991, North Carolina mental health and substance abuse in 1994, North Dakota mental health and substance abuse in 2002, Ohio mental health and substance abuse in 1989, Oklahoma mental health and substance abuse in 1996, Oregon mental health and substance abuse in 1994, Pennsylvania mental health and substance abuse in 1986, Rhode Island mental health and substance abuse in 1994, South Carolina neither mental health nor substance abuse, South Dakota mental health in 1994 but no substance abuse waiver, Tennessee mental health and substance abuse in 1994, Texas mental health in 1993 with substance abuse in 1998, Utah mental health in 1991 but no substance abuse waiver, Vermont mental health and substance abuse in 1996, Virginia mental health and substance abuse in 1992, Washington State mental health in 1993 but no substance abuse waiver, West Virginia neither mental health nor substance abuse, Wisconsin mental health and substance abuse in 1984, and Wyoming with neither mental health nor substance abuse. Table 4 shows implementation by state and year of Medicaid waivers as well as inclusion (or not) of mental health and-or substance abuse within the waivers.

Medicaid waivers pertaining to substance abuse treatment are shown in Figures 1 and 2 which depict representative years in the study period. As the figures show, few states had Medicaid waivers pertaining to substance abuse in 1993. However, as noted, there was substantial increase in Medicaid waivers (including those pertaining to substance abuse treatment) during the middle 1990s. By the year 2004 (Figure 2), most states had Medicaid managed care waivers that addressed substance abuse treatment.

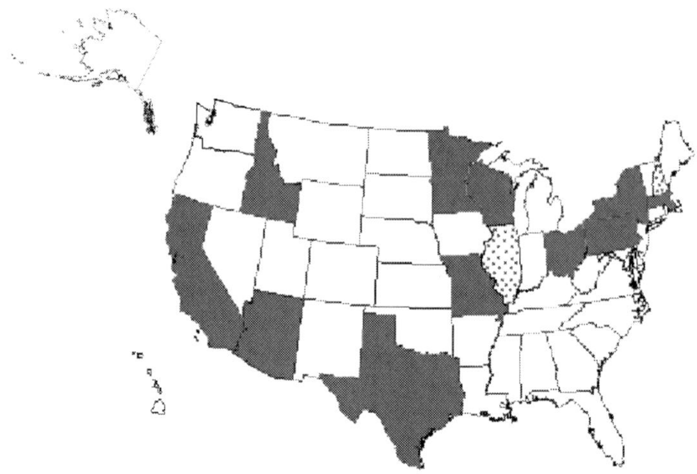

Figure 1. States with Medicaid waivers involving substance abuse: 1993

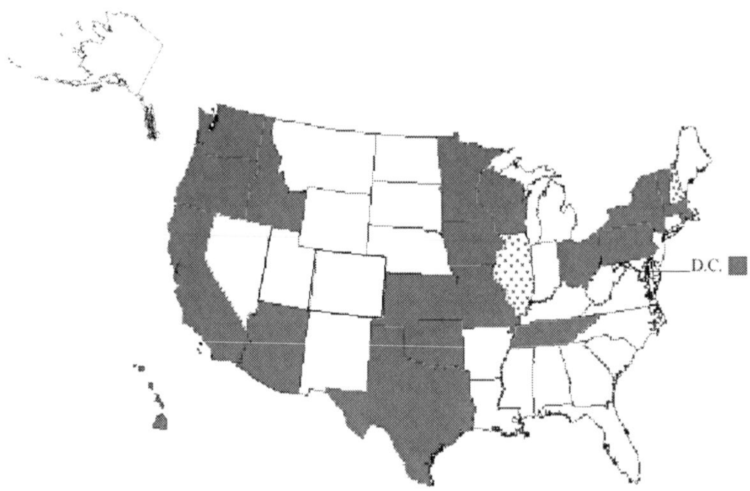

Figure 2. States with Medicaid waivers involving substance abuse: 2000.

Table 4. Medicaid waivers by state and year

State	'82	'83	'84	'85	'86	'87	'88	'89	'90	'91	'92	'93	'94	'95	'96	'97	'98	'99	'00	'01	'02	Total
AL							2									2						2
AK																						0
AZ	7																					1
AR												1		1	4		1					4
CA	1	1,2				1					1		1,2,2,7	1,2,2	1,1	1	1,7					17
CO	2	1												2	1							4
CT														3								1
DE															5				11			2
DC													1,1	7								3
FL										1		3			2			2				4
GA												1,3	2			1						4
HI													7									1
ID												3										1
IL																						0
IN													1									1
IA									2					3,3				3				4
KS			1,3											1								3
KY					1												1					2
LA											1											1
ME													1					9				2
MD										2,2						7						3
MA											3					7						2
MI	1	3														2	3					4
MN				3,7			4							7								4
MS												1										1
MO						3								3			7					3
MT												1		3								2
NE														1,3								2
NV														10								1

Table 4. (Continued)

State	'82	'83	'84	'85	'86	'87	'88	'89	'90	'91	'92	'93	'94	'95	'96	'97	'98	'99	'00	'01	'02	Total
NH																						0
NJ														1					1			2
NM															1	3						2
NY										3	3			1		7			7			5
NC										1			3		5,9		1		1,9			7
ND													1								11	2
OH								3												3		2
OK														5	7							2
OR													1,2,7									3
PA					3								3	3		3						4
RI													7									1
SC																						0
SD												1	2									2
TN													7									1
TX												2	1	1,2			3	3				6
UT	1									2										1		3
VT															7							1
VA											1,3				1,3							4
WA												1,2										2
WV											1				1							2
WI			3										3		7	11		7				5
WY																						0
Total	5	4	3	2	2	2	2	1	1	6	7	11	21	22	15	10	8	5	5	2	1	135

MH = mental health; SA = substance abuse

1=1915(b), neither MH nor SA
2=1915(b), MH only
3=1915(b), MH and SA
4=1915(b), SA only
5=1115, neither MH nor SA
6=1115, MH only
7=1115, MH and SA
8=1115, SA only
9=1932(a), neither MH nor SA
10=1932(a), MH only
11=1932(a), MH and SA
12=1932(a), SA only

From the national summary of state Medicaid managed care programs at web sites maintained by the Centers for Medicare and Medicaid Services.

Table 5 summarizes coverage of substance abuse treatment by state Medicaid programs for the year 2000. Notice that virtually all states included hospital detoxification and outpatient substance abuse treatment within services provided to their categorically eligible Medicaid clients and nearly all states included such services for their medically needed Medicaid populations. However, there was marked variation among states in use (or not) of Medicaid waivers pertaining to substance abuse services.

Table 6 provides information about Medicaid waivers, inclusion of mental health and-or substance abuse services, and the covered populations as of June 30, 2002. The table shows that Medicaid waivers were used to establish numerous programs covering assorted populations. Behavioral health services were included in some programs for some populations but were by no means universal.

Table 7 shows Medicaid managed care programs as of June 30, 2002. States had adopted numerous systems using assorted mechanisms for financing and overseeing provision of services. The Medicaid managed care programs might or might not include substance abuse and-or mental health treatments. Moreover, various treatment modalities were included in the managed care programs but some might have remained fee-for-service. For example, a Medicaid managed care program could encompass inpatient substance abuse treatment whereas outpatient might be fee-for-service.

Table 5. State Medicaid substance abuse coverage as of 2000

State	Program Type	Inpatient Detoxification	Outpatient Substance Abuse	Waiver	Type
AL	Cat. Needy	Yes	Yes	1915(b)	MH
	Med. Needy	No	No		
AK	Cat. Needy	Yes	Yes	None	
	Med. Needy	No	No		
AR	Cat. Needy	No	No	1915(b)	SA
	Med. Needy	No	No		
AZ[1]	Cat. Needy	Yes		1115	MH and SA
	Med. Needy	No			
CA	Cat. Needy	Yes	Yes	1115 and	MH and SA[2]
	Med. Needy	Yes	Yes	1915(b)	
CO	Cat. Needy	Yes	Yes	1915(b)	MH[3]
	Med. Needy	Yes	Yes		
CT	Cat. Needy	Yes	Yes	1915(b)	MH and SA[4]
	Med. Needy	Yes	Yes		
DC	Cat. Needy	Yes	Yes	1115	MH and SA[5]
	Med. Needy	Yes	Yes		
DE	Cat. Needy	Yes	Yes	1932(a)	MH and SA[6]
	Med. Needy	No	No		
FL	Cat. Needy	Yes	Yes	1915(b)	MH and SA[7]
	Med. Needy	Yes	Yes		
GA	Cat. Needy	No	Yes	1915(b)	MH and SA[8]
	Med. Needy	No	Yes		
HI	Cat. Needy	Yes	Yes	1115	MH and SA[9]
	Med. Needy	Yes	Yes		

Table 5 (Continued)

ID	Cat. Needy	No	No	1915(b)	MH and SA[10]
	Med. Needy	No	No		
IA	Cat. Needy	Yes	Yes	1915(b)	MH and SA
	Med. Needy	Yes	Yes		
IL	Cat. Needy	Yes	Yes	None	[11]
	Med. Needy	Yes	Yes		
IN	Cat. Needy	Yes	Yes	1915(b)	Neither MH
	Med. Needy	No	No		nor SA[12]
KS	Cat. Needy	Yes	Yes	1915(b)	MH and SA[13]
	Med. Needy	Yes	Yes		
KY	Cat. Needy	Yes	Yes	1915(b)	Neither MH
	Med. Needy	Yes	Yes		nor SA[14]
LA	Cat. Needy	No	Yes	1915(b)	Neither MH
	Med. Needy	No	Yes		nor SA[15]
MA	Cat. Needy	Yes	Yes	1915(b)	MH and SA[16]
	Med. Needy	Yes	Yes	1115	
MD	Cat. Needy	Yes	Yes	1915(b)	MH and SA[17]
	Med. Needy	Yes	Yes	1115	
ME	Cat. Needy	Yes	Yes	1915(b)	Neither MH
	Med Needy	Yes	Yes	1932(a)	nor SA[18]
MI	Cat. Needy	Yes	Yes	1915(b)	MH and SA[19]
	Med. Needy	Yes	Yes		
MN	Cat. Needy	Yes	Yes	1915(b)	MH and SA[20]
	Med. Needy	Yes	Yes	1115	
MO	Cat. Needy	Yes	Yes	1915(b)	MH and SA[21]
	Med. Needy	No	No	1115	
MS	Cat. Needy	No	Yes	1915(b)	Neither MH
	Med. Needy	No	No		nor SA[22]
MT	Cat. Needy	Yes	Yes	1915(b)	MH and SA[23]
	Med. Needy	Yes	Yes		
NC	Cat. Needy	Yes	Yes	1915(b),1115,	MH and SA[24]
	Med. Needy	Yes	Yes	1932(a)	
ND	Cat. Needy	Yes	Yes	1915(b), 1932(a)	MH and SA[25]
	Med. Needy	Yes	Yes		
NE	Cat. Needy	Yes	Yes	1915(b)	MH and SA[26]
	Med. Needy	Yes	Yes		
NH	Cat. Needy	No	Yes	None	MH and SA[27]
	Med. Needy	No	Yes		
NJ	Cat. Needy	Yes	Yes	1915(b)	Neither MH
	Med. Needy	Yes	Yes		nor SA[28]
NM	Cat. Needy	Yes	Yes	1915(b)	MH and SA[29]
	Med. Needy	No	No		
NV	Cat. Needy	Yes	Yes	1932(a)	MH[30]
	Med. Needy	No	No		
NY	Cat. Needy	Yes	Yes	1915(b), 1115	MH and SA[31]
	Med. Needy	Yes	Yes		
OH	Cat. Needy	Yes	Yes	1915(b)	MH and SA[32]
	Med. Needy	Yes	Yes	1115	
OK	Cat. Needy	Yes	Yes	1115	MH and SA
	Med. Needy	Yes	Yes		(limited)[33]

OR	Cat. Needy	Yes	Yes	1115	MH and SA[34]
	Med. Needy	No	Yes		
PA	Cat. Needy	Yes	Yes	1915(b)	MH and SA[35]
	Med. Needy	Yes	Yes		
RI	Cat. Needy	Yes	Yes	1115	MH and SA[36]
	Med. Needy	Yes	Yes		
SC	Cat. Needy	Yes	Yes	None	MH and SA[37]
	Med. Needy	Yes	Yes		
SD	Cat. Needy	Yes	No	1915(b)	MH[38]
	Med. Needy	No	No		
TN	Cat. Needy	Yes	Yes	1115	MH and SA[39]
	Med. Needy	Yes	Yes		
TX	Cat. Needy	No	No	1915(b)	MH and SA[40]
	Med. Needy	No	No		
UT	Cat. Needy	Yes	Yes	1915(b)	MH[41]
	Med. Needy	Yes	Yes		
VA	Cat. Needy	Yes	No	1915(b)	MH and SA[42]
	Med. Needy	Yes	No		
VT	Cat. Needy	Yes	Yes	1115	MH and SA[43]
	Med. Needy	Yes	Yes		
WA	Cat. Needy	No	Yes	1915(b)	MH[44]
	Med. Needy	No	Yes		
WI	Cat. Needy	Yes	Yes	1915(b)	MH and SA[45]
	Med. Needy	Yes	Yes		
WV	Cat. Needy	Yes	Yes	1915(b)	Neither MH
	Med. Needy	Yes	Yes		nor SA
WY	Cat. Needy	Yes	Yes	1915(b)	Neither MH
	Med. Needy	No	No		nor SA[46]

MH = mental health; SA = substance abuse

From the Centers for Medicare and Medicaid Services (CMS) National summary of state Medicaid managed care programs http://cms.hhs.gov/medicaid/managedcare/ and from Medicaid Managed Care: A Guide for States, fifth edition, 2001, National Academy for State Health Policy.

Footnotes to Table 5:

1. National Academy for State Health Policy Medicaid Managed Care: A Guide for States as of 6/30/2000 showed neither service provided but CMS (then the Health Care Financing Administration) data files showed mental health and substance abuse services both covered.
2. Medi-Cal substance abuse services excluded from managed care.
3. Almost all public sector substance abuse treatment services paid for by the Alcohol and Drug Abuse Division included under a managed care arrangement.
4. Statewide managed care program that covered acute mental health and substance abuse services but the state also had a number of non-managed care arrangements to deliver public sector substance abuse services.
5. All public sector mental health services, aside from those provided to children with special health care needs excluded from managed care programs. All substance abuse services funded by the DC substance Abuse Authority excluded from managed care programs.
6. State offered a limited mental health and substance abuse benefit under managed care (30 inpatient days and 20 outpatient visits). Adults requiring services beyond that basis package remained in the fee-for-service system for substance abuse services.

7. Other than in the Tampa Bay area, mental health and substance abuse treatment services were excluded from managed care plans and are provided on a fee-for-service basis.
8. Medicaid mental health and substance abuse services excluded from managed care and remained fee-for-service.
9. Department of Health contracted for public sector mental health and substance abuse services provided in a non-managed care environment but had to meet same data reporting requirements as managed care organizations.
10. Idaho operated one statewide non-Medicaid substance abuse managed care program. Medicaid mental health and substance abuse services remained under the traditional fee-for-service system.
11. Illinois operated an integrated, voluntary Medicaid managed care program that includes some (unspecified) mental health and substance abuse. Medicaid recipients who chose not to enroll in the voluntary program or who lived in areas not covered by the program received mental health and substance abuse services through Medicaid fee-for-service.
12. The state 's Medicaid Agency excluded behavioral health benefits (not clear if substance abuse was included) from the mandatory health maintenance organization managed care program for low income pregnant women, children, and families.
13. Kansas excluded all behavioral health from managed care and all mental health and substance abuse services remained in the fee-for-service system according to State Profiles 2000. Its waiver only provided authority to do Primary Care Case Management (PPCM).
14. Kentucky 's Medicaid managed care efforts covered physical health services. Mental health and substance abuse services were not covered by managed care and remained in the fee-for-service system.
15. All Medicaid mental health and substance abuse services remained in the traditional fee-for-service system.
16. Medicaid beneficiaries had two options: join a Managed Care Organization and receive all their health needs or see a physician in a Behavioral Health Plan carve-out.
17. Public sector behavioral health services delivered through two separate systems: 1) a capitated system for physical health which included substance abuse services; and 2) a "specialty" mental health program comprised of a managed fee-for-service system which incorporated both Medicaid and State general funds.
18. Maine excluded all mental health and substance abuse services from managed care.
19. Michigan operated four Medicaid managed care programs: 1) for physical health services with limited outpatient mental health benefits, 2) specialty program for behavioral health and developmental disabilities, 3) voluntary program for children, and 4) for child welfare services. Hospital based detoxification was only substance abuse service that remained fee-for-service.
20. One managed care program provided substance abuse services (CCDTF).
21. Missouri operated two managed care programs and both included behavioral health coverage. One program was a managed fee-for-service substance abuse carve-out program.
22. All Medicaid mental health and substance abuse services were under a traditional fee-for-service system and excluded from managed care.
23. Montana cancelled its managed behavioral health program in March of 1999. Mental health and substance abuse services were then under a fee-for service system.
24. North Carolina 's Medicaid waiver to operate a specialty behavioral health program for children and adolescents expired in March of 1999. Mental health and substance abuse services funded by the state were excluded from managed care.
25. North Dakota had a statewide PCCM and also an HMO in Grand Forks County. With the exception of these programs all other behavioral health services were under fee-for-service.
26. Nebraska had two behavioral health managed care programs. One was a Medicaid waiver program and was a carve-out covering all mental health and substance abuse services on a capitated bass. The other was a non-Medicaid managed care carve-out covering uninsured and under insured.

27. New Hampshire operated two publicly funded managed care programs that provided behavioral health services. One was a physical health Medicaid voluntary HMO covering some mental health and substance abuse services. The second program was specifically designed for persons with severe mental illness and was supported by State Mental Health Authority funding.
28. All behavioral health services were provided on a fee-for-service basis and excluded from New Jersey 's Medicaid managed care program.
29. New Mexico operated two managed behavioral health programs. One was a Medicaid managed care program and the second was a non-Medicaid program for uninsured adults.
30. Nevada operated a non-waiver Medicaid managed care program in Clark and Washoe counties. Medicaid mental health and substance abuse services remained fee-for-service in all other areas of the state.
31. New York provided limited managed behavioral health services to the Medicaid population through a Prepaid Mental Health Plan. Supplemental Security Income (SSI) beneficiaries also received inpatient detoxification. All other behavioral health services continued to be available through the Medicaid fee-for-service program.
32. Ohio did have a 1959(b) waiver in the past but currently operated only one Medicaid managed care program under a Section 1115 waiver and integrated physical and behavioral health services in an HMO operating in 16 of the State 's 88 counties.
33. Oklahoma had one Medicaid waiver program with two separate and distinct initiatives. One was a fully capitated model implemented in 3 of the state 's most populated areas. Everywhere else, Medicaid mental health and substance abuse services remained in the traditional fee-for-service system.
34. Oregon 's statewide Medicaid managed care program covered behavioral health services for both Medicaid and non-Medicaid populations. All substance abuse services were fully integrated with physical health and mental health services were provided through a specialty carve-out.
35. Pennsylvania had a separate behavioral health program operated by counties. In counties where this program had not yet been implemented enrollees could receive care through the voluntary HMO program.
36. Rhode Island operated one managed care program that includes behavioral health services.
37. South Carolina operated a Medicaid physical health managed care program, the voluntary HMO program, with limited behavioral health benefits and one Prior Authorization Program for Medicaid substance abuse services.
38. South Dakota operated one statewide Medicaid managed care program, a primary care case management program that requires referrals for in- and outpatient services including behavioral health.
39. Tennessee operated one managed care program with a behavioral health care carve-out.
40. Texas had three managed care programs that include some behavioral health services. Each covered a different geographic area.
41. Utah operated one public sector Medicaid managed care program for mental health services. Substance abuse services were not under any managed care at this time.
42. Virginia operated two Medicaid managed care programs: a mandatory HMO and a primary care case management program. The state Medicaid agency contracted directly with primary care physicians for a range of mental health services and substance abuse residential treatment.
43. Vermont operated two managed care programs with behavioral health components. The first was a primary care case management program which provided acute mental health and substance abuse benefits. The second provided long-term behavioral health care to seriously mentally ill patients.
44. Washington operated two managed care programs which provided behavioral health services. A carve-out program covered the Medicaid population for community inpatient and outpatient mental health and rehabilitation services. The second plan was a physical health managed care program with limited behavioral health benefits and was for non-Medicaid individuals.

45. Wisconsin piloted a number of managed care plans designed around specifically defined populations. Currently it operated seven managed behavioral health care programs. Substance abuse and mental health services provided outside these pilot projects were delivered under the fee-for-service system.
46. Wyoming had excluded behavioral health services from managed care. State Medicaid mental health and substance abuse services remained under traditional fee-for-service.

Methodology Regarding Impact of Medicaid Managed Care on Severity of Substance Abuse Treatment Clients

National data were used to examine the impact of Medicaid managed care on severity of clients in treatment for substance abuse. Data were obtained from the Treatment Episode Data Set maintained by the U.S. Substance Abuse and Mental Health Services Administration (described subsequently). The dependent variable was the Deck severity measure (Deck and McFarland, 2002; McCamant et al., 2007; McFarland, Deck et al., 2005). Predictors were state, year (nested within state), and indicators for Medicaid managed care. The methodology included use of hierarchical linear models as will be described.

Treatment Episode Data Set

The Treatment Episode Data Set (TEDS) is a database containing information on annual admissions to substance abuse treatment (McCarty et al., 1998). The system focuses on programs that receive at least some public (state or Federal) funding. The unit of analysis for the TEDS system is the admission. Of course, clients may have more than one admission in a given year. TEDS data are analogous to cumulative treated incidence (McFarland, 1996).

The TEDS data base includes the Minimum Data Set and the Supplemental Data Set. Domains of the Minimum Data Set are: provider identifier, client identifier, codependency / collateral status, transaction type (*e.g.,* admission versus transfer), admission date, number of prior treatment admissions, source of referral, date of birth, gender, race, ethnicity, education, employment, substance use (alcohol and other drugs) to include primary substance of abuse, secondary substance of abuse, tertiary substance of abuse, route of administration for primary substance of abuse, route of administration for secondary substance of abuse, route of administration for tertiary substance of abuse, frequency of use for primary substance of abuse, frequency of use for secondary substance of abuse, frequency of use for tertiary substance of abuse, age at first use for primary substance of abuse, age at first use for secondary substance of abuse, age at first use for tertiary substance of abuse, type of treatment service planned (*e.g.,* outpatient, intensive outpatient, residential, or hospital), and methadone planned (yes or no). Supplemental data elements include details on primary substance of abuse, details on secondary substance of abuse, details on tertiary substance of abuse, diagnosis according to American Psychiatric Association Diagnostic and Statistical Manual of Mental Disorders,

Table 6. Medicaid waivers, services, and populations as of June 30, 2002

	Authority and Implementation Date Waiver Type					MH and-or SA Covered Service		Covered
State	1915(b)	1115	1932(a)	Voluntary[1]	Plan Title	Yes	No	Population
Alabama	9/1/88		Converted 6/1/99		Maternity Care Program	2		a, b, f, h
Alabama				10/1/96	Partnership Hospital Program, Inpt. Svcs. Only		7	a, b, c, d, e, f, h
Alabama	1/1/97				Patient 1st	1		a, b, c, d, e, f, h
Alaska					NO WAIVERS			
Arizona		10/1/82			Arizona HealthCare Cost Containment System	1(a), 4(a) 10, 11		a, b, c, d, e, f
Arkansas	3/1/98				Non-Emergency Transportation		15	
Arkansas	11/1/96				Primary Care Physician	4		a, b, c, e, f, h
California		11/1/98			Altamed Senior Buenacare PACE[2]	3, 6		d, f
California	10/1/95				Caloptima		9	a, b, c, d, e, f, h
California		4/1/95			Center for Elders Independence (PACE)	3, 6		d, f
California	1/1/96				Central Coast Alliance for Health		9	a, b, c, d, e, f, h
California	11/30/87				Health Plan of San Mateo	9, 10		a, b, c, d, e, f, h
California	4/24/92				Hudman (plan for placement in freestanding nursing facilities)	4, 6		?
California	3/1/97				Managed Care Network (People with Complex Social Needs)	8, ?		a, b, c, d, e, f, h

Table 6. (Continued)

	Authority and Implementation Date Waiver Type					MH and-or SA Covered Service		
State	1915(b)	1115	1932(a)	Voluntary[1]	Plan Title	Yes	No	Covered Population
California	4/1/95				MediCal Mental Health Field Test (San Mateo Co.)	3		a, b, c, d, e, f, h
California	3/15/95				MediCal Specialty Mental Health Services Consolidation	3		a, b, c, d, e, f, h
California		11/1/83			On Lok Senior Health Services	3, 6, 10, 11		d, f
California	5/1/94				Partnership Health Plan of California	1, 11, 10		a, b, c, d, e, f, h
California				1/1/72	Prepaid Health Plan Program		9	a, b, c, d, e, f, h
California	7/1/84				Primary Care Management Program	12	8	a, b, c, d, e, f, h
California	4/1/94				Sacramento Geographic Managed Care	4	9	a, b, c, d, e, f, h
California	10/17/98				San Diego Geographic Managed Care		9	a, b, c, d, e, f, h
California	9/1/83				Santa Barbara Health Initiative	10, 22	9	a, b, c, d, e, f, h
California	9/21/82				Selective Provider Contracting Program		7	a, b, c, d, e, f, h
California		1/1/85			Senior Care Action Network (Social HMO)	13	9	a, b, c, d, e, f, h
California		5/1/94			Sutter Senior Care	3, 6		d, f
California	1/23/96				Two-Plan Model Program		9	a, b, c, d, e, f, h
Colorado	5/1/83				Managed Care Program		9	a, b, c, d, e, f,

Table 6. (Continued)

	Authority and Implementation Date Waiver Type					MH and-or SA Covered Service		
State	1915(b)	1115	1932(a)	Voluntary[1]	Plan Title	Yes	No	Covered Population
Colorado	7/1/95				Mental Health Capitation Program	3, 14		a, b, c, d, e, f,
Connecticut	10/1/95				Husky A (Access)	3, 10		a, b, c, e, h
Delaware		1/1/96			Diamond State Health Plan	3, 6		a, b, c, d, e, f, g
District of Columbia	4/1/94				D.C. Medicaid Managed Care Program	10, 11	9	a, b, c, h, i
District of Columbia				2/1/96	Health Services for Children with Special Needs	1(a), 4(a), 10, 11		e
Florida	10/1/92				Managed Health Plan	1, 4		a, b, c, d, e, f, h
Florida	3/1/96				Prepaid Mental Health Plan	3, 14		a, b, c, e, f,
Florida	4/1/99				Statewide Inpatient Psychiatric Program[3]	1		?
Georgia	10/1/93				Georgia Better Health Care	1, 4		a, c, d, e, f,
Georgia	10/1/97				Non-Emergency Transportation Broker Program	15		?
Georgia	11/1/94				Preadmission Screening and Annual Resident Review	16		?
Hawaii		8/1/94			Hawaii Quest	1(a), 4(a), 10, 11		a, b, c, g
Idaho	10/1/93				Healthy Connections	3, 4		a, b, c, d, e, f, h, i

Table 6. (Continued)

State	Authority and Implementation Date Waiver Type				Plan Title	MH and-or SA Covered Service		Covered Population
	1915(b)	1115	1932(a)	Voluntary[1]		Yes	No	
Illinois[4]				11/1/74	Voluntary Managed Care	3, 6		a, b, c, h
Indiana	7/1/94				Hoosier Health Care			a, b, c, h
Iowa[5]	12/1/86		Converted 4/1/01		Iowa Medicaid Managed Health Care			?
Iowa	1/1/99				Iowa Plan for Behavioral Health	1(a), 4(a), 10, 11, 17		?
Kansas	1/1/84				KMMC: Health Connect Kansas	3, 6		a, b, c, e, f,
Kansas	12/1/95				KMMC: Healthwave 19			a, b, c,
Kentucky	6/1/98				Human Services Transportation	15	15	?
Kentucky		11/1/97			Kentucky Health Care Partnership Program		9	a, b, c, d, e, f, h
Kentucky	2/1/82		Converted 4/1/00		Kentucky Patient Access and Care Program		9	a, b, c,
Louisiana	6/1/92				Community Care		9	a, b, c, e, f, h
Maine			5/1/99		MaineCare Primary Care Case Management		9	a, b, c, h
Maryland		6/2/97			HealthChoice	10, 18	9	a, b, c, e, f, h
Massachusetts		7/1/97			Mass Health MCO (Comprehensive Benefits) Full Cap.	1(a), 4(a), 10, 11		a, b, c, e, f, g, h

Table 6. (Continued)

	Authority and Implementation Date Waiver Type					MH and-or SA Covered Service		
State	1915(b)	1115	1932(a)	Voluntary[1]	Plan Title	Yes	No	Covered Population
Massachusetts		7/1/97			(MH/SA) PHP- Full Capitation	1(a), 4(a), 10, 11, 14, 19, 23		a, b, c, e, f, g, h
Michigan				9/1/98	Children 's Special Health Care Services	11	9	c, e, h
Michigan	7/1/97				Comprehensive Health Plan	11	9	a, b, c, d, e, f, h, i
Michigan	10/1/98				Specialty Community Mental Health Services Program	1(a), 10, 11, 14, 21, 19		a, b, c, d, e, f, h
Minnesota	1/1/88				Consolidated Chemical Dependency Treatment Fund	4, 4(a), 10, 20		?
Minnesota				9/1/01	Disability Health Options	3, 6		?
Minnesota				3/1/97	Senior Health Options Program	1(a), 4(a), 10, 11		d
Minnesota		7/1/95			MinnCare Program for Families and Children	3, 6		g, i,
Minnesota		7/1/85			Prepaid Medical Assistance Program	1(a), 4(a), 10, 11		a, b, c, d, h
Mississippi	10/1/93				HealthMACS[6]		9	a, b, c, h
Missouri		9/1/98			MC+ Managed Care/1115	1(A), 4(A), 10, 11		a, b, c, h
Missouri		10/1/95			MC+ Managed Care/1915(b)	3, 6		a, b, c, h

Table 6. (Continued)

State	Authority and Implementation Date Waiver Type				Plan Title	MH and-or SA Covered Service		Covered Population
	1915(b)	1115	1932(a)	Voluntary[1]		Yes	No	
Montana	1/1/94				Passport to Health	1(A), 4(A), 10, 11		a, b, c, d, e, f,
Nebraska	7/1/95				Health Connection Combined Waiver Program		9	a, b, c, d, e, f, h
Nebraska					ASO Non-Risk Fee-For-Service	1(A), 4(A), 10,11		a, b, c, d, e, f, h
Nevada			12/1/98		Mandatory Health Maintenance Program	3, 11, 21		a, b, c,
Nevada				4/1/97	Voluntary Health Maintenance Program	1(a), 4(a),10, 11		a, b, c,
New Hampshire				3/2/83	Voluntary Managed Care Program	3, 6		a, b, c, h, i
New Jersey	10/1/00				Care 2000+(1915(b). NOTE: MH/SA Svcs only for clients of the Div. Of Developmental Disabilities.		9	a, b, c, d, e, f,
New Jersey			9/1/95		Care 2000+(1932). NOTE: MH/SA Svcs only for clients of the Div. Of Developmental Disabilities.		9	a, b, c, d, e, f, h
New Mexico	7/1/97				SALUD!	3, 6		a, b, c, d, e, f, h
New York	7/1/96				Non-Emergency Transportation	15	15	?
New York				4/1/96	Office of Mental Health/Partial Cap. Program	11		?

Table 6. (Continued)

	Authority and Implementation Date Waiver Type					MH and-or SA Covered Service		
State	1915(b)	1115	1932(a)	Voluntary[1]	Plan Title	Yes	No	Covered Population
New York		3/31/01			Partnership Plan-Family Health Plus. NOTE: Limited inpatient MH to 30 days, outpatient to 60 visits. None on SB.	1(a), 4(a), 10, 11		?
New York		3/1/97			Partnership Plan Medicaid Managed Care Program	3, 6		a, b, c, d, e, f, g
North Carolina	7/1/98				Access II/III 1915b		9	a, b, c, d, e, f,
North Carolina			1/1/99		Access II/III 1932(a)		9	a, b, c, d, e, f,
North Carolina	4/1/91				Carolina ACCESS 1915(b)		9	a, b, c, d, e, f,
North Carolina			1/1/99		Carolina ACCESS 1932		9	a, b, c, d, e, f
North Carolina	7/1/96				HealthCare Connection (1915)b NOTE: Statement of services clearly says MH and SA are excluded from Inpatient and Clinic Services.		9	a, b, c, e, f
North Carolina			7/1/96		HealthCare Connection (1932)a NOTE: Statement of services clearly says MH and SA are excluded from Inpatient and Clinic Services.		9	a, b, c, e, f
North Dakota	1/1/94		Converted 7/1/01		Access and Care Program FFS and Full Cap.	1(a), 4(a), 10, 11		a, b, c, h
Ohio	7/1/01				PremierCare	3, 6		a, b, c, h
Oklahoma		1/1/96			SoonerCare MCO Full Cap.	1(a), 4(a) 10, 11		a, b, c, d, e, f, g, h,
Oregon		2/1/94			Oregon Health Plan MH and SA PHP Full Cap.	1(a), 10, 11, 21		a, b, c, d, e, f, g

Table 6. (Continued)

State	Authority and Implementation Date Waiver Type 1915(b)	1115	1932(a)	Voluntary[1]	Plan Title	MH and-or SA Covered Service Yes	No	Covered Population
Oregon		2/1/94			Oregon Health Plan MCO (comprehensive benefits)	1(a), 4(a), 10, 11		a, b, c, d, e, f, g
Oregon	9/1/94				Transportation Program	15	15	?
Pennsylvania	2/1/94				Family Care Network PCCM Provider FFS	1(a), 4(a), 10, 11		a, c, e
Pennsylvania	2/1/97				HealthChoices MH/SA PHP Full Cap.	1(a), 4(a), 10, 11, 14, 17, 19, 23		a, b, c, d, e, f,
Pennsylvania				1/1/72	Voluntary HMO Contracts	1(a), 4(a), 10, 11		a, b, c, d, e, f,
Rhode Island		8/1/94			Rite Care	1(a), 4(a), 10, 11		a, b, c, g, h
South Carolina				8/1/96	Health Maintenance Organization	10, 11		a, b, c, e, h
South Carolina				5/1/96	Physicians Enhanced Program		?	a, c, e, f, h
South Dakota				7/1/96	Dental Program		?	a, b, c, d, e, f,
South Dakota	9/1/93				Prime	3		a, b, c, e, f, h
Tennessee		1/1/94			TennCare	1(a), 4(a), 10, 11, 14, 19		a, b, c, d, e, f, g, h, i
Texas	9/1/94				Lonestar Select I		7	?
Texas	3/10/95				Lonestar Select II. NOTE: Selectively contracts with free standing psychiatric hospitals for inpatient care of children.	1		?

Table 6. (Continued)

State	Authority and Implementation Date Waiver Type				Plan Title	MH and-or SA Covered Service		Covered Population
	1915(b)	1115	1932(a)	Voluntary[1]		Yes	No	
Texas	11/1/99				NorthSTAR (MH/SA) PHP Full Cap.	1(a), 4(a),10 11, 17, 19, 23		a, b, c, d, e, f, h, i
Texas	8/1/93				STAR PCCM Provider FFS and MCO Full Cap.	1(a), 4(a), 10,11		a, b, c, d, e, f, h
Texas	1/1/98				STAR+PLUS	3, 6		d, e, f
Utah	7/1/82				Choice of Health Care Delivery	24	9	a, b, c, d, e, f
Utah	7/1/01				Non-Emergency Transportation	15	15	?
Utah	7/1/91				Prepaid Mental Health Program	1, 2, 14, 21		a, b, c, d, e, f
Utah				10/1/00	Voluntary PCCM/MCO Program	24	9	a, b, c, d, e, f
Vermont		1/1/96			Vermont Health Access PCCM Provider FFS	1(a), 4(a), 10, 11		a, b, c, d, e, f, g,
Virginia	3/1/92				Medallion	3, 6		a, b, c, d, e, f, g,
Virginia	1/1/96				Medallion II	1, 4, 11		a, b, c, d, e, f, g,
Washington	10/1/93				Health Options		9	a, b, c
Washington	7/1/93				The Integrated Mental Health Services	1, 2, 14		a, b, c, d, e, f,

Table 6. (Continued)

	Authority and Implementation Date Waiver Type					MH and-or SA Covered Service		
State	1915(b)	1115	1932(a)	Voluntary[1]	Plan Title	Yes	No	Covered Population
West Virginia	9/1/96				Mountain Health Trust		9	a, b, c
West Virginia	6/1/92				Physician Assured Access System		9	a, b, c, e, f,
Wisconsin		7/1/99			BadgerCare (SCHIP) MCO Full Cap.	1(a), 4(a),10, 11		?
Wisconsin				4/1/93	Children Come First (MH/SA) PHP Full Cap.	1(a), 4(a),10, 11		i
Wisconsin				7/1/94	Independent Care	1(a), 4(a), 10, 11		e, f
Wisconsin	8/1/84		Converted 4/1/99		Medicaid HMO Program	1(a), 4(a), 10, 11		a, b, c, g, h,
Wisconsin		1/1/96			Wisconsin Partnerships Program	1(a), 4(a), 10, 11		d, f
Wisconsin				3/1/97	Wraparound Milwaukee (MH/SA) PHP Full Cap.	1(a), 4(a), 10, 11, 14, 21		i
Wyoming					No Managed Care Program			

Table 6. (Continued)

Data from Centers for Medicare and Medicaid Services (CMS), including the National summary of state Medicaid managed care programs and from Medicaid Managed Care: A Guide for States, fifth edition, 2001, Portland, ME: National Academy for State Health Policy

Key to Covered Services

1 Hospital Inpatient Mental Health
1(a) Inpatient Mental Health
2. Hospital Outpatient Mental Health
3 Hospital In- and Outpatient Mental Health
4 Hospital Inpatient Substance Abuse
4(a) Inpatient Substance Abuse
5 Hospital Outpatient Substance Abuse
6 Hospital In- and Outpatient Substance Abuse
7 Inpatient Hospital
8 Outpatient Hospital
9 In- and Outpatient Hospital
10 Outpatient Substance Abuse
11 Outpatient Mental Health
12 Specialty Mental Health
13 Mental Health
14 Residential Mental Health
15 Non-emergency Transportation
16 Mental Health/Retardation Rehab.
17 Detoxification
18 Primary Mental Health
19 Residential Substance Abuse Rehab.
20 Halfway House
21 Mental Health Rehabilitation
22 Inpatient Substance Abuse
23 Opiate Treatment Program
24 Inpatient Medical Detoxification
25 Plan Services Description vague

Key to Covered Population

a Family Coverage
b Poverty level Pregnant Women
c Poverty Level Children
d Aged
e Supplemental Security Income Children
f Supplemental Security Income Adults
g 1115 Expansion
h Children's Health Insurance Program Expansion
i Other
? Plan listed in Centers for Medicare and Medicaid Services files but not in state Medicaid Managed Care Overview

Footnotes to Table 6:

[1] Plans listed under the voluntary column do not indicate a waiver authority as none is required by the Federal government.

[2] PACE (Program of All inclusive Care for Elders) is a non-Federal program for the frail elderly. If the potential participant meets the eligibility requirements for enrollment into the PACE program, which is 55 years and older, lives in the plans approved service area, and is certified for nursing facility level of care and elects to enroll in the PACE program, the participant will remain enrolled in the program unless he or she chooses to voluntarily dis-enroll from the plan or is involuntarily dis-enrolled by the plan with DHS approval. PACE programs do not require a Waiver.

[3] This plan is not in Medicaid Managed Care: A Guide for States, fifth edition, 2001, National Academy for State Health Policy.

[4] National Academy of State Health Policy Medicaid Managed Care: a Guide for States, fifth edition, 2001 shows a PACE plan implemented in 1995 but the CMS files do not show it.

[5] Iowa is not shown in the National Academy of State Health Policy Medicaid Managed Care: a Guide for States, fifth edition, 2001.

[6] Mississippi's HealthMACS program was dropped from the 2002 CMS database as Mississippi no longer had a capitated managed care program with HMO plans as they were taken over by the Department of Insurance for financial reasons.

Table 7. State Medicaid managed care programs as of June 30, 2002

State	Program Title	Operating authority	Service area	Implementation date	Service delivery	Payment system	MH covered	SA Covered
Alabama	Maternity Care	1932	County	June 1, 1999	PCCM	FFS	No	No
Alabama	Partnership Hospital Program	Voluntary, no authority	Region	Oct. 1, 1996	Med. Only PHP	Full Capitation	No	No
Alabama	Patient 1st	1915(b)	Statewide	Jan. 1,1997	PCCM	FFS	Inpatient	No
Arkansas	Primary Care Phys	1915(b)	Statewide	Nov. 1, 1996	PCCM	FFS	No	Inpatient
Arizona	AHCCCS	1115	Statewide	Oct. 1, 1982	MCO (comp. Benefits)	Full Capitation	In and Out	In and Out
Arizona	AHCCCS	1115	Statewide	Oct. 1, 1982	(MH/SA) PHP	Full Capitation	In and Out+	In and Out+
California	Altamed Senior Buenacare	1115	County	Nov. 1, 1998	LTC MCO	Full Capitation	In and Out	In and Out
California	Center for Elders Independence	1115	County	April 1, 1995	LTC MCO	Full Capitation	In and Out	In and Out
California	Central Coast Alliance for Health	1915(b)	County	January 1, 1996	HIO	Full Capitation	No	No
California	Health Plan of San Mateo	1915(b)	County	Nov. 30, 1987	HIO	Full Capitation	No	Outpatient
California	Hudman	1915(b)	Statewide	April 24, 1992	[1]			
California	Managed Care Network	1915(b)	County	March 1, 1997	PCCM	FFS	No	No
California	Medi-Cal Mental Health care Field Test(San Mateo County)	1915(b)	County	April 1, 1995	[2]	FFS	Yes	?
California	Medi-Cal Specialty Mental Health Services Consolidation	1915(b)	Statewide (Except Solano and San Mateo)	March 15, 1995	[3]	FFS	Yes	?

Table 7. (Continued)

State	Program Title	Operating authority	Service area	Implementation date	Service delivery	Payment system	MH covered	SA Covered
California	On Lok Senior Health Services	1115	County	Nov. 1, 1983	LTC- MCO	Full Capitation	In and Out	In and Out
California	Partnership Health Plan of California	1915(b)	County	May 1, 1994	HIO	Full Capitation	In and Out Solano Co. only	Out
California	Prepaid Health Plan Program	Voluntary	County	Jan. 1, 1972	MCO (Comprehensive Benefits)	Full Capitation	No	No
California	Prepaid Health Plan Program	Voluntary	County	Jan. 1, 1972	PHP (Only for Emotional Support)	Full Capitation	Yes	No
California	Primary Care Case Management Program	1915(b)	County	August 1, 1984	Medical-only PHP	Full Capitation	Specialty MH	No
California	Sacramento Geographic Managed Care	1915(b)	County	April 1, 1994	MCO (Comprehensive Benefits)	Full Capitation	No	Inpatient
California	San Diego Geographic Managed Care	1915(b)	County	Oct. 17, 1998	MCO (Comprehensive Benefits)	Full Capitation	No	No
California	Santa Barbara Health Initiative	1915(b)	County	Sept. 1, 1983	HIO	Full Capitation	No	In and Out
California	Selective Provider Contracting Program	1915(b)	Statewide	Sept. 21, 1982	[4]		No	No
California	Senior Care Action Network	1115	County	Jan. 1, 1985	Social HMO	Full Capitation	Mental Health[5]	No
California	Sutter Senior Care	1115	County	May 1, 1994	Long Term Care MCO	Full Capitation	In and Out	In and Out

Table 7. (Continued)

State	Program Title	Operating authority	Service area	Implementation date	Service delivery	Payment system	MH covered	SA Covered
California	Two-Plan Model Program	1915(b)	County	Jan. 23, 1996	MCO (Comprehensive Benefits)	Full Capitation	No	No
Colorado	Mental Health Capitation Program	1915(b)	Statewide	July 1, 1995	Mental Health PHP	Full Capitation	In and Out, Rehab., Residential Support	No
Connecticut	Husky A	1915(b)	Statewide	Oct. 1, 1995	MCO (Comprehensive Benefits)	Full Capitation	In and Out	Out
Delaware	Diamond State Health Plan	1115	Statewide	Jan. 1, 1996	MCO (Comprehensive Benefits)[6]	Full Capitation	In and Out	In and Out
District of Columbia	D.C. Medicaid Managed Care Program	1915(b)	Statewide	April 1, 1994	MCO (Comprehensive Benefits)[7]	Full Capitation	Out	Out
Florida	Managed Health Care	1915(b)	Statewide	Oct. 1, 1992	PCCM Provider[8]	FFS	Inpatient	Inpatient
Florida	Prepaid Mental Health	1915(b)	County	March 1, 1996	Mental Health PHP	Full Capitation	In and Out, Rehab. Support	No
Florida	Statewide Inpatient Psychiatric Program	1915(b)	Statewide	April 1, 1999	[9]		Inpatient	No
Georgia	Georgia Better Health Care	1915(b)	Statewide	Oct. 1, 1993	PCCM Provider	FFS	Inpatient	Inpatient
Georgia	PASARR[10]	1915(b)	Statewide	Nov. 1, 1994	Mental Health PHP	Full Capitation	[11]	No
Hawaii	Hawaii QUEST	1115	Statewide	Aug. 1, 1993	MCO (Comprehensive Benefits)	Full Capitation	In and Out	In and Out

Table 7. (Continued)

State	Program Title	Operating authority	Service area	Implementation date	Service delivery	Payment system	MH covered	SA Covered
Idaho	Healthy Connections	1915(b)	County	Oct. 1, 1993	PCCM Provider	FFS	In and Out	Inpatient
Illinois	Voluntary Managed Care	Voluntary	County	Nov. 1, 1974	MCO (Comprehensive Benefits)	Full Capitation	In and Out	In and Out
Indiana	Hoosier Healthwise	1915(b)	Statewide	July 1, 1994	PCCM Provider	FFS	No[12]	No
Iowa	Iowa Medicaid Managed Health Care	1932	County	Dec. 1, 1986	MCO (Comprehensive Benefits)	Full Capitation	No	No
Iowa	Iowa Plan for Behavioral Health	1915(b)	Statewide	Jan. 1, 1999	(MH/SA PHP	Full Capitation	In and Out	In and Out, Detox.
Kansas	KMMC: Health Connect Kansas	1915(b)	Statewide	Jan. 1, 1984	PCCM Provider	FFS	In and Out	In and Out
Kansas	KMMC: Health Wave [19]	1915(b)	County	Dec. 1, 1995	MCO (Comprehensive Benefits)	Full Capitation	No	No
Kentucky	Kentucky Health Care Partnership Program	1115	Region	Nov. 1, 1997	MCO (Comprehensive Benefits)	Full Capitation	No	No
Kentucky	Kentucky Patient Access and Care Program	1932	Region	Apr. 1, 2000	PCCM Provider	FFS	No	No
Louisiana	Community Car	1915(b)	Parish	June 1, 1992	PCCM Provider	FFS	No	No
Maine	MaineCare Primary Care Case Management	1932	Statewide	May 1, 1999	PCCM Provider	FFS	No	No
Maryland	HealthChoice	1115	Statewide	June 1, 1997	MCO (Comprehensive Benefits)	Full Capitation	Primary MH	Outpatient

Table 7. (Continued)

State	Program Title	Operating authority	Service area	Implementation date	Service delivery	Payment system	MH covered	SA Covered
Massachusetts	Mass Health	1115	Statewide	July 1, 1997	PCCM Provider	FFS	No	No
Michigan	Childrens Special Health Care Services	Voluntary	Statewide	Sept. 1, 1998	MCO (Comprehensive Benefits)	Full Capitation	Outpt.	No
Michigan	Comprehensive Health Plan	1915(b)	County	July 1, 1997	MCO (Comprehensive Benefits)	Full Capitation	Outpt.	No
Michigan	Specialty Community Mental Health Services Program	1915(b)	Statewide	Oct. 1, 1998	Dev. Disabled, Mental Health and Substance Abuse PHP	Full Capitation	[13] In and Out	In and Out
Minnesota	CCDTF[14]	1915(b)	Statewide	Jan. 1, 1988	County Case Manager	FFS	No	In and Out, Rehab., Half-way house
Minnesota	Minnesota Disability Health Options	Voluntary	County	Sept. 1, 2001	MCO (Comprehensive Benefits)	Full Capitation	In and Out	In and Out
Minnesota	Senior Health Options Program	Voluntary	County	March 1, 1997	MCO (Comprehensive Benefits)	Full Capitation	In and Out	In and Out
Minnesota	MinnesotaCare Program for Families and Children	1115	Statewide	July 1, 1995	MCO (Comprehensive Benefits)	Full Capitation	In and Out	In and Out
Minnesota	Prepaid Medical Assistance Program	1115	County	July 1, 1985	MCO (Comprehensive Benefits)	Full Capitation	In and Out	In and Out
Mississippi	HealthMACS[15]	1932	Statewide	June 28, 1998	PCCM Provider	FFS	No	No

Table 7. (Continued)

State	Program Title	Operating authority	Service area	Implementation date	Service delivery	Payment system	MH covered	SA Covered
Missouri	MC+Managed Care/1915(b)	1915(b)	City, County	Sept. 1, 1998	MCO (Comprehensive Benefits)	Full Capitation	In and Out	In and Out
Montana	Passport to Health	1915(b)	Statewide	Jan. 1, 1994	PCCM Provider	FFS	In and Out	In and Out
Nebraska	Health Connection Combined Waiver Program	1915(b)	Statewide	July 1, 1995	PCCM Provider	FFS	No	No
Nebraska	Health Connection Combined Waiver Program	1915(b)	Statewide	July 1, 1995	MCO (Comprehensive Benefits)	Full Capitation	No	No
Nebraska	Health Connection Combined Waiver Program	1915(b)	Statewide	July 1, 1995	ASO (non-risk)	FFS	In and Out	In and Out, Opiate Treatment
Nevada	Mandatory Health Maintenance Program	1932	County	Dec. 1, 1998	MCO (Comprehensive Benefits)	Full Capitation	In and Out, Rehab.	No
Nevada	Voluntary Health Maintenance Program	1932	County	April 1, 1997	MCO (Comprehensive Benefits)	Full Capitation	In and Out, Rehab.	No
New Hampshire	Voluntary Managed Care Program	Voluntary	Statewide	March 2, 1983	MCO (Comprehensive Benefits)	Full Capitation	In and Out	In and Out
New Jersey	New Jersey Care 2000+(1915b)	1915(b)	Statewide	Oct. 1, 2000	MCO (Comprehensive Benefits)	Full Capitation	[16]	
New Jersey	New Jersey Care 2000+(1915b)	1932	Statewide	Sept. 1, 1995	MCO (Comprehensive Benefits)	Full Capitation	[17]	

Table 7. (Continued)

State	Program Title	Operating authority	Service area	Implementation date	Service delivery	Payment system	MH covered	SA Covered
New Mexico	SALUD!	1915(b)	Statewide	July 1, 1997	MCO (Comprehensive Benefits)	Full Capitation	In and Out	In and Out
New York	Office of Mental Health/Partial Capitation Program	Voluntary	County	April 1, 1996	Mental Health PHP	Partial Capitation	Outpt[18]	No
New York	Partnership Plan-Family Health Plus	1115	Statewide	Sept. 4, 2001	MCO (Comprehensive Benefits)	Full Capitation	In and Out[19]	In and Out
New York	Partnership Plan Medicaid Managed Care Program	1115	Statewide	Oct. 1 1997	MCO (Comprehensive Benefits)	Full Capitation	In and Out	In and Out
North Carolina	Access II/III 1915b	1915(b)	County	July 1, 1998	PCCM Provider	FFS	No	No
North Carolina	Access II/III1932(a)	1932	County	Jan. 1, 1999	PCCM Provider	FFS	No	No
North Carolina	Carolina ACCESS 1915(b)	1915(b)	Statewide	Apr. 1, 1991	PCCM Provider	FFS	No	No
North Carolina	Carolina ACCESS 1932	1932	Statewide	Jan. 1, 1999	PCCM Provider	FFS	No	No
North Carolina	Health Care Connection (1915)b	1915(b)	County	July 1, 1996	MCO (Comprehensive Benefits)	Full Capitation	No	No[20]
North Carolina	Health Care Connection (1932)a	1932	County	July 1, 1996	MCO (Comprehensive Benefits)	Full Capitation	No	No[21]
North Dakota	North Dakota Access and Care Program	1932	Statewide	Jan. 1, 1994	PCCM Provider	FFS	In and Out	In and Out

Table 7. (Continued)

State	Program Title	Operating authority	Service area	Implementation date	Service delivery	Payment system	MH covered	SA Covered
Ohio	Premier Care	1915(b)	County	July 1, 2001	MCO (Comprehensive Benefits)	Full Capitation	In and Out	In and Out
Oklahoma	SoonerCare	1115	County, Region	Jan. 1, 1996	MCO (Comprehensive Benefits)	Full Capitation	In and Out	In and Out
Oregon	Oregon Health Plan	1115	Statewide	Feb. 1, 1994	(MH/SA) PHP	Full Capitation	In and Out+[22]	In and Out+
Oregon	Oregon Health Plan	1115	Statewide	Feb. 1, 1994	MCO (Comprehensive Benefits)	Full Capitation	In and Out	In and Out
Pennsylvania	Family Care Network	1915(b)	County	Feb. 1, 1994	PCCM Provider	FFS	In and Out	In and Out
Pennsylvania	HealthChoices	1915(b)	County	Feb. 1, 1997	MCO (Comprehensive Benefits)	Full Capitation	No	No
Pennsylvania	HealthChoices	1915(b)	County	Feb. 1, 1997	(MH/SA) PHP	Full Capitation	In and Out+	In and Out+
Pennsylvania	Voluntary HMO Contracts	Voluntary	County	Jan. 1, 1972	MCO (Comprehensive Benefits)	Full Capitation	In and Out	In and Out
Rhode Island	Rite Care	1115	Statewide	Aug. 1, 1994	MCO (Comprehensive Benefits)	Full Capitation	In and Out	In and Out
South Carolina	Health Maintenance Organization	Voluntary	County	Aug. 1, 1996	MCO (Comprehensive Benefits)	Full Capitation	Outpt	Outpatient.
South Dakota	PRIME	1915(b)	Statewide	Sept. 1, 1993	PCCM Provider	FFS	In and Out	No

Table 7. (Continued)

State	Program Title	Operating authority	Service area	Implementation date	Service delivery	Payment system	MH covered	SA Covered
Tennessee	TennCare	1115	Statewide	Jan. 1, 1994	MCO (Comprehensive Benefits)	Full Capitation	No	No
Tennessee	TennCare	1115	Statewide	Jan. 1, 1994	(MH/SA) PHP	Full Capitation	In and Out+	In and Out+
Texas	Lonestar Select I	1915(b)	Metropolitan Statistical Areas	Sept. 1, 1994	[23]	Solely Reimbursement Arrangement	No	No
Texas	Lonestar Select II	1915(b)	Metropolitan Statistical Areas	March 10, 1995	[24]	Solely Reimbursement Arrangement	Yes	Yes?
Texas	NorthSTAR	1915(b)	Region	Nov. 1, 1999	(MH/SA)PHP	Full Capitation	In and Out+	In and Out+
Texas	STAR	1915(b)	County	August 1, 1993	PCCM Provider	FFS	In and Out	In and Out
Texas	STAR+PLUS	1915(b)	County	Jan. 1, 1998	MCO (Comprehensive Benefits)	Full Capitation	In and Out	In and Out
Texas	STAR+PLUS	1915(b)	County	Jan. 1, 1998	PCCM Provider	FFS	In and Out	In and Out
Utah	Choice of Health Care Delivery	1915(b)	County	July 1, 1982	MCO (Comprehensive Benefits)	Full Capitation	No	Inpatient, Medical Detox.
Utah	Prepaid Mental Health	1915(b)	County	July 1, 1991	(MH/SA)PHP	Full Capitation	In and Out+	No
Utah	Voluntary PCCM/Managed Care Organization Program	1932	County	October 1, 2000	PCCM Provider	FFS	No	No

Table 7. (Continued)

State	Program Title	Operating authority	Service area	Implementation date	Service delivery	Payment system	MH covered	SA Covered
Utah	Voluntary PCCM/Managed Care Organization Program	1932	County	October 1, 2000	MCO (Comprehensive Benefits)	Full Capitation	No	InpatientMedical Detox.
Vermont	Vermont Health Access	1115	Statewide	January 1, 1996	PCCM Provider	FFS	In and Out	In and Out
Virginia	Medallion	1915(b)	City, County	March 1, 1992	PCCM Provider	FFS	In and Out	Inpatient
Virginia	Medallion II	1915(b)	City, County	January 1, 1996	MCO (Comprehensive Benefits)	Full Capitation	In and Out	Inpatient
Washington	Healthy Options	1915(b)	Statewide	October 1, 1993	PCCM Provider	FFS	No	No
Washington	Integrated Mental Health Services	1915(b)	County	July 1, 1993	(MH) PHP	Full Capitation	In and Out+	No
West Virginia	Mountain Health Trust	1915(b)	County	Sept. 1, 1996	MCO (Comprehensive Benefits)	Full Capitation	No	No
West Virginia	Physician Assured Access System	1915(b)	Statewide	June 1, 1992	PCCM Provider	FFS	No	No
Wisconsin	Badger Care (SCHIP)	1115	Statewide	July 1, 1999	MCO (Comprehensive Benefits)	Full Capitation	In and Out	In and Out
Wisconsin	Children Come First	Voluntary	County	April 1, 1993	(MH/SA) PHP	Full Capitation	In and Out+	In and Out
Wisconsin	Independent Care	Voluntary	County	July 1, 1994	MCO (Comprehensive Benefits)	Full Capitation	In and Out	In and Out
Wisconsin	Medicaid HMO Program	1932	Statewide	March 31, 1997	MCO (Comprehensive Benefits)	Full Capitation	In and Out	In and Out

Table 7. (Continued)

State	Program Title	Operating authority	Service area	Implementation date	Service delivery	Payment system	MH covered	SA Covered
Wisconsin	Wisconsin Partnership Program	1115	County	January 1, 1996	MCO (Comprehensive Benefits)	Full Capitation	In and Out	In and Out
Wisconsin	Wraparound Milwaukee	Voluntary	County	March 1, 1997	(MH/SA) PHP	Full Capitation	In and Out+	In and Out

From the national summary of state Medicaid managed care programs, as of June 30, 2002, Centers for Medicare and Medicaid Services (CMS) accessed 3 February 2004.

HIO = Health Insuring Organization
MCO = Managed Care Organization
PACE = Program of All inclusive Care for the Elderly
PCCM = Primary Care Case Management
PAHP = Prepaid Ambulatory Health Plan
PHP = Prepaid Health Plan
PIHP = Prepaid Inpatient Health Plan

Footnotes to Table 7:

1. This waiver is a mechanism for placement in freestanding nursing facilities rather than hospital based distinct part nursing facilities unless waiver exemptions allow residents to remain in distinct part nursing facilities.
2. Case rate funding mechanism for most specialty mental health services with fee-for-service for therapy. Not clear if substance abuse is covered.
3. Mechanism to allow fee-for-service payment for mental health services statewide. Not clear if substance abuse is covered.
4. This waiver allows California selectively to contract with hospitals to provide acute inpatient care to all Medi-Cal beneficiaries. This waiver does not differentiate by beneficiary aid code.
5. Included services stated as "mental health" with no indication as to level or type.
6. This program offers very limited health and substance abuse benefits. Most of the mental health and substance abuse services are fee-for-service.
7. This program offers very limited health and substance abuse benefits. Most of the mental health and substance abuse services are fee-for-service.
8. PCCM enrollees in six counties receive mental health services through a capitated arrangement. Enrollees are allowed to choose either the fee-for-service or a capitated plan. If the enrollee fails to make a choice, they are mandatory enrolled into a capitated health plan.

9. The program is a fee-for-service per diem all inclusive rate.
10. Pre-admission Screening and Annual Resident Review
11. Services included: Mental Health/Mental Retardation Rehabilitation (setting not specified).
12. Inpatient psychiatric hospital and outpatient psychiatric services are generally carved-out. However, when these services are provided by an acute care hospital or a primary care provider, they are included. The same coverage condition applies to inpatient and outpatient substance abuse services.
13. This Michigan plan provides the most extensive list of services of any state plan: Inpatient mental health, Mental health rehabilitation, Mental health residential, Mental health support, Mental health clinic, Outpatient mental health (partial hospitalization), Outpatient substance abuse, Personal care, Residential substance abuse rehabilitation
14. Consolidated Chemical Dependency Treatment Fund
15. Mississippi no longer has capitated managed care programs with HMO plans as they have been taken over by the Department of Insurance for financial reasons.
16. Mental health and substance abuse services provided for enrollees who are clients of the Division of Developmental Disabilities.
17. Mental health and substance services provided for enrollees who are clients of the Division of Developmental Disabilities.
18. Included services are "Mental Health Continuation Day Treatment, Mental Health Intensive Psychiatric Rehabilitation, Mental Health Outpatient". Terminology is not consistent with other plans' description of services.
19. This plan specifically limits inpatient mental health to 30 days per year and outpatient mental health to 60 days per year. No such limits are specified for substance abuse services, either in or outpatient.
20. This plan's list of Included Services specifically states "Inpatient Hospital Except for Mental Health and Substance Abuse".
21. This plan's list of Included Services specifically states "Inpatient Hospital Except for Mental Health and Substance Abuse".
22. A Plus sign (+) indicates that the plan covers more than just inpatient and outpatient mental health services or substance abuse services, *e.g.*, Rehabilitation, Day Treatment, Residential, Support, etc.
23. This program enables Texas selectively to contract with general acute care hospitals including children's hospitals. Under selective contracting arrangements, providers must bid a discount from their Medicaid reimbursement rates. Then, the state accepts or negotiates those bids so that qualified providers may serve the Medicaid population for a period of three years.
24. This program enables the state to contact selectively with freestanding psychiatric facilities for inpatient services to children. Under this program, providers must bid all inclusive per diem rates for Medicaid reimbursement. The State then either accepts or negotiates those rates so that providers may serve the under 21 Medicaid population for a period of 3 years.

psychiatric problem (yes/no), pregnancy status, veterans status, living arrangements, source of income, health insurance, expected source of payment for treatment, details on employment status, details on criminal justice status, marital status, and days between first contact and first service. All states are required to submit the Minimum Data Set and some states also provide the supplemental information. Pertinent items from the Minimum Data Set include race and ethnicity data, treatment modality (*e.g.,* inpatient, residential, outpatient, and-or methadone), referral source (which includes data on legal status), treatment history (*i.e.,* number of previous admissions), education, employment status, and substance use. Supplemental data of interest include insurance status (such as Medicaid) and psychiatric co-morbidity. Substantial information is available on the universe of programs eligible to report to the TEDS system and on response rates. Data from TEDS have been used in several studies (see, *e.g.,* Hopfer et al., 2000).

Data from TEDS for 1992 through 2002 were employed. The TEDS data provided information on the severity of clients receiving services. The severity indicator was constructed from TEDS data items such as "frequency of use" and "age at first use" as described by McCamant et al. (2007). Owing to the massive sample sizes, a one percent random sample was employed.

Data Analyses

Hierarchical linear models were used in the data analysis. There were two levels to the model – subjects (lower level) and states (upper level). Using the Bryk and Raudenbusch (1992, 1996) formulation of hierarchical models the approach was as follows. Let "y_{ij}" be the dependent variable (*i.e.,* the severity measure). In this two-level analysis, "y_{ij}" is the severity for subject "j" in state "i". Let the vector of predictor variables be denoted by "$\underline{x}_{ij}$". These predictors include the policy-relevant indicators pertaining to Medicaid managed care. Then the equation to be estimated is:

$$y_{ij} = a_i + \underline{b}_i ' \underline{x}_{ij} + e_{ij} \qquad (1)$$

where "a_i" is an intercept (for each state), "$\underline{b}_i$" is a vector of coefficients (for each state), and "e_{ij}" is an error term. This level of the hierarchical model serves to "nest" the subjects within the states.

Now, at the upper level of the model, the characteristics of each state can modify lower level parameters. For example, let

$$b_{1i} = c + \underline{d} ' \underline{z}_i + f_i \qquad (2)$$

where "c" is an intercept, "$\underline{z}_i$" is a vector of state characteristics, "$\underline{d}$" is a vector of upper level coefficients to be estimated, and "f_i" is an error term. In effect, this level of the hierarchy allows for interactions of individual level factors with other co-variates.

Time (i.e., the several study years) was incorporated into this model. For example, indicators were constructed for each of the study years and included in the vector of predictor variables "$\underline{x}_{ij}$". Alternative approaches modeled linear or quadratic functions of time by including the appropriate polynomial (of time) among the predictor variables (Murray, 1998; Murray et al., 1998). As noted, the hierarchical framework facilitates the construction of interaction terms. By including time in the model, attention is directed to "condition by time" interaction terms where "condition" refers to Medicaid managed care versus fee for service.

IMPACT OF MEDICAID MANAGED CARE ON SEVERITY OF CLIENTS IN SUBSTANCE ABUSE TREATMENT

Table 8 shows the demographics of admitted persons (*i.e.,* admissions) in the Treatment Episode Data Set during selected study years. Notice that the severity measure shows no obvious pattern with respect to year. If anything, the severity score increased with time (indicating that more severely impaired clients were admitted in later study years). Parenthetically, it should be noted that the severity score is approximately Gaussian in distribution in this data set.

Numerous analyses of variance and hierarchical models were fitted to these data. As expected, given the massive sample sizes, demographics such as gender and race / ethnicity were highly statistically significant predictors of severity. Also expected were highly statistically significant variation for both state and year.

However, the indicator(s) for Medicaid substance abuse treatment managed care, while statistically significant, explained microscopic fractions of the variance. For example, in a model with a simple yes / no indicator for Medicaid substance abuse treatment managed care, state accounted for 7.1 percent of variance, year accounted for 0.076 percent of variance, and the Medicaid substance abuse managed care indicator accounted for 0.0086 percent of variance. Moreover, the coefficient was such that, if anything, Medicaid managed care for substance abuse treatment was associated with elevated degrees of client severity.

It is instructive to consider the possible impact of Medicaid substance abuse treatment managed care on the overall client severity measure obtained from the TEDS data. Let the (unknown) average Deck severity score for Medicaid clients in fee for service substance abuse treatment be "x", the (unknown) average Deck severity score for non-Medicaid clients in fee for service substance abuse treatment be "y", and the overall average Deck severity score for substance abuse treatment clients (both Medicaid and non-Medicaid) in fee for service be "z". Notice that "z" can be obtained from the TEDS data.

Now suppose the average Deck severity score differs by "d" units for Medicaid clients in managed care versus Medicaid clients in fee for service substance abuse treatment. Then the average Deck severity score for Medicaid clients in "state-years" with Medicaid substance abuse treatment managed care will be "x + d". Suppose that the average Deck severity score for non-Medicaid clients is "y" in both Medicaid fee for service state-years and in Medicaid managed care state-years. In other words, suppose that Medicaid managed care has no impact on non-Medicaid substance abuse treatment clients. Further suppose that Medicaid clients represent "p" percent of all substance abuse treatment clients. Then the overall average Deck severity score in state-years with fee for service Medicaid substance abuse treatment will be the quantity $z = (px + (1 - p)y)$. Analogously, in state-years with managed care Medicaid substance abuse treatment, the overall average Deck severity score will be (p(x + d) + (1 -

p)y). Subtracting these two quantities shows that the impact of Medicaid substance abuse treatment managed care on overall (Medicaid and non-Medicaid) client severity is given by "pd". In other words, overall average Deck severity for both Medicaid and non-Medicaid clients in Medicaid managed care state-years is "z + pd".
Recall that at the beginning of the study period, there were some 11 states with Medicaid managed care pertaining to substance abuse treatment (Figure 1) whereas by the end of the study period all but 18 states had Medicaid managed care pertaining to substance abuse treatment (Figure 2). In other words, the fraction of state-years with Medicaid managed care for substance abuse treatment increased from 11 of 51 (22 percent) to 32 of 51 (64 percent). Therefore, on average roughly 43 percent of the state-years included Medicaid managed care for substance abuse treatment.

Accordingly, the average Deck severity is z + (.43 pd).

The variance due to Medicaid managed care is

$$(.43((z - (z + (.43\ pd)^2) + (.57((z + pd) - (z + (.43\ pd)^2))$$

$$= ((.43)^3)(pd)^2) + ((.57)^3)(pd)^2)$$

$$= (.079507 + .185193)(pd)^2)$$

$$= .2647\ (pd)^2)$$

A conservative estimate is that over the study years Medicaid clients represented ten percent of substance abuse treatment clients (*i.e.,* $p = 0.1$). If $p = 0.1$, then variance due to Medicaid managed care is 0.002647 (d^2). From Table 8, the overall variance is approximately $(0.2)^2 = .04$. Then the variance due to Medicaid managed care is

$$(0.002647\ (d^2) / 0.04 = 0.066175\ (d^2) = (d^2) * 6.6175 \text{ percent}$$

The observed variance explained by Medicaid managed care is 0.0086 percent which corresponds to a value for "d" of 0.036. As noted, the sign for "d" is positive because, if anything, substance abuse treatment clients in Medicaid managed care appeared to have slightly higher Deck severity scores (worse severity) than did comparable clients in fee for service. Now from McCamant et al. (2007), the smallest odds ratio for baseline Deck severity score as a predictor of relapse 12 months after completion of treatment was 3.264 (for alcohol use among Drug Abuse Treatment Outcomes Study participants). Note that the Deck severity score lies between zero and one. Therefore, the impact on odds of relapse of change in Deck severity score "d" can be computed by 3.264^{d}. In this case d = 0.036 so that the odds of relapse are given by $3.264^{0.036} = 1.0435$. In other words, increase in Deck severity score of 0.036 units will increase odds of relapse at 12 months following treatment by roughly four percent. Put differently, Medicaid managed care was (at most) associated with minimally increased severity of Medicaid clients in substance abuse treatment. There was no evidence for "cream skimming" in this nation-wide project.

Table 8. Demographics of admissions in Treatment Episode Data Set

	1992	1994	1996	1998	2000	2002
N	13,798	14,956	14,751	15,023	14,539	17,124
Age (std dev)	32.5 (10.2)	33.0 (10.2)	33.3 (10.6)	33.3 (10.8)	33.7 (11.1)	34.1 (11.4)
Gender						
Female	3,752 (27%)	4,374 (29%)	4,336 (29%)	4,486 (30%)	4,437 (30%)	5,121 (30%)
Male	10,046 (73%)	10,582 (71%)	10,415 (71%)	10,537 (70%)	10,102 (70%)	12,003 (70%)
Race						
White	8,788 (64%)	9,160 (61%)	9,165 (62%)	9,374 (62%)	9,152 (63%)	10,768 (63%)
African American	3,485 (25%)	3,956 (27%)	3,820 (26%)	3,638 (24%)	3,485 (24%)	4,277 (25%)
Other	1,525 (11%)	1,840 (12%)	1,766 (12%)	2,011 (13%)	1,902 (13%)	2,079 (12%)
Primary Substance						
None	161 (1%)	171 (1%)	141 (1%)	113 (1%)	95 (1%)	130 (1%)
Alcohol	8,205 (60%)	7,834 (53%)	7,430 (51%)	7,206 (48%)	6,627 (46%)	7,573 (45%)
Cocaine/Crack	2,391 (17%)	2,825 (19%)	2,422 (17%)	2,346 (16%)	2,015 (14%)	2,247 (13%)
Marijuana	883 (6%)	1,335 (9%)	1,834 (12%)	2,074 (14%)	2,252 (16%)	2,643 (16%)
Heroin	1,702 (12%)	2,116 (14%)	2,165 (15%)	2,363 (16%)	2,598 (18%)	2,687 (16%)
Methamphetamine	66 (1%)	62 (<1%)	46 (<1%)	39 (<1%)	44 (<1%)	951 (6%)
Other	320 (2%)	523 (4%)	615 (4%)	762 (5%)	821 (6%)	697 (4%)
Severity (std dev)	.398 (.200)	.410 (.200)	.410 (.199)	.407 (.196)	.399 (.194)	.413 (.197)

In other words, with regard to severity and Medicaid managed care for substance abuse treatment, it appears that there was little if any relationship. Indeed, if anything, Medicaid managed care was associated with elevated severity for individuals in the national data set. Therefore, the present project found no evidence for "cream skimming" in the conversion of Medicaid fee for service to managed care.

Of course, the study had numerous limitations related to the advantages and disadvantages of the national information systems. First, the data systems emphasize publicly funded facilities and clients. Obviously, the national data sets under-count clients and providers who are solely in the private sector (Alexander and Lemak, 1997; Alexander et al., 1998; D'Aunno and Vaughn, 1995; Friedmann, Alexander, and D'Aunno, 1999). It is worth recalling, however, that in 1997, for example, some 64 percent of funds for substance abuse treatment came from the public sector (Coffey et al., 2000). In other words, the national data bases pertain to the vast majority of alcohol and drug abuse treatment.

A second consideration with the national data systems is their universality. On the one hand, the systems attempt to capture information on most of the substance abuse treatment in the United States. On the other hand, the national systems must, perforce, rely on some fifty states plus tens of thousands of facilities to supply data. To cite but one potential problem, differences in response rates from state to state presumably reflect states' varying requirements for data submission from facilities receiving public funds. However, the national data system includes a "cross-walk" inventory of state reporting requirements designed to address these issues. Furthermore, the analytic component of the project relied chiefly on longitudinal approaches designed to facilitate the examination of year to year changes. Indeed, program staff in the Office of Applied Studies at SAMHSA advise analyses of change over time within states that take into account possible inconsistencies in state reporting procedures.

Finally, it was unfortunate that reporting on health insurance status for people in the Treatment Episode Data Set was markedly incomplete. While the TEDS Minimum Data Set items were complete for the vast majority of admissions, the Supplemental Data were often missing. In particular, more than half the admissions had missing data on health insurance (including Medicaid status). Therefore, it was not possible to focus the study on Medicaid clients. However, it can be argued (Deck and McFarland, 2002) that there is considerable interest in the impact of Medicaid managed care on public sector substance abuse clients in general. With these caveats in mind, it is fair to say that Medicaid managed care for substance abuse treatment appears to have had no adverse selection impact on public sector clients receiving care for addictions.

Conclusion

Medicaid underwent substantial change over the last several years as fee for service was largely replaced by managed care. Because changes were implemented on a state-by-state and year-by-year basis this Medicaid transition provides an invaluable "natural experiment" examining the impact of organization and financing on health care. This chapter carefully catalogued these changes as well as the numerous Medicaid waivers that facilitated much of the transition to managed care. Focusing on substance abuse treatment, these data were used to address the contention that managed care encouraged "cream skimming" wherein providers select less severe clients. No evidence was found for decline in substance abuse treatment client severity as Medicaid managed care was implemented. The next chapters now examine Medicaid managed care for special populations including adolescents and individuals involved with the criminal justice system. Challenges of research and evaluation are addressed.

ACKNOWLEDGMENT

Supported in part by grant number R21 AA 014050 from the National Institute on Alcohol Abuse and Alcoholism.

REFERENCES

Alexander, J. A., and Lemak, C. H. (1997). The effects of managed care on administrative burden in outpatient substance abuse treatment facilities. *Medical Care, 35*, 1060-1068.

Alexander, J. A., and Lemak, C. H. (1997). Managed care penetration in outpatient substance abuse treatment units. *Medical Care Research and Review, 54*(4), 490-507.

Alexander, J. A., Lemak, C. H., and Campbell, C. I. (2003). Changes in managed care activity in outpatient substance abuse treatment organizations, 1995-2000. *Journal of Behavioral Health Services and Research, 30*, 369-381.

Alexander, J. A., Wheeler, J. R., Nahra, T. A., and Lemak, C. H. (1998). Managed care and technical efficiency in outpatient substance abuse treatment units. *Journal of Behavioral Health Services and Research, 25*(4), 377-396.

American Managed Behavioral Healthcare Association and the National Association of State Alcohol and Drug Abuse Directors (1999). Public substance abuse and managed behavioral healthcare. *Behavioral Healthcare Tomorrow*, 25-30.

Babigian, H. M., Cole, R. E., Reed, S. K., Brown, S. W., and Lehman, A. F. (1991). Methodology for evaluating the Monroe-Livingston capitation system. *Hospital and Community Psychiatry, 42*(9), 913-919.

Babigian, H. M., and Marshall, P. E. (1989). Rochester: A comprehensive capitation experiment. *New Directions in Mental Health Services*(43).

Bergman, G. T. (1999). *A second generation of managed behavioral health programs emerge*. Rockville, MD: U.S. Department of Health and Human Services, Substance Abuse and Mental Health Services Administration, Managed Behavioral Healthcare Updates Series.

Bien, T. H., Miller, W. R., and Tonigan, J. S. (1993). Brief interventions for alcohol problems: A review. *Addiction, 88*, 315-336.

Bryk, A. S., and Raudenbush, S. W. (Eds.). (1992). *Hierarchical linear models: Applications and data analysis methods*. Newbury Park, CA: Sage Publications.

Bryk, A. S., Raudenbush, S. W., and Congdon, R. T. (Eds.). (1996). *HLM: Hierarchical Linear and Nonlinear Modeling with the HLM/2L and HLM/3L Programs*. Lincolnwood, IL: SSI Scientific Software International.

Callahan, D. (1995). Once again reality: The lesson from the SUPPORT study Special Supplement. *Hastings Center Report, 24*, S33-S36.

Chang, C. F., Kiser, L. J., Bailey, J. E., Martins, M., Gibson, W. C., Schaberg, K. A. et al. (1998). Tennessee's failed managed care program for mental health and substance abuse services. *Journal of the American Medical Association, 279*, 864-869.

Coffey, R. M., Mark, T., King, E., Harwood, H., McKusick, D., Genuardi, J. et al. (2000). *National estimates of expenditures for mental health and substance abuse treatment, 1997 (SAMHSA Publication Number SMA-00-3499)*. Rockville, MD: U.S. Department of Health and Human Services, Substance Abuse and Mental Health Services Administration.

Cole, R. E., Reed, S. K., Babigian, H. M., Brown, S. W., and Fray, J. (1994). A mental health capitation program: I. Patient outcomes. *Hosp Community Psychiatry, 45*(11), 1090-1096.

D'Aunno, T., and Vaughn, T. E. (1995). An organizational analysis of service patterns in outpatient drug abuse treatment units. *Journal of Substance Abuse, 7*, 27-42.

Deck, D. D., McFarland, B. H., Titus, J. M., Laws, K. E., and Gabriel, R. M. (2000). Access to substance abuse treatment services under the Oregon Health Plan. *Journal of the American Medical Association, 284*(16), 2093-2099.

Deck, D. D., and McFarland, B. H. (2002). Medicaid managed care and substance abuse treatment. *Psychiatric Services, 53,* 802.

Draper, D. A., and Gold, M. R. (2003). Provider risk sharing in Medicaid managed care plans. *Health Affairs, 22*, 159-167.

Draper, D. A., Hurley, R. E., and Short, A. C. (2004). Medicaid managed care: The last bastion of the HMO? *Health Affairs, 23*, 155-167.

Egnew, R. C. (1996). Refining the concept of public/private partnerships. *Behavioral Healthcare Tomorrow, 5*, 37-39.

Etheridge, R. M., Craddock, S. G., Dunteman, G. H., and Hubbard, R. L. (1995). Treatment services in two national studies of community-based drug abuse treatment programs. *Journal of Substance Abuse, 7*, 9-26.

Ettner, S. L., Argeriou, M., McCarty, D., Dilonardo, J., and Liu, H. (2003). How did the introduction of managed care for the uninsured in Iowa affect the use of substance abuse services? *Journal of Behavioral Health Services and Research, 30*, 26-40.

Ettner, S. L., Denmead, G., Dilonardo, J., Cao, H., and Belanger, A. J. (2003). The impact of managed care on the substance abuse treatment patterns and outcomes of Medicaid beneficiaries: Maryland's HealthChoice Program. *Journal of Behavioral Health Services and Research, 30*, 41-62.

Finney, J. W. (1995). Enhancing substance abuse treatment evaluations: Examining mediators and moderators of treatment effects. *Journal of Substance Abuse Treatment, 7*, 135-150.

Finney, J. W., and Monahan, S. C. (1996). The cost-effectiveness of treatment for alcoholism: A second approximation. *Journal of Studies on Alcohol, 57*, 229-243.

Finney, J. W., and Moos, R. H. (2002). Psychosocial treatments for alcohol use disorders. In P. E. Nathan and J. M. Gorman (Eds.), *A guide to treatments that work* (2nd ed.). New York: Oxford University Press.

Fleming, M. F., Barry, K. L., Manwell, L. B., Johnson, K., and London, R. (1997). Brief physician advice for problem alcohol drinkers – a randomized controlled trial in community-based primary care practices. *Journal of the American Medical Association, 277*, 1039-1045.

Friedmann, P. D., Alexander, J. A., and D'Aunno, T. A. (1999). Organizational correlates of access to primary care and mental health services in drug abuse treatment units. *Journal of Substance Abuse Treatment, 16*(1), 71-80.

Galanter, M., Keller, D. S., Dermatis, H., and Egelko, S. (2000). The impact of managed care on substance abuse treatment: A report of the American Society of Addiction Medicine. *Journal of Addictive Disease, 19*, 13-34.

Galanter, M., Keller, D. S., Dermatis, H., Egelko, S., and American Society of Addiction Medicine (2001). The impact of managed care on substance abuse treatment: a problem in need of solution. A report of the American Society of Addiction Medicine. *Recent Developments in Alcoholism, 15*, 419-436.

Goldman, W., McCulloch, J., and Sturm, R. (1998). Cost and use of mental health services before and after managed care. *Health Affairs, 17*, 40-52.

Gustafson, J. S., Anderson, R., Sheehan, K., McGencey, S., Reda, J., O'Donnell, C. et al. (1999). *State resources and services related to alcohol and other drug problems: Fiscal years 1996 and 1997*. Washington, D.C.: National Association of State Alcohol and Drug Abuse Directors, Inc.

Hopfer, C. J., Mikulich, S. K., and Crowley, T. J. (2000). Heroin use among adolescents in treatment for substance use disorders. *Journal of the American Academy of Child and Adolescent Psychiatry, 39*, 1316-1323.

Horgan, C. (2001). Substance abuse: The nation's number one health problem. Princeton, NJ: Robert Wood Johnson Foundation.

Humphreys, K., and Moos, R. H. (1996). Reduced substance-abuse-related health care costs among voluntary participants in Alcoholics Anonymous. *Psychiatric Services, 47*, 709-713.

Hurley, R. E., and Somers, S. A. (2003). Medicaid and managed care: A lasting relationship? *Health Affairs, 22*, 77-88.

Iglehart, J. K. (1999). The American health care system: Medicaid. *New England Journal of Medicine, 340*, 403-408.

Institute of Medicine (1990). *Broadening the base of treatment for alcohol problems*. Washington, DC: National Academy Press.

Institute of Medicine (Ed.). (1996). *Managing managed care: Quality improvement in behavioral health*. Washington, DC: National Academy Press.

Laws, K., Gabriel, R., and McFarland, B. H. (2002). Integration and its discontents: Substance abuse treatment in the Oregon Health Plan. *Health Affairs, 21*, 284-289.

Lewin-VHI (1995). *States as payers: Managed care for Medicaid populations, the states and private sector: Leading health care reform*. Washington, DC: National Institute for Health Care Management.

Maglione, M., and Ridgely, M. S. (2006). Is conventional wisdom wrong? Coverage for substance abuse treatment under Medicaid managed care. *Journal of Substance Abuse Treatment, 30,* 285-290.

Manski, C. F., Pepper, J. V., and Petrie, C. V. (2001). *Informing America's policy on illegal drugs. What we don't know keeps hurting us*. Washington, DC: National Academy Press.

Mark, T. L., Buck, J. A., Dilonardo, J. D., Coffey, R. M., and Chalk, M. (2003). Medicaid expenditures on behavioral health care. *Psychiatric Services, 54*, 188-194.

Mark, T. L., Levit, K. R., Buck, J. A., Coffey, R. M., and Vandivort-Warren, R. (2007). Mental health treatment expenditure trends, 1986-2003. *Psychiatric Services, 58*, 1041-1048.

McCamant, L. E., Zani, B. G., McFarland, B. H., and Gabriel, R. M. (2007). Prospective validation of substance abuse severity measures from administrative data. *Drug and Alcohol Dependence, 86*, 37-45.

McCarty, D., and Argeriou, M. (2003). The Iowa Managed Substance Abuse Care Plan: Access, utilization, and expenditures for Medicaid recipients. *Journal of Behavioral Health Services and Research, 30*, 18-25.

McCarty, D., Dilonardo, J., and Argeriou, M. (2003). State substance abuse and mental health managed care evaluation program. *Journal of Behavioral Health Services and Research, 30*, 7-17.

McCarty, D., McGuire, T. G., Henrick, H. J., and Field, T. (1998). Using state information systems for drug abuse services research. *The American Behavioral Scientist, 41*, 1090-1106.

McFarland, B., and George, R. (1995). Ethics and managed care. *Child and Adolescent Psychiatric Clinics of North America, 4*, 885-901.

McFarland, B. H. (1994). Health maintenance organizations and persons with severe mental illness. *Community Mental Health Journal, 30*, 221-242.

McFarland, B. H. (1996). Comparing period prevalences with application to drug utilization. *Journal of Clinical Epidemiology, 49*, 473-482.

McFarland, B. H. (2000). Overview of Medicaid managed behavioral health care. In R. R. Goetz, B. H. McFarland and K. V. Ross (Eds.), *What the Oregon Health Plan can teach us about managed mental health care. New Directions for Mental Health Services, No. 85* (pp. 17-22). San Francisco: Jossey-Bass.

McFarland, B. H., Deck, D. D., McCamant, L. E., Gabriel, R. M., and Bigelow, D. A. (2005). Outcomes for Medicaid clients with substance abuse problems before and after managed care. *Journal of Behavioral Health Services and Research, 32*(4), 351-367.

McFarland, B. H., Lierman, W. K., Penner, N. R., McCamant, L. E., and Zani, B. G. (2003). Employee benefits managers' opinions about addiction treatment. *Journal of Addictive Diseases, 22*, 15-29.

McFarland, B. H., McCamant, L. E., and Barron, N. M. (2005). Outcomes for clients of public substance abuse treatment programs before and after Medicaid managed care. *Journal of Substance Abuse Treatment, 28*, 149-157.

McFarland, B. H., and Minkoff, K. (1996). Utilization management. In K. Minkoff and D. Pollack (Eds.), *Managed mental health care in the public sector: A survival manual.* Amsterdam: Harwood Academic Publishers.

McKusick, D., Mark, T. L., King, E., Harwood, R., Buck, J. A., Dilonardo, J. et al. (1998). Spending for mental health and substance abuse treatment, 1996. *Health Affairs, 17*, 147-157.

McLellan, A. T., Cacciola, J. S., and Fureman, I. (1996). The Addiction Severity Index and the Treatment Services Review. In L. I. Sederer and B. Dickey (Eds.), *Outcomes assessment in clinical practice*. Philadelphia: Williams and Wilkins.

Mechanic, D. (Ed.). (1999). *Mental health and social policy: the emergence of managed care, 4th edition*. Boston, MA: Allyn and Bacon.

Miller, W. R., and Hester, R. K. (1986). Inpatient alcoholism treatment: Who benefits? *American Psychologist, 41*, 794-805.

Moos, R. H., and Finney, J. W. (1995). Substance abuse treatment programs and processes: Linkages to patients' needs and outcomes. *Journal of Substance Abuse, 7*, 1-8.

Murray, D. M. (Ed.). (1998). *Design and analysis of group-randomized trials. Monographs in epidemiology and biostatistics (vol. 27)*. New York: Oxford University Press.

Murray, D. M., Hannan, P. J., Wolfinger, R. D., Baker, W. L., and Dwyer, J. H. (1998). Analysis of data from group randomized trials with repeat observations on the same groups. *Statistics in Medicine, 17*, 1581-1600.

National Academy for State Health Policy (2001). *Medicaid Managed Care: A Guide for States, fifth edition, 2001*, Portland, Maine: National Academy for State Health Policy, 2001.

National Institute on Drug Abuse (1999). *Principles of drug addiction treatment: A research-based guide*. Rockville, MD: United States Department of Health and Human Services.

O'Brien, C., and McLellan, A. (1996). Myths about the treatment of addiction. *Lancet, 347*, 237-240.

Office of Applied Studies (2001). *Growth of managed care in substance abuse treatment. DASIS Report*. Rockville, MD: Office of Applied Studies, Substance Abuse and Mental Health Services Administration.

Parish, D. C. (1997). Another indication for screening and early intervention: Problem drinking. *JAMA, 277*, 1079-1080.

Pettinati, H. M., Meyers, K., Jensen, J. M., Kaplan, F., and Evans, B. D. (1993). Inpatient vs. outpatient treatment for substance dependence revisited. *Psychiatric Quarterly, 64*, 173-182.

Policy Resource Center and George Washington University Center for Health Policy Research (1996). *SAMHSA Managed Care Tracking System: Final report. Prepared under contract with the Substance Abuse and Mental Health Services Administration and the Health Resources and Services Administration [contract No. 240-OA-45(5)]*. Rockville, MD: Substance Abuse and Mental Health Services Administration.

Reed, S. K., and Babigian, H. M. (1994). Postmortem of the Rochester capitation experiment. *Hospital and Community Psychiatry, 45*(8), 761-764.

Reed, S. K., Hennessy, K. D., and Babigian, H. M. (1995). Setting capitation rates for comprehensive care of persons with disabling mental illness. *Psychiatric Services, 46*(2), 127-129.

Reed, S. K., Hennessy, K. D., Mitchell, O. S., and Babigian, H. M. (1994). A mental health capitation program: II. Cost-benefit analysis. *Hospital and Community Psychiatry, 45*(11), 1097-1103.

Scott, M. A., Snowden, L. R., and Libby, A. M. (2002). Alcohol and juvenile justice contacts: A comparison of fee-for-service and capitated Medicaid mental health services. *Journal of Studies on Alcohol, 63*(1), 44-48.

Sosin, M., and D'Aunno, T. (2001). The organization of substance abuse managed care. *Recent Developments in Alcoholism, 15*, 27-49.

Steenrod, S., Brisson, A., McCarty, D., and Hodgkin, D. (2001). Effects of managed care on programs and practices for the treatment of alcohol and drug dependence. *Recent Developments in Alcoholism, 15*, 51-71.

Stein, B., Reardon, E., and Sturm, R. (1999). Substance abuse service utilization under managed care: HMOs versus carve-out plans. *Journal of Behavioral Health Services and Research, 26*, 451-456.

Substance Abuse and Mental Health Services Administration (1998). *Substance abuse and mental health statistics source book 1998 (Analytic Series A-4)*. Rockville, MD: Substance Abuse and Mental Health Services Administration Office of Applied Studies.

Sullivan, E., and Fleming, M. (1997). *A guide to substance abuse services for primary care clinicians*. Rockville, MD: Center for Substance Abuse Treatment.

Talbott, J. A., and Hales, R. E. (2001). *Textbook of Administrative Psychiatry: New Concepts for a Changing Behavioral Health System, Second Edition*. Arlington, VA: American Psychiatric Publishing, Inc.

Timko, C., Finney, J. W., Moos, R. H., and Moos, B. S. (1995). Short-term treatment careers and outcomes of previously untreated alcoholics. *Journal of Studies on Alcohol, 56*, 597-610.

Tonigan, J. S., Toscova, R., and Miller, W. R. (1996). Meta-analysis of the literature on Alcoholics Anonymous: Sample and study characteristics moderate findings. *Journal of Studies on Alcohol, 57*, 65-72.

Walsh, D. C., Hingson, R. W., Merrigan, D. M., Levenson, S. M., Cupples, L. A., Heeren, T. et al. (1991). A randomized trial of treatment options for alcohol-abusing workers. New England Journal of Medicine, 325, 775-782.

Weisner, C., McCarty, D., and Schmidt, L. (1999). New directions in alcohol and drug treatment under managed care. American Journal of Managed Care, 5, SP57-SP69.

Zwick, W. R., and Berman, M. (1992). Spectrum of services for the alcohol abusing patient. In J. L. Feldman and R. J. Fitzpatrick (Eds.), Managed mental health care. Washington, DC: American Psychiatric Press, Inc.

In: Medicaid and Treatment for People... ISBN 978-1-61470-742-4
Editors: B.H. McFarland, D. McCarty et al, pp.111-121© 2011 Nova Science Publishers, Inc.

Chapter 5

Medicaid Managed Care for Adolescent Substance Abuse Treatment Clients

David Hughes, Virginia Mulkern and Sarah Guckenburg
All authors are affiliated with Human Services Research Institute, Cambridge, MA, USA

Abstract

Adolescents are substantially over-represented in Medicaid but little is known about substance abuse treatment for this population. In 1997, the federal Substance Abuse and Mental Health Services Administration (SAMHSA) funded the Human Services Research Institute to conduct a multi-site study examining the impact of managed care on the services received and outcomes achieved for adolescents with substance abuse disorders in managed care and fee for service environments. Study sites included Massachusetts, New York, Oregon, Pennsylvania, Puerto Rico, Tennessee, and Washington state. Interviews were completed for 1,568 youth at treatment entry. Follow-up interviews were conducted after six months. Administrative data on treatment utilization also were analyzed. This chapter summarizes the methods and results of this large study. Implementation of managed care varied substantially by site with numerous mechanisms involved. There were few if any differences by managed care versus fee for service on the self-report measures. Administrative data showed complex patterns of utilization changes during the study period. While not obviously detrimental to young Medicaid clients in treatment for substance abuse problems, managed care apparently did little if anything to improve outcomes for this population.

Introduction

The transition from fee for service to managed care in the public sector occurred largely since the mid-1990s after it was nearly complete in private insurance. The process began with states seeking to control Medicaid costs, which had been rising rapidly in the 1980s, by making use of the (then) Health Care Financing Administration (HCFA) "waiver" regulations to implement managed care programs for general health care. Within a few years nearly every state operated some form of Medicaid managed care program (Lewin Group, 1998). Between 1991 and 1998, the number of Medicaid recipients enrolled in managed care programs increased six-fold, from 2.7 to 16.6 million (Kaiser Commission on Medicaid and the Uninsured, 1999).

Initially, states implementing Medicaid managed care programs tended to retain behavioral health benefits under fee for service arrangements, especially for beneficiaries whose eligibility was based on disability (*e.g.,* recipients of Social Security Disability Insurance) (Callahan et al., 1995). As the states gained experience managing general health care for clients in the Aid to Families with Dependent Children/Temporary Assistance to Needy Families (AFDC/TANF) system, however, they began to manage behavioral health benefits and to enroll persons with disabilities in managed care programs. Typically these systems were structured as carve-out programs, *i.e.,* specialty programs established to manage mental health and substance abuse benefits separately from general health care (Frank et al., 1996).

These programs may be operated by private for-profit managed care organizations (MCOs), by public agencies at the state, county or even city level, or by some combination of private for-profit and public non-profit organization. In most respects managed care programs are heterogeneous, with much variation in characteristics such as relationship to general health care benefits (*e.g.,* integrated versus carve-out), techniques of utilization management, manner and extent of risk sharing, specifics of benefits packages, and provisions of the contracts between public agencies and private MCOs, and between MCOs and providers (Gold and Hurley, 1997; Lewin Group, 1998; Rosenbaum et al., 1998; Rosenthal, 1999). This heterogeneity characterized the managed care programs included in the present study as well (Mulkern, 1999).

The states implemented these programs in advance of much empirical evidence concerning their effects (Mechanic et al., 1995). The (then) HCFA required, as a condition of receiving a waiver, that states obtain an independent evaluation, and the health services research community, including federal funding agencies and private foundations demonstrated considerable interest in these policy initiatives. The pace of implementation, however, combined with the considerable challenges for research design resulted in findings beyond the level of case studies being relatively sparse, as indicated below (Leff and Woocher, 1998). The Substance Abuse and Mental Health Services Administration (SAMHSA) multi-site study described in this report provides some of the most comprehensive data on public sector managed care for adolescents with substance use disorders to date.

SAMHSA's Managed Care and Vulnerable Populations project had two broad goals: to enhance knowledge about the range of managed behavioral health care services provided to individuals with psychiatric and substance abuse disorders, and to enhance knowledge about the outcomes of persons served under managed care and fee for service conditions. Six sites and one Coordinating Center were funded via cooperative agreements to design and implement a multi-site study using common data collection instruments and design protocols. Study sites included Massachusetts, New York, Oregon (plus Washington state), Pennsylvania, Puerto Rico, and Tennessee (plus Mississippi). In the Pacific Northwest, Oregon was the managed care site and Washington state was the fee for service site. In the South, Mississippi provided fee for service administrative data. The project had sub-studies including:

1. A survey of the structural characteristics of the managed care initiatives at each site
2. A prospective study examining outcomes among samples of individuals in managed care and fee for service programs at each site
3. An analysis of system level service utilization and costs using extant administrative data bases

This chapter has two main sections. The first section highlights methods of the study, and the second section summarizes the main findings. Analysis strategies are included in the results section.

METHODS

Implementation Study

The goal of the implementation study was to determine the way in which the managed care intervention had been implemented at each site. In order to understand the information collected on service utilization and client outcomes at each site, and to compare these data across sites, it was crucial to have a clear understanding of:

- How adolescents moved through these systems and who paid for what types of services under what conditions
- The managed care initiatives at each site and how they changed during the study period
- The degree to which contractual elements were implemented at each managed care site
- The evolving nature of the fee for service comparison programs
- The effect of changes such as welfare reform, state health care reform, and changes in the criminal justice systems on the managed care initiative

The project developed the protocols, manuals and frameworks for the sites as they conducted key informant interviews, analyzed secondary data and reviewed documents. Materials included a key informant interview protocol, a key informant interview manual, and a conceptual and coding framework.

Managed Care Organization Data

Managed care varied considerably in implementation and was hardly a unitary concept. Rather, it represented a collection of financial and utilization management strategies that were bundled together in various ways within different sorts of organizational contexts. The Coordinating Center developed an instrument to "unbundle" some of this complexity and to provide a way of categorizing various managed care initiatives in terms of several domains that may be related to variations in service use, costs and outcomes. The domains included:

- Characteristics of the managed care contract
- Organizational arrangements
- Services covered
- Characteristics of enrollees included
- Benefit design and medical necessity criteria
- Benefit coverage determination procedures
- Network composition
- Risk sharing arrangements
- Capitation arrangements
- Accountability mechanisms

Separate protocols were developed to collect information on the contract between the state and the managed care organization, between the managed care organization and the behavioral health sub-contractor (if applicable) and between the managed care or managed behavioral health care company and providers. Administration manuals were developed for each level of the instrument. A glossary of terms was also developed.

Prospective Outcome Study

The prospective outcome study compared outcomes for clients in managed care and fee for service conditions at each site. Clients were interviewed twice. The data collection interval was approximately six months with a protocol for common data collection. Interviews were conducted with 1,568 individuals. Table 1 summarizes the baseline interview numbers by site.

Table 1. Baseline interviews completed by target population and overall

Site	Managed Care N (%)	Fee for Service N (%)
Massachusetts	155 (53%)	138 (47%)
New York	2 (1%)	201 (99%)
Oregon / Washington state	149 (46%)	176 (54%)
Pennsylvania	102 (33%)	203 (67%)
Puerto Rico	134 (72%)	52 (28%)
Tennessee	256 (100%)	0 (0%)
Total	798	770

Note: Oregon was the managed care site and Washington state was the fee for service site in the Pacific Northwest.

Utilization Study Using Administrative Data

The utilization sub-study was designed to examine differences in service utilization patterns for persons receiving services in managed care and fee for service environments. Data sources used were Medicaid, Managed Care encounter and state Block Grant files.

In order to reconcile different coding schemes across the various databases in each state, the Coordinating Center, in collaboration with the sites, created a number of tools. These included:

- *Common service taxonomies.* Sites mapped their local coding schemes to the general study categories.
- *Algorithmic definition charts.* Each site prepared detailed tables that included how they mapped local variables (*e.g.,* procedure code, diagnosis, provider specialty, other local coding conventions) onto the common coding categories.
- *Common eligibility categories.* Sites performed a similar mapping procedure with eligibility categories.

RESULTS

Implementation Study

Analysis for Implementation Study

The implementation study was conducted during 1999. Study sites collected information using a combination of methods including (1) key informant interviews, (2) document review, and (3) analyses of extant data from multiple data systems.

The Cross-Site Implementation Study report (Adolescent Managed Care Study Group, 2001) summarizes service delivery issues that were identified in the site implementation reports.

Results for Implementation Study

The goals of the adolescent implementation study were to assess state systems for serving adolescents with substance abuse problems and to examine the impact of managed care on these systems. The resulting reports pointed to service systems in disarray. Often, the implementation of managed care had little, if any, overall impact on the most significant problems faced by systems that served youth, including lack of resources, fragmented services, and little formal evaluation or oversight of treatment effectiveness.

Some of the promises of managed care included increased access to comprehensive and appropriate services, improved quality of care, and coordination of services. Some states reported that access to services, in particular, increased under managed care. However, informants also reported that managed care arrangements may have limited access to services, compromised quality of care, and complicated service coordination.

Problems in the substance abuse treatment system were only a microcosm of larger systemic problems, informants said. They pointed to the need for a comprehensive framework for all child and adolescent services, based on cross-disciplinary needs assessments, joint planning, and blended funding. Youth require developmentally and culturally appropriate services coordinated along a continuum of care. Because a substantial proportion of youth enter substance abuse treatment through the juvenile justice system, many informants believed that all adolescents who come in contact with the juvenile justice system should be screened for substance abuse and mental health disorders.

Prospective Outcome Study

Analysis for Outcome Study

This sub-study assessed possible differences in client level outcomes for clients receiving services in managed care and fee for service conditions. Since persons were not randomized into managed care and fee for service conditions, possible compositional differences between conditions were assessed by residualizing outcomes on demographics and clinical variables prior to analysis using ordinary least squares regressions. The unstandardized residuals were used in further analysis. To test for significant overall differences between managed care and fee for service, after controlling for demographic and clinical differences, a hierarchical random effects model was employed. The statistical software used for this analysis was Comprehensive Meta-Analysis, with the DerSimonian and Laird (1986) algorithm for hierarchical random effects. Variable domains included Alcohol Use, Drug Use, Marijuana Use, Symptomatology, Criminal Justice Involvement, and Risky Behaviors.

Results for Outcome Study

Alcohol Use: Alcohol use was measured via two variables – one question that asked about alcohol use during the past six months (with seven categories ranging from no use to daily use) and a question that asked about the number of times in the past six months in which five or more drinks were consumed (also with seven categories ranging from "never" to "daily"). The mean score between these two questions was taken as the outcome measure at baseline and at follow-up. No differences between managed care and fee for service conditions were detected at the cross-site level and only Oregon - Washington state showed a significant difference at the site level favoring fee for service.

Drug Use: Overall drug use was operationalized from ten questions dealing with use of marijuana, powdered cocaine, crack cocaine, methamphetamine, other amphetamines, barbiturates and sedatives, inhalants, hallucinogens, opiates, and other drug use. All of these questions were asked about the previous six-month period of time and all of them were based on a seven-point scale ranging from "no use" to "daily use". The mean score of these ten items was created at baseline and at follow-up. No differences between managed care and fee for service conditions were detected at the cross-site and site level.

Marijuana Use: The third outcome used was marijuana alone. This question also had the same seven-point scale as the other drug questions. Marijuana was employed as a separate outcome measure from the drug composite score because a cluster analysis showed a large group of marijuana users and it was felt important to look at this drug separately. No differences between managed care and fee for service conditions were detected at the cross-site and site level.

Criminal Justice Involvement: Criminal justice involvement was taken from three questions. These questions asked about drug crime, property crime, and crime against another person in the past six months. If the respondent answered yes to any of the three questions, then he or she was coded as being involved in the criminal justice system. No differences between managed care and fee for service conditions were detected at the cross-site and site level.

Mental Health Symptomatology: Overall mental health symptoms were operationalized using the raw score on the Youth Self Report (YSR) scale. The YSR scale is a general test of overall symptomatology designed for adolescents and young adults. No differences between managed care and fee for service conditions were detected at the cross-site level and only Pennsylvania showed a significant result (favoring managed care) at the site level.

Risky Behavior: This scale combined questions dealing with risky drug use as well as sexual behavior. It was the sum of seven items: injecting drugs, ever sharing needles, sharing needles with many individuals, going to a "shooting gallery", going to a crack house, number of sexual partners, and the use of condoms. All of the items asked about the previous six-month period of time. No differences between managed care and fee for service conditions were detected at the cross-site and site level.

The results of this evaluation suggested that managed care in the public sector did not significantly affect self-reported short-term outcomes for adolescents with substance abuse disorders in treatment. Thus, if policymakers implemented managed care for the purpose of achieving better outcomes, the evidence here does not indicate success. The results of the implementation study suggested that managed care is one of many different influences on the delivery of adolescent substance abuse treatment and that managed care and fee for service alike rely on a system of adolescent substance abuse treatment that is complex, under-resourced and fragmented. Thus, it is not surprising that managed care did not make an impact, positive or negative, on the outcomes of adolescents with substance use disorders.

Population Administrative Data Study

Analysis for Administrative Data

Data from Medicaid, managed care companies and state substance abuse authority databases were analyzed to assess service utilization patterns for individuals receiving services in managed care and fee for service conditions.

Aggregate Analyses: Claims and encounter data were aggregated and analyzed according to:

1. Number of people in each category eligible to receive services each month
2. The number of people receiving each type of service in each month
3. The number in specific demographic and clinical categories receiving each type of service in each month
4. Expenditures for each service provided in each month

Data were divided into two groups:

Group I: Fee for service pre-implementation (months 1–24) to Fee for service post-implementation (beyond month 24)

Group II: Fee for service (months 1–24) to Managed Care (months 25–42)

Meta-analyses of the risk differences between Groups I and II by month and by site were conducted by categories of services and, for selected services, for subcategories of gender, ethnicity, and diagnosis. A meta-regression model was also used to examine the effect of site, diagnosis, age, race, and condition in months 1 through 24 on the outcome variables for months post 24. Rates by month for each outcome and classification were computed using a random effects model. Individual program results were precision weighted to control for group size and variability.

Variable domains included:

- Service Measures:
  - Penetration Rate: Number of consumers receiving service divided by number eligible
  - Utilization Rate: Number of units (visits/days) of service provided divided by number of consumers eligible.

- Service Categories:
  - Inpatient services
  - Partial / day treatment
  - Outpatient medication treatment
  - Outpatient services (excluding medication)

- Factors and covariates for meta regression: Each of the outcome variables was calculated by the following subgroup classifications of the data:
  - Month: 1–24, pre and 25–36, 25–42, and 25–48 (where data was available)
  - Site
  - Condition: Managed care or Fee for service

RESULTS FOR ADMINISTRATIVE DATA

Penetration (Number of Persons Receiving Service)

All the states were serving significantly fewer youth than the conservative "need" rate of 3.5% or 35 per 1000 who are dependent on drugs and/or alcohol and in need of treatment (SAMHSA, 2002). Oregon and Washington state came the closest at 14 and 18 per 1000, respectively. In addition, Washington and New York had dramatic increases in access within the fee for service system. However, New York, Tennessee, and Mississippi were below the 10 per 1000, or 1% access rate. There were falling access rates in Oregon, Tennessee and Mississippi.

The pattern of the regression results suggested at least strong regional variation in access levels for substance abuse services by adolescents in the Medicaid system. With data from more states, smaller time units (*e.g.,* quarterly or monthly data), and more data from the pre- and post-managed care time periods, the estimates would have been more stable. In addition, numbers were insufficient to examine youth access by explanatory variables (*e.g.,* age, race, gender) and other characteristics affecting need for services (*e.g.,* type of drug use, degree of dependence) and enabling to access services (*e.g.,* provider availability). Unfortunately, such detail was beyond the scope of this project. In this analysis, the level of detail was the best that could be achieved in coordination between the project staff and Medicaid officials.

- *Inpatient services:* Prior to the implementation of managed care, the proportions of people in both groups (those who would remain in fee for service and those who would be enrolled in managed care) were comparable and declining slightly for both throughout the period. Post managed care rates for the managed care group continued to decline, while they increased for the fee for service group.
- *Partial / day treatment:* At the beginning of the period prior to managed care implementation, rates were notably higher for the group that would be enrolled in managed care. They were declining throughout the period for both groups, but more rapidly for the managed care group. Post implementation, they leveled off at approximately the same amount, at about 10 percent of each group.
- *Outpatient medication treatment:* Prior to managed care implementation, penetration rates were comparable for the two groups and level through the period. With managed care, medication treatment increased significantly while declining slightly for fee for service consumers. Exploratory subgroup analysis of differences for racial groups produced the important suggestion that during the pre-managed care period, penetration rates for managed care non-whites were lower, whereas post managed care they were higher for managed care non-whites.
- *Outpatient services:* The percent of persons using any outpatient service was level and comparable for the two groups prior to managed care. Following implementation, the rate climbed considerably for the fee for service group while, for the managed care group, it declined temporarily then rose to the pre-managed care level.

Utilization (Amount of Service Received)

- *Inpatient services:* As expected given the relatively low penetration rate for this service, the average amount of inpatient service received by individuals in both groups was low, less than one-tenth of a day in any month. The rate was slightly higher for the fee for service group in the pre-implementation period, and it remained level for both groups across the pre- and post-implementation periods.
- *Partial / day treatment:* The average amount of this service received, roughly comparable in the pre-implementation period, increased significantly for the fee for service group following implementation and declined slightly for the managed care group over the same period.
- *Outpatient medication treatment:* Prior to managed care, people in the managed care group, compared to those in fee for service, were receiving more of the service; following managed care, the average amount declined for both, but more for the managed care group. The penetration and utilization patterns combined suggest that managed care was providing medication to proportionately more people, but less intensively, *i.e.,* with fewer and/or briefer visits.
- *Outpatient services:* Following implementation, outpatient services increased significantly for the fee for service group while declining slightly for the managed care group.

Conclusion

The results of this evaluation suggested that managed care in the public sector did not significantly affect short-term self-reported outcomes for adolescents with substance abuse disorders in treatment. Administrative data revealed complex patterns of service utilization changes. Implementation analyses showed that numerous varieties of managed care arrangements were adopted. Thus, if policymakers implemented managed care for the purpose of achieving better outcomes, the evidence here does not indicate success. Moreover, the implementation study suggested that managed care is but one of many different influences on the delivery of adolescent substance abuse treatment and that managed care and fee for service alike rely on a system of adolescent substance abuse treatment that is complex, under-resourced and fragmented. Thus, it is not surprising that managed care did not make an impact, positive or negative, on the outcomes of adolescents with substance use disorders. The next chapters address Medicaid managed care for another special population – namely people involved with the criminal justice system.

Acknowledgments

In 1997, the federal Substance Abuse and Mental Health Services Administration funded the Human Services Research Institute to conduct a multi-site study examining the impact of managed care on the services received and outcomes achieved for adolescents with substance abuse disorders in managed care and fee for service environments.

References

Adolescent Managed Care Study Group. (2001). Falling through the cracks: Meeting the needs of adolescents with substance abuse problems in managed care and fee-for-service systems. Cambridge, MA: Human Services Research Institute.

Callahan, J. J., Shepard, D. S., Beinecke, R. H., Larson, M. J., and Cavanaugh, D. (1995). Mental health/substance abuse treatment in managed care: The Massachusetts Medicaid experience. Health Affairs, 14, 173-184.

DerSimonian, R., and Laird, N. (1986). Meta-analysis in clinical trials. Controlled Clinical Trials, 7, 177-188.

Frank, R. G., Huskamp, H. A., McGuire, T. G., and Newhouse, J. P. (1996). Some economics of mental health 'carve-outs'. Archives of General Psychiatry, 53, 933-937.

Gold, M., and Hurley, R. (1997). The role of managed care "products" in managed care "plans." Inquiry, 34, 29-37.

Kaiser Commission on Medicaid and the Uninsured (1999). The Medicaid program at a glance. Washington, DC: Kaiser Family Foundation.

Leff, H. S., and Woocher, L. S. (1998). Trends in the evaluation of managed mental health care. Harvard Review of Psychiatry, 5, 344-347.

Lewin Group (1998). SAMHSA Managed Care Tracking System. Fairfax, VA: Lewin Group.

Mechanic, D., Schlesinger, M., and McAlpine, D. D. (1995). Management of mental health and substance abuse services: State of the art and early results. Milbank Quarterly, 73, 19-55.

Mulkern, V. (1999). Managed behavioral health care in the public sector: A study of utilization, cost and outcomes. Cleveland, OH: Association for Health Services Research Annual Meeting.

Rosenbaum, S., Shin, P., Zakheim, M., Shaw, K., and Teitelbaum, J. (1998). Negotiating the new health system: A nationwide study of Medicaid managed care contracts. Washington DC: Center for Health Policy Research, George Washington University.

Rosenthal, M. B. (1999). Risk sharing in managed behavioral health care. Health Affairs, 18, 204-213.

Substance Abuse and Mental Health Services Administration. (2002). 2001 National Household Survey on Drug Abuse. Rockville, MD: U.S. Department of Health and Human Services.

In: Medicaid and Treatment for People… ISBN 978-1-61470-742-4
Editors B.H. McFarland, D. McCarty, et al., pp.123-161© 2011 Nova Science Publishers, Inc.

Chapter 6

Medicaid Managed Care and Drug Court Outcomes

***Douglas A. Bigelow*[1], *Michael Finigan*[2], *Shannon Carey*[2], *and Bentson H. McFarland*[3]**

[1] Department of Psychiatry, Oregon Health and Science University, Portland, OR
[2] NPC Research, Inc., Portland, OR , USA
[1] Departments of Psychiatry and Public Health and Preventive Medicine, Oregon Health and Science University, Portland, OR,USA

Abstract

Medicaid managed care and drug courts both grew dramatically during the 1990s. Yet heretofore there has been little or no evaluation of potential impact of Medicaid managed care on drug court participants. This chapter defines drug court, briefly reviews the history of this innovation, and describes one of earliest of such programs. The chapter reviews development of Medicaid managed care in Oregon and shows how there might be impact of Medicaid managed care on substance abuse treatment services for drug court participants. Using before versus after (Medicaid managed care) analyses the project described here tested hypotheses about possible managed care influences on drug court participants. Study subjects included individuals eligible for (but not necessarily participants in) drug court before versus after Medicaid managed care. Under managed care, less time was invested in treatment, especially for participants who chose but did not complete the drug court program. However, there were no more drug court program failures in the managed care period. Moreover, managed care had no effect on measures of recidivism, such as survival time to first arrest and days in the community for drug court participants. Analyses focused on Medicaid eligible drug court participants suggested, overall, that managed care had no impact on this group's numbers of arrests during follow-up, time to first follow-up arrest, or days in the community during follow-up. In summary, implementation of Medicaid managed care appeared not to be detrimental for drug court participants.

INTRODUCTION

The last decades have seen dramatic growth in drug courts (as shown in Figure 1). Drug courts may be defined as programs in which "components of the criminal justice and substance abuse treatment systems work together to try and use the coercive power of the court to promote abstinence and prosocial behavior" (Belenko, 1998). A more formal definition of drug court is outlined in Table 1 (National Association of Drug Court Professionals, 1997). Florida is generally acknowledged as the first state to implement a drug court program in 1989 (Belenko, 1998; Drug Strategies, 1999; Finn and Newlyn, 1993; Terry, 1999). Oregon's drug court system started shortly thereafter in 1991 (General Accounting Office, 1997). Now there are numerous drug courts operating in most if not all states (Bureau of Justice Assistance Drug Court Clearinghouse, 2007; Drug Court Clearinghouse and Technical Assistance Project, 1998; Drug Courts Program Office, 1998; Huddleston et al., 2008). In an early review, Belenko (1998) concluded that "drug courts generate savings, at least in the short term, from reduced jail or prison time, reduced criminality and lower criminal justice cost and drug use is substantially reduced." More recently, the Government Accountability Office found that drug courts are effective at reducing recidivism (Government Accountability Office, 2005). Similar conclusions have been reached by other reviewers (see, *e.g.,* National Institute of Justice, 2006; Sanford and Arrigo, 2005; Wilson, 2007). Treatment services provided to participants in a drug court program have been described (Schwartz and Schwartz, 1998) and overall recommendations about drug abuse treatment services for drug court participants are available (*e.g.,* Center for Substance Abuse Treatment, 1997; Chandler et al., 2009; National Association of Drug Court Professionals, 1997; National Institute on Drug Abuse, 2006; Peters et al., undated).

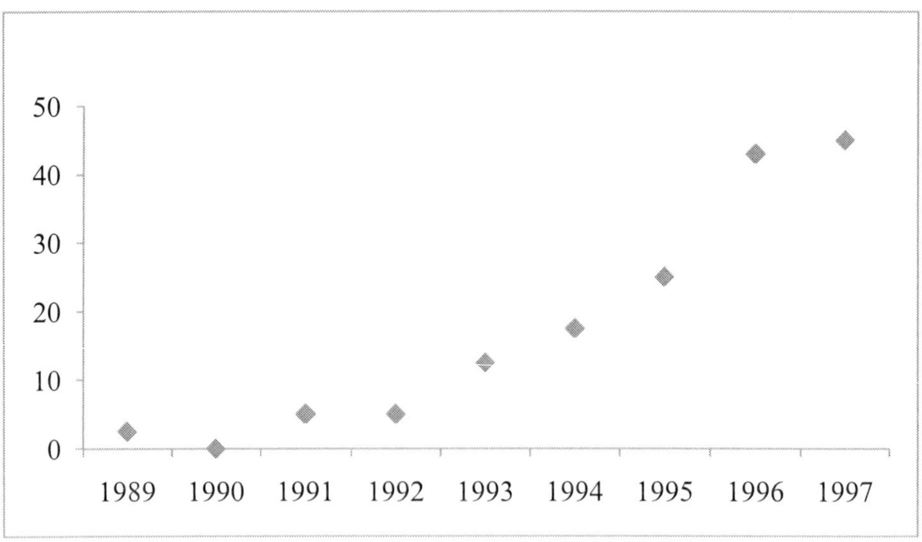

Figure 1. Drug courts established by year.

Table 1. Key components of drug courts

1. Integrate drug treatment with justice system
2. Prosecution and defense counsel promote public safety
3. Eligible participants identified early
4. Access to a continuum of drug treatment
5. Abstinence monitored frequently
6. Coordinated response to non-compliance
7. Judicial interaction with each participant
8. Monitoring and evaluation of program effectiveness
9. Interdisciplinary continuing education
10. Partnerships among drug courts and agencies

Source: NADCP (1997)

On the other hand, much less has been written about Medicaid, managed care and drug courts. This topic is of interest for several reasons. First, it is likely that substantial numbers of drug court participants are (or could become) Medicaid clients. Second, funding is a key component of a drug court's "sustainability plan" (Reilly and Pierre-Lawson, 2008). Third, some drug courts have used their discretionary funds to match federal Medicaid dollars (Reilly and Pierre-Lawson, 2008). Fourth, numerous state Medicaid programs now include managed care for substance abuse treatment services.

Managed care may be defined as the provision of services in accordance with medical necessity which, in turn, is the "health care service that will effectively and efficiently address the patient's medical condition" (McFarland and George, 1995). Numerous managed care mechanisms have evolved that seek to limit treatment services to those deemed "medically necessary" (Kihlstrom, 1997; McFarland and Minkoff, 1996; Mechanic et al., 1995). The impact has been dramatic. For example, in the commercial sector a survey of 1,043 large employers showed that from 1988 to 1997, the value of general health care (*i.e.,* medical-surgical) benefits declined by seven percent whereas the value of addiction treatment benefits dropped by 71 percent (Galanter, 1998).

Managed Care and Public Sector Behavioral Health Services

Managed care also arrived in the public sector (Alexander and Lemak, 1997a, 1997b; McFarland and Minkoff, 1996). A report from the Substance Abuse and Mental Health Services Administration (Bergman, 1999; SAMHSA, 1998) showed that 49 states have either implemented or have considered some form of managed care in their Medicaid behavioral health programs. The fraction of Medicaid clients enrolled in managed care programs rose from 10 percent in 1991 to 48 percent in 1997 (Iglehart, 1999). It should be noted that Medicaid enrollment itself rose during the 1990s from 11 percent of the U.S. in 1993 to 15 percent in 1998 (Iglehart, 1999). Medicaid is especially important for minority group members who during the 1990s comprised some 27 percent of the U.S. population but 46 percent of Medicaid enrollees (United States Bureau of the Census, 1998). It should be noted too that in some states block grant funded substance abuse treatment programs have also been converted to managed care (American Managed Behavioral Healthcare Association and the National Association of State Alcohol and Drug Abuse Directors, 1999; Bergman, 1999; SAMHSA, 1998).

Reports from the private sector indicate that managed care strategies such as prior authorization and-or utilization review can shift the locus of treatment for people with drug abuse problems away from inpatient programs and into residential and-or outpatient care (Flaherty and Kim, 1997; McFarland and George, 1995; Miller, 1994; Silverman, 1994; Wilson, 1993). Lo and Woodward (1993) found that costs of care for Medicare beneficiaries with substance abuse problems were lower in freestanding facilities versus hospital programs (but health status outcomes were not available). Zwick and Bermon (1992) pointed out that health maintenance organizations (which are, by definition, paid on a capitated basis) typically emphasize outpatient over inpatient substance abuse treatment. Callahan et al. (1995) and Frank et al. (1996; 1997) found that the introduction of managed care into the Massachusetts Medicaid program led to a dramatic drop in use of inpatient substance abuse programs with a modest increase in use of outpatient or residential services. Similar results were obtained in Minnesota (Institute of Medicine, 1996). However, client level outcome data were not available for the Massachusetts or Minnesota Medicaid enrollees. To summarize, managed care approaches (and, presumably, financial changes like capitation) serve to minimize high cost service delivery (such as 28 day hospital or residential treatment programs) while (perhaps) increasing use of outpatient services.

Reviews of the literature comparing inpatient with outpatient care (McLellan et al., 1996; Miller and Hester, 1986) suggest that this shift to outpatient treatment should have relatively little impact on client outcomes (although work by Walsh et al., 1991 might raise some concerns). The Institute of Medicine's (1990) conclusions can be summarized by saying that "there is no overall advantage in terms of outcome for residential or inpatient treatment over outpatient treatment" (Scott, 1996). On the other hand, an observational study based on the Drug Abuse Treatment Outcome Studies (DATOS) population raised the possibility that longer term residential treatment may be preferable to other therapies for individuals with severe cocaine dependence (Simpson et al., 1999).

Furthermore, there is considerable geographic variation in modality of treatment for people with drug abuse problems. For example, the 1992 National Drug and Alcoholism Treatment Unit Survey (NDATUS) provided a one day census of clients in substance abuse treatment programs across the country (National Clearinghouse for Alcohol and Drug Information, 1997). Nationally, some 11 percent of clients were in residential rehabilitation programs. However, this figure ranged from a high of 32 percent in Minnesota to a low of six percent in Kentucky (the figure for Oregon was seven percent). Presumably, managed care approaches instituted in states that historically made considerable use of high cost services would have relatively little impact on client outcomes.

Less clear is the impact of organizational and-or financial system changes on clients receiving drug abuse treatment in states that have made limited use of inpatient or residential programs. This issue is especially pertinent for programs in the public sector where funding limitations have minimized use of the more expensive services (Kunnes et al., 1993). In this regard, Humphreys and Moos (1996) found that clients with substance abuse problems treated in Alcoholic Anonymous (AA) programs with rather little professional participation appeared to fare better than comparable clients in more expensive programs that had extensive professional involvement. However, Humphreys and Moos (1996) cautioned that their results should not be taken to imply that "individuals with alcohol problems attend AA rather than more expensive outpatient treatment." Indeed, an observational study in Philadelphia raised the possibility that conversion from fee for service to capitated Medicaid may be detrimental for clients with drug abuse problems (Institute of Medicine, 1996).

Also pertinent here is the work on brief interventions for people with substance abuse problems (Bien et al., 1993). Indeed, "brief interventions can be effective compared with no treatment and they can be quite cost-effective compared with more intensive treatment" (Institute of Medicine, 1990; Scott, 1996). Whether or not interventions can be "too brief" for some clients is a matter of considerable interest. Observational studies (see, *e.g.,* Moos et al., 1995 or Timko et al., 1995) suggest that longer duration of enrollment in treatment is associated with improved outcomes for people with substance abuse problems. However, randomized trials are less clear on this point (see, *e.g.,* Bien et al., 1993 and Miller and Hester, 1986 for reviews). Work comparing 12 hours per week with six hours per week in a four week cocaine treatment program at the Philadelphia Veterans Affairs Medical Center suggested that the two degrees of treatment intensity yielded similar client outcomes (Alterman et al., 1996; Institute of Medicine, 1996).

Managed Care and Drug Courts

The Center for Substance Abuse Treatment (1997) referred to managed health care as one of the "critical planning issues for courts". Perhaps in an ideal world there would be "co-funding of coordinated drug court systems" (Tauber, 1994) in which the treatment funds would flow through the court. In the real world, however, it is likely that managed care systems will influence provision of treatment services to drug court participants (CSAT, 1997). Indeed, in their recent survey of drug courts, Reilly and Pierre-Lawson (2008) found explicit connections between Medicaid managed care systems and drug courts in Louisiana, New York, Pennsylvania, and Rhode Island. In the managed care era, services such as a five-week inpatient program for drug court participants (Schwarz and Schwarz, 1998) will inevitably be regarded with skepticism. For example, it could be hypothesized that less intensive treatment for drug court participants might be as efficacious as more costly programs (Humphreys and Moos, 1996; Miller and Hester, 1986). Certainly, managed care administrators (McFarland and George, 1995) not infrequently take the position that treatment should occur in the "least restrictive setting" (which is often the least costly setting).

A more subtle issue is the "spillover" effect of managed care. It can be argued that treatment providers' practice patterns are influenced as much by the overall managed care environment as by the circumstances of the individual client (Alexander and Lemak, 1997a). For example, providers who are at financial risk in a capitated payment system may adopt a practice style involving low intensity services. When these providers serve a drug court participant it is conceivable that the drug court client will also receive low intensity services (even if funding for the drug court client is based on a fee for service system or comes from a block grant). In other words, the implementation of managed care in a community of providers may alter treatment practices for all clients (not just those who are in managed care). Numerous studies on geographic variation in provision of health services provide at least some evidence for this contention (Ashton et al., 1999; Wennberg, 1999).

These considerations are of interest because a literature exists indicating that "treatment works" for people with drug abuse problems (Finney and Monahan, 1996; Holder, 1998; O'Brien and McLellan, 1996) and more treatment works better than less (Onken et al., 1997.) In other words, the provision of drug abuse treatment services can have an impact on an individual's behavior where the behavior of interest includes criminal activity and substance use. Specifically, treatment is believed to reduce substance use, crime, illness, health care costs, social dysfunction, and social costs chiefly due to reduced crime (Belenko et al., 2005; Gerstein and Harwood, 1990; McLellan et al., 1996; Prendergast et al., 2000). Moreover, time in treatment is generally thought to be positively related to treatment outcome. Modality (*e.g.,* directive, faith-based, 12-step) and intensity (*e.g.,* brief, outpatient, intensive outpatient, residential) have complex relationships to outcome mediated by client characteristics (*e.g.,* addiction severity, aging, readiness) and context (social support and pressure, incentives, recovery environment).

Drug courts have been instituted to facilitate treatment for drug abusing clients. In exchange for the possibility of dismissed charges or reduced sentences, defendants agree to be assigned to drug court programs where prosecutors, defense attorneys, and treatment providers collaborate, presided over by a judge. One of the strategies of drug court is to get offenders into drug treatment, keep them there, and ensure compliance with treatment regimens — which both humanizes the criminal justice system and also adds an involuntary component to the treatment protocol. Drug courts provide supervision, treatment, testing, sanctions and incentives (NADCP, 1997).

Some evidence has been found for the efficacy of more molecular components of drug courts such as graduated sanctions for positive urine tests (Harrell et al., 1998) and frequent judicial status hearings (Marlowe et al., 2003; Marlowe et al., 2004). The Government Accountability Office (GAO) issued another in a series of reports on adult drug courts in February 2005 (GAO-05-219). For the first time, the GAO found evidence for recidivism reductions during the length of the program and for some financial benefits. On average, between 27 and 66 percent of drug court participants completed the program. Limited evidence suggested net cost benefit, mainly due to reduced recidivism.

Changes in financing and organization of treatment services may affect outcomes of drug courts by influencing time in (and other characteristics of) treatment. Managed care represented a major financing and organizational change. The major functions of Managed Care Organizations (MCO) include utilization control, cost containment, and stabilization of government expenditures. MCOs primarily use revenues from pre-payment to contract with independent providers. MCOs receive capitated payments for "covered lives" somewhat like insurance companies receive premium payments. MCOs have been able to make reductions in expenditures for unnecessary procedures, supplies, and equipment in the otherwise unorganized and unmanaged employer-financed private sector as well as reducing prices by wielding increased purchasing power (Aaron, 2002). In the public sector, MCOs also came to supplement the public payer's role as financial and utilization manager.

"Utilization management" always raises questions of "dosage" and "quality." In addition, utilization management is not cost-free; its costs are met by diverting expenditures for direct services to reporting, review and approval, administrative activities and to the MCO itself. If this diversion is an issue in the private sector, it is much more so in the public sector where financing is thin and clienteles are both chronic and vulnerable. Furthermore, the administration of public health insurance has historically cost no more than a third as much, while still monitoring more closely and managing utilization to a greater degree, than has the employer-financed private insurance sector (Bodenheimer, 2002). Public health insurance has done a better job of managing growth in per capita expenditures (Altman and Levitt, 2002; Bodenheimer, 2002). So, potential gains in efficiency seem smaller and potential losses in outcome seem greater when managed care organizations are added to the public sector (see Rothbard et al., 2002.

It is likely that managed care has had some effect on the provision of treatment services to drug court participants. As noted, in the managed care era, services such as a five-week inpatient program for drug court participants (Schwarz and Schwarz, 1998) are not favored. For drug court as for other treatment programs, providers' practice patterns are likely to be influenced as much by the overall managed care environment as by the circumstances of the individual client (Alexander and Lemak, 1997). For example, providers who are at financial risk in a capitated payment system may adopt a practice style involving low intensity services for all clients. Moreover, some agency treatment resources may be converted to cash flow management and similar overhead expenditures. If managed care affects pattern of practice, especially time in treatment, did the advent of managed care have an impact on the outcomes of drug court clients?

In other words, the provision of drug abuse treatment services can have an impact on an individual's behavior where the behavior of interest includes criminal activity and substance use. Several factors may influence the nature and extent of the drug abuse treatment services provided. These influences will, of course, include court mandates but they will also include the offender's individual characteristics and the treatment provider's practice patterns. It is hypothesized that managed care (and, especially, the replacement of fee for service with capitated Medicaid) can influence the treatment provider's delivery of services. The intensity and duration of treatment may, in turn, have an impact on criminal recidivism.

It should be noted that the influence of managed care may operate in several ways. Offenders who rely on their health insurance to pay for their court ordered treatment may find that the insurer has some influence on the services provided. Another, and perhaps more likely, scenario is that the climate of managed care has an "all pervasive" influence on treatment providers. It may well be the case that clinicians operating in a managed care environment (especially one in which the provider is at financial risk) find that their "standards of practice" emphasize low intensity (and, perhaps, short duration) treatments. Conversely, providers operating in a fee for service environment may endorse high intensity and-or long duration care.

To assess the impact of managed care on time in treatment and outcomes of one drug court, this study took advantage of a "natural experiment," a longstanding drug court program spanning "eras" before and after implementation of managed behavioral health care in the public sector.

PUBLIC SECTOR MANAGED BEHAVIORAL HEALTH CARE IN OREGON

Oregon has relied heavily on Medicaid to pay for public sector substance abuse treatment services and, to a limited extent, on block grants derived from federal and state funds (Cutler et al., 1992). Moreover, Oregon's public substance abuse treatment system was radically changed in 1995 when fee for service Medicaid was replaced entirely by managed care (using prepayment or capitation from the state to the MCO). The director of the Multnomah County (greater Portland) drug court outpatient treatment program (InAct, Inc.) noted the substantial impact of this new approach to Medicaid financing in Oregon (Moore, personal communication, 1998).

This dramatic change is part of a larger approach to health care reform known as the Oregon Health Plan that is described in some detail by Pollack et al. (1994), McFarland et al. (1997) and Cutler et al. (1998). Briefly, in 1994 the eligibility criteria for the Oregon Medicaid program were expanded to include the working poor, enlarging the eligible pool by about 50%. Simultaneously, Medicaid clients in 1994 were enrolled in fully capitated MCOs. Over a dozen MCOs elected to participate in the Medicaid program.

During 1995, the MCOs assumed responsibility for delivering substance abuse treatments to their enrollees who were Medicaid clients (Ross and McFarland, 2000). Block grant programs in Oregon (never very extensive) were dramatically reduced. The MCOs, for the most part, entered into numerous financial arrangements with pre-existing private not for profit agencies who would continue delivering substance abuse treatment services to Medicaid clients. These financial arrangements included discounted fee for service, case rate payment systems, and sub-capitation programs (in which the agencies assumed financial risk). In addition, the state implemented placement criteria similar to those of the American Society for Addiction Medicine (1996).

Under the pre-1995 fee for service system, providers had no financial incentive to reserve more intensive treatment modalities (*e.g.,* residential programs) for more severe clients. Under managed care, an incentive exists at the MCO level to deny more costly services for less seriously impaired clients. Indeed, the incentive exists for an MCO manager (who may have been recruited from the insurance industry and know little of behavioral health) to deny inappropriately or to discourage intensity, duration, and comprehensiveness.

Therefore, the potential exists for managed care to influence (in either direction) both efficiency and effectiveness. To assess these impacts, McFarland and associates have done a series of studies on capitated payment and managed care as these payment systems were rolled out in Oregon over a 20-year period. Bigelow et al. (1991) studied a cohort of state mental hospital patients identified for intensive community services to be delivered under a supplementary contract with a major county provider and a cohort of hospital dischargees from an earlier period. This contract introduced outcome objectives (decreased hospital utilization and improved quality of life) for specified individuals, as well as mandated and funded services for them. Patients served under this contract did receive more services across the comprehensive range of services offered; bed utilization decreased threefold; and quality of life was better in most domains in contrast to the comparison group. System change objectives were also achieved — converting state institution capacity to intensive community capacity. Although not the purpose of the study, it demonstrated the efficacy of goal-directed, client-specific contracting.

Upon discharge from involuntary state hospitalization, a group of 200 patients received outpatient services financed by a risk-adjusted capitated payment to providers in a 1988-89 demonstration project. McFarland et al. (1995) found that use of the state mental hospital by these patients appeared to decline, while outpatient service utilization was modest and unrelated to risk. Although this study continued to demonstrate the efficacy of focusing services on individuals, establishing outcomes goals for those individuals, and designating responsibility for meeting the goals, the project also began to suggest that utilization (input) and benefit (outcome) might not be related in a simple way.

McFarland and service system researchers at five sites nationwide examined the impact of managed care upon publicly financed services for vulnerable populations. In Oregon, outpatient service utilization by seriously and persistently mentally ill persons decreased, but neither client satisfaction nor outcomes decreased (Bianconi et al., 2006). Rothbard et al., (2004) found reduced costs attributable to reduced hospital utilization, with no differences in ambulatory utilization, under managed care. Again, the effect of utilization management did not seem adverse, despite apparent administrative inefficiency (extra layers and tasks) and system disruption in the managed care system.

After the statewide introduction of Medicaid managed substance abuse treatment in 1995, access for Medicaid-eligible persons increased (Deck et al., 2000). Also after that introduction of managed care, access to mental health services by Medicaid-enrollees receiving substance abuse services did not change (Bigelow et al., 2004). Yet again, the effect of utilization management through MCOs did not seem adverse. Moreover, before versus after studies (including non-Medicaid comparison groups) suggested that outcomes for Oregon Medicaid clients in substance abuse treatment did not change with the introduction of managed care (McFarland, Deck, et al., 2005). Altogether, results of the managed care research program suggest that managed care increased the numbers of persons able to get services while the amount of service per client either remained stable or declined somewhat, but satisfaction and outcomes were unaffected. The impact on efficiency was positive and on effectiveness, neutral. It remained to be seen whether or not there would be similar findings with regard to drug court participants.

DRUG COURT IN OREGON

Oregon operates "diversion model" drug court programs as depicted in the flow chart (Figure 2). Eligibility criteria focus on individuals with possession of controlled substance charge(s). Exclusion criteria are distribution of controlled substance or manufacture of controlled substance charges. Offenders with other, non-drug charges can also be eligible provided that probation conditions do not interfere with drug court program participation. Arrestees who are eligible for and agree to participate in drug court are diverted out of the standard criminal justice system and into the mandated treatment program. In Oregon, defendants participating in drug court agree that if they fail the program they will be tried based solely on the police report (*i.e.,* a "stipulated facts" trial).

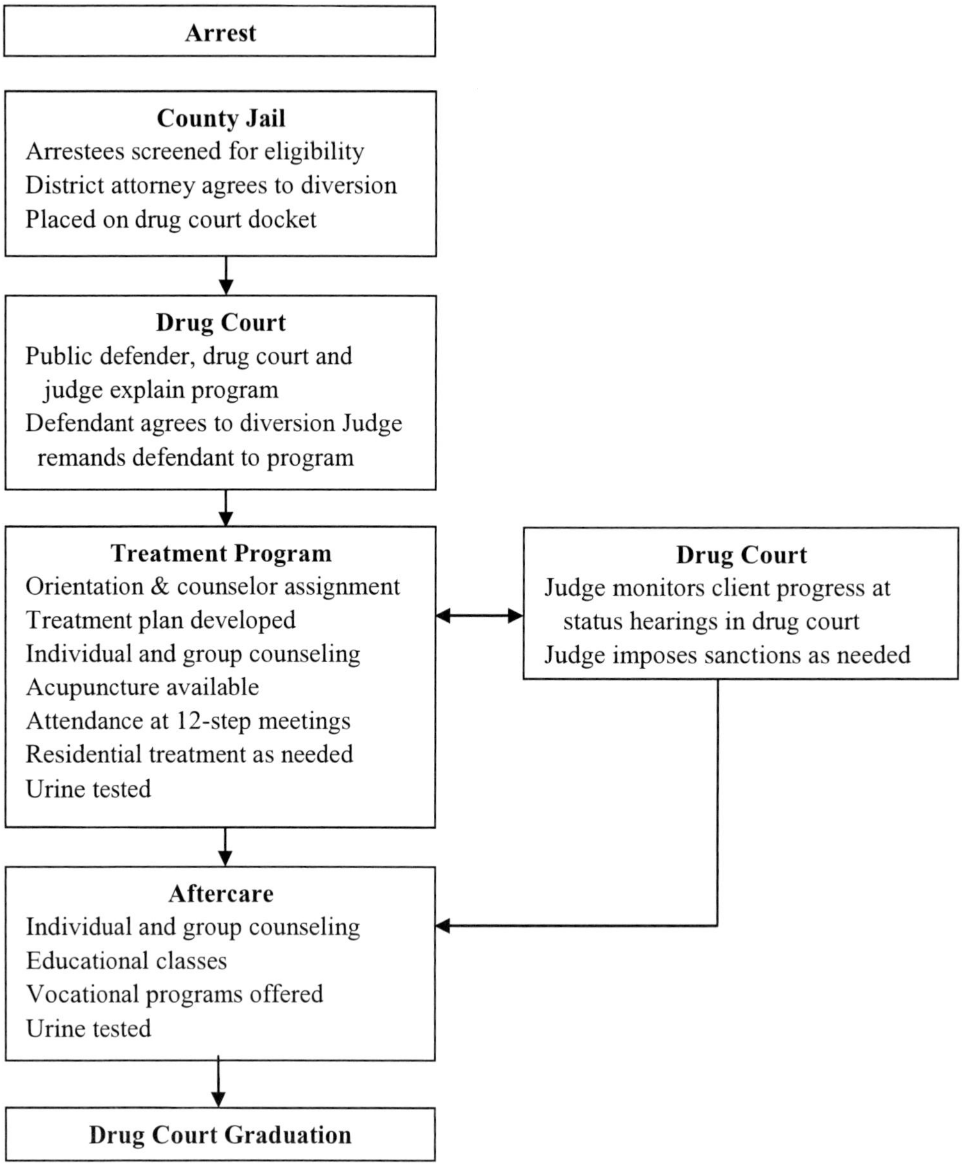

Figure 2. Flow chart for Oregon drug court programs

As shown in Table 2, the Oregon drug court program lasts roughly 12 months, has phases ranging from greater to lesser intensity, and has both required and optional components. In particular, residential treatment is an option. Oregon drug court programs involve frequent court appearances (typically on a monthly basis but more often as needed). Both scheduled and random urinalyses are required. The program assumes that participants will experience relapses and there are various contingencies for addressing relapse. These "graduated sanctions" include increasing the frequency of court appearances, increasing urinalysis requirements, greater attendance at 12-step programs, residential treatment, etc.

Table 2. Oregon drug court treatment program phases

Phase I: Detoxification
- Goals
  - Stop using drugs
  - End physical dependence
- Activities
  - Psychosocial assessment
  - Treatment plan
  - Urine testing
  - Court appearances
  - Acupuncture available
  - Residential available
- Average stay: 2 - 6 weeks

Phase II: Stabilization
- Goals
  - Accept philosophy and principles of drug free living
  - Remain drug free
- Activities
  - Individual counseling
  - Group counseling
  - Wellness curriculum
  - Fellowship meetings
  - 12-step program
  - Urine testing
  - Court appearances
  - Acupuncture available
  - Residential available
- Average stay: 3 - 6 months

Phase III: Aftercare
- Goals:
  - Obtain pre-employment skills
  - Secure employment
  - Remain drug free
- Activities
  - Literacy education
  - Educational courses
  - Vocational training
  - Job search assistance
  - Urine testing
  - Court appearances
- Average stay: 8 - 12 months

Finigan (1998) has described the Multnomah County (greater Portland, Oregon) S.T.O.P. (Sanction, Treatment, Opportunity, Progress) Drug Diversion Program. This drug court was established in 1991 by the Honorable Judge Harl Haas and is one of the oldest programs in the country (Belenko, 1999). The drug court used treatment provided under fee for service before 1995 and managed care after 1995.

Arrestees who are eligible for and agree to participate in drug court are diverted out of the standard criminal justice system and into the mandated treatment program. Defendants agree that if they fail the program they will be tried based solely on the police report (*i.e.,* a "stipulated facts" trial). Treatment is provided by InAct Inc., which is a private, not for profit agency responsible for multi-phased outpatient services. Roughly 25 percent of InAct participants are Medicaid clients. Residential treatment is provided by two not for profit agencies (Comprehensive Options for Drug Abusers or CODA and the Volunteers of America or VOA). Specialized programs are also available for women and Hispanics. Aftercare services include literacy programs. The Multnomah County drug court program accounts for the vast majority of drug court participants in Oregon.

Roughly 900 to 1,100 defendants are eligible each year for the Multnomah County program and some 400 to 700 participate. Historically, drug court participants have been, on average, 33 years old, 28% female, 23% non-white, and have had 2.5 prior arrests.

It is worth noting that the demographic data on participants in the Oregon program suggest that these offenders are similar to drug court participants nationally. Data from the Drug Court Program Office in the U.S. Department of Justice indicate that, nationally, drug court participants have median age between 26 and 35, are 23 percent female, and have had a median of one to three prior felony convictions (Drug Courts Program Office, 1998). In other words, Oregon participants appear to be reasonably representative of national drug court participants.

OUTCOMES OF OREGON DRUG COURT

Drug court programs in Oregon have been evaluated with respect to their impact on crime (Finigan, 1998). Drug court participants were compared to offenders who were eligible for drug court but who were instead dealt with in the criminal justice system. Subjects for the evaluation were chosen from the years 1994 and 1995 (at which time the Multnomah County drug court program had been in operation for several years). During those years in the greater Portland, Oregon area about 2,400 persons per year were arrested with drug offenses as the primary charge and another 4,400 per year were arrested with drug offenses as secondary charge(s). Roughly 1,100 per year were eligible for drug court and about 400 to 500 per year were drug court participants. Random samples of 150 drug court graduates and 150 drug court participants who did not graduate were selected for the evaluation. The 150 comparison group subjects were matched to participants on age, gender, ethnicity, and prior criminal justice history. In general, the comparison group had not entered the drug court program due to bench warrants. Participant and comparison groups were followed for two years from the "index" date. For participants, the index date was the date of graduation or termination from drug court. For comparison subjects, the index date was the day they became eligible for drug court. Information on subsequent arrests was obtained from the state law enforcement data system. Briefly, the participants had an arrest rate of 59 new arrests per 100 persons in the 24-month follow-up period versus 153 arrests per person during the 24-month follow-up period for the comparison group. This difference (0.295 versus 0.765 arrests per person per year) is highly significant statistically ($p < .001$). Therefore, the drug court program participants have lower arrest rates during follow-up than do comparison subjects. Following the initial evaluation, there have been detailed analyses of expenditures in the Multnomah County drug court (Carey and Finigan, 2003) and as well as a ten-year study on the program (Finigan et al., 2007).

Also of interest is the possibility that there was a "dose-response" impact of drug court participation. Figure 3 shows the follow-up arrest rate for four groups of Oregon subjects: comparison (labeled "none" in the figure), those whose duration of enrollment was less than a third of the program, those who remained enrolled for more than a third of the program but failed to graduate, and the graduates. Notice that the follow-up arrest rate appears to decrease as a function of enrollment duration. Of course, there are numerous issues of selection bias here that confound the possible "dose-response" relationship. Nonetheless, these data are at least consistent with the notion that longer duration in the treatment program leads to lower arrest rates during the follow-up period. Therefore, it is reasonable to hypothesize that if managed care reduces duration (or, perhaps, intensity) of drug abuse treatment then there might be a subsequent rise in criminal recidivism for drug court participants.

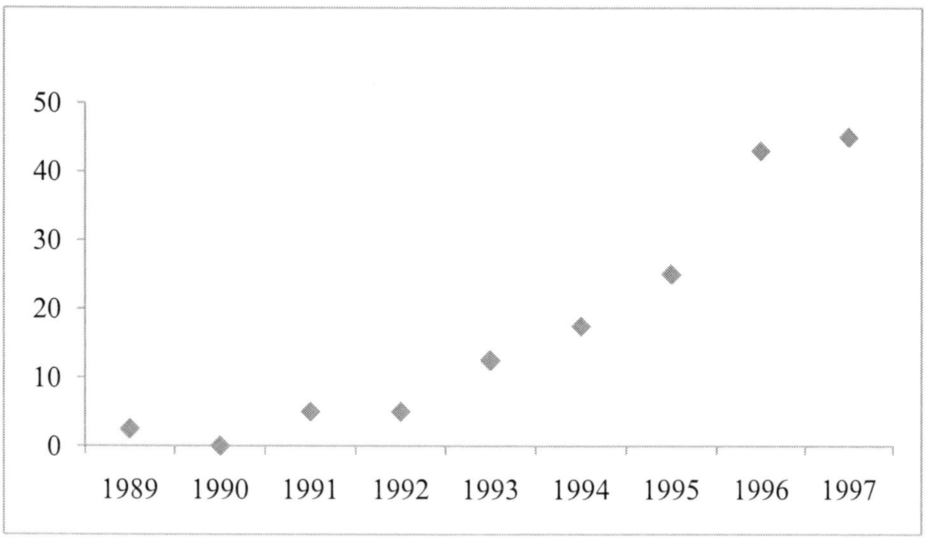

Figure 3. Follow-up arrest rate (per 100 persons per 24 months) by duration in Oregon drug court program.

Hypotheses Regarding Medicaid Managed Care and Drug Court

It is hypothesized that managed care, which replaced fee for service with capitated Medicaid, influenced the treatment provider's delivery of services by increasing access but reducing intensity and duration. Many feared that this change would depress outcomes.

However, previous findings by McFarland et al. (2005; 2005), led to the expectation that the change in intensity and duration of treatment would improve efficiency but not at the expense of effectiveness.

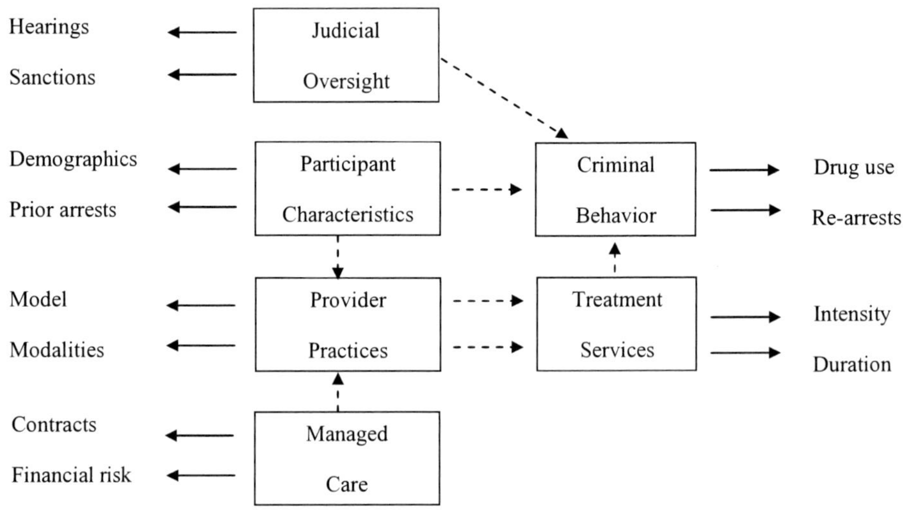

Figure 4. Influence diagram

Figure 4 is an influence diagram incorporating these ideas. In the figure, dashed arrows show possible influences. For example, participant characteristics influence behavior such as drug use and criminal activity. Participant characteristics may also influence provider practices. Judicial actions are also believed to influence participant behavior. Moreover, treatment can (hopefully) modify participant actions. Managed care may influence providers who, in turn, can have influence on participants. In the figure, solid arrows point to measures of the underlying concepts. For example, criminal behavior is measured by re-arrests. Figure 4 is, of course, an ideal situation in which data are available for all concepts. Nonetheless, numerous measures were available to test at least some of the influences suggested by the diagram.

With this background, the following hypotheses were addressed.

Hypothesis 1: Proportion eligible for Medicaid increased under managed care.
Hypothesis 2: Time in treatment decreased under managed care.
Hypothesis 3: Treatment failure was not increased by managed care
Hypothesis 4: Managed care did not increase arrests.
Hypothesis 5: Managed care did not decrease time until first arrest or booking.
Hypothesis 6. Managed care did not reduce days in the community.

METHODS

Measures

Data sources available for this project included the following:

Law Enforcement Data System (LEDS): Police agencies in Oregon enter data on encounters and arrests into a statewide database. This system can be linked to state behavioral health and Medicaid data bases (Finigan, 1998; McFarland and Blair, 1995).

Offender Profile System: This database provides reliable information about both the offender and the offense. Especially useful are data on incarceration and release from jail or prison. The system includes extensive demographic data and inmate risk assessment measures.

Inmate Status Information System (ISIS): This database of parole and probation violation information is maintained by the Multnomah County (greater Portland, Oregon) department of community corrections. The data system includes post-release employment and housing information.

Sheriff's Warrant Information System (SWIS): This system records the status of county jail inmates. The data base includes information on "psychiatric alerts" and use of jail psychiatric treatment beds. This data base can be linked with state mental health and Medicaid information systems (McFarland and Blair, 1995).

Department of Corrections (DOC) data system: The Oregon Department of Corrections maintains an extensive data base on offenders. This system can be linked with state alcohol and drug and Medicaid data bases.

Client Process Monitoring System (CPMS): Oregon's publicly funded behavioral health programs use a computer system known as CPMS. All state licensed alcohol and/or drug abuse treatment systems are required to report intake and exit data on all clients to the state substance abuse treatment agency. All the agencies serving drug court clients are required to report information to CPMS. The system operates "on-line" in many provider organizations while a few providers upload data in batch mode to the state's mainframes.

The information collected by CPMS includes admission date, termination date, demographics, primary drug of abuse, evidence of poly-substance abuse, typical route of drug administration, frequency of drug use, age at first drug use, treatment outcomes, drug or alcohol tests administered, and results of alcohol or drug testing. The system also records modality of treatment (*e.g.,* outpatient, intensive outpatient, residential, or methadone).

In addition, all inpatient psychiatric programs in Oregon that serve publicly funded clients participate in the CPMS system. Therefore, the CPMS database includes psychiatric admission dates, discharge dates, and diagnoses for publicly funded clients. The CPMS database can be linked to criminal justice and Medicaid information systems (see, *e.g.,* McFarland and Blair, 1995; McFarland et al., 1995).

Medicaid Management Information System (MMIS): The state Medicaid agency operates a Medicaid Management Information System known as MMIS. In the fee for service era this system was used chiefly to process providers' claims. Now the system is an encounter database. As such it is used to record client demographics, eligibility, outpatient diagnoses and procedures, and inpatient admissions (including diagnoses, procedures, lengths of stay, etc.). The system is used as part of the agency's quality assurance program. The system also includes data on providers such as administrative information (dates contracts were signed, capitation rate calculations, aggregate client demographics, etc.) and financial transactions (records of pre-payments, etc.). The MMIS system also contains pharmacy data (including dates of drug dispensings, generic name of the drug, strength of the drug, and number of pills dispensed). Medicaid clients are identified by a unique alphanumeric identifier known as the "prime" number. This identifier is also included in other state databases.

For purposes of these analyses, subjects were categorized with respect to Medicaid eligibility. That is, subjects who were known to be eligible for the Medicaid program (during specific time periods to be described subsequently) were identified as "yes" with regard to Medicaid. Of course, these Medicaid eligible subjects may or may not have made use of the Medicaid program (*i.e.,* they may or may not have enrolled with a Medicaid managed care system and-or may or may not have received Medicaid-funded health care services).

Conversely, other subjects who were known not to be Medicaid eligible (during specific time periods) were categorized as "no" with regard to Medicaid. Individuals in the "no" category had at one time been Medicaid clients, but not within the specific time periods of interest for the present study.

Still other subjects were classified as "unknown" with respect to Medicaid. The "unknown" cases were subjects without a match in the Medicaid database. A separate chapter describes the challenges of data linkage for individuals who may (or may not) have involvement with both Medicaid and criminal justice systems.

State Vital Statistics database: This system contains birth and death certificates.

Vital statistics information (particularly death certificates) can be linked with other databases.

Metropolitan Public Defender database: This system identified offenders arrested for drug offenses. As noted, defendants were eligible for the Multnomah County drug court program by reason of arrest on charges of Possession of Controlled Substance I or II.

Multnomah County District Attorney Computerized Tracking System: This database includes a case number; criminal charge(s); felony/misdemeanor; class of felony or misdemeanor (A, B, C); arrest date; date of birth, gender; police-recorded ethnicity; criminal justice and law enforcement database identification numbers; and sentence including jail time, prison time, as well as probation, parole, and conditions of probation.

In principle, then, the following information was available: dates of enrollment and termination for publicly funded substance abuse treatment; modality of substance abuse treatment (regular outpatient, intensive outpatient, residential, methadone); provider ratings of client level of function (including abstinence) at termination; dates of enrollment and termination in publicly funded mental health services; type of mental health treatment; dates of admission and discharge for publicly funded psychiatric hospitalizations; discharge diagnoses for publicly funded psychiatric hospitalizations; dates of law enforcement contacts; dates of jail admission and discharge; and nature of charges pending for persons booked into jail . The psychiatric hospital data encompassed general hospital psychiatric services, private psychiatric hospitals, and the state mental hospitals. The following information was also available (again, in principle): dates of Medicaid enrollment and disenrollment; dates of psychotropic drug dispensings, generic name of prescribed medication, strength of medication, and numbers of pills dispensed; as well as dates of admission and discharge for all hospitalizations and all hospital discharge diagnoses. Theoretically, this data set included virtually all the measures of treatment effectiveness recommended by the Institute of Medicine (1996) for studies on managed care and drug abuse treatment services. Moreover, these data systems have been used in several studies (see, *e.g.,* McKenzie et al., 1999).

Subjects

Subjects selected for the study were eligible for drug court during the Medicaid fee-for-service (FFS) era or during the Medicaid managed care (MC) era. Eligible defendants included both individuals who actually entered the drug court program ("participants") as well as persons who were eligible for but did not enter the drug court program ("comparison" subjects) instead choosing criminal court trial. Thus the project employed a two-by-two (payment type by court type) design. A comparison before and after the implementation of managed care is the closest available design to a randomized trial of managed care. To explore further the effect of managed care, pre- versus post- comparisons are also made within two drug court subgroups: graduates and treatment failures.

Both Medicaid and non-Medicaid eligibles were included because (a) managed care was expected to affect entire programs and clienteles, not just Medicaid eligibles and (b) Medicaid eligibility was unknown in many cases (as is discussed subsequently). Persons under age 18 at the time they became eligible for drug court and undocumented aliens were excluded.

The study encompassed two time periods (Figure 5). Subjects were sampled from the "fee-for-service (pre-managed care) era" from January 1, 1992 through December 31, 1993. By the start of this fee-for-service (FFS) period the drug court program had been in operation for several months. The end of this FFS sampling period preceded by 16 months the conversion from fee for service to managed care (*i.e.,* May 1, 1995). Thus the FFS (pre-managed care) selection period was bracketed by fee-for-service.

Fee for Service Era					Managed Care Era					
9 9 1	1992	1993	1994	1995	1996	1997	1998	1999	2000	2001
	Pre-Managed Care sample			Managed Care start		Post-Managed care sample				

Figure 5. Sampling Frame.

Subjects were sampled from the "managed care era" from January 1, 1997 through December 31, 1998. By the start of this managed care (MC) period, substance abuse treatment programs had been functioning under MC for more than 18 months (since May 1, 1995). At the end of the MC sampling period, managed care would continue for several more years. Thus the managed care selection period was bracketed by managed care.

Table 3: Subjects by index and closing years

Year	Medicaid era	Index	Closing
1991	FFS	163	0
1992	FFS	485	393
1993	FFS	361	617
1994	FFS	0	0
1995	MC	0	0
1996	MC	148	0
1997	MC	479	443
1998	MC	303	486
Total		1939	1939

FFS = fee for service
MC = managed care

Subjects were selected from a list maintained by the Metropolitan Public Defender (MPD) of all defendants eligible for the Multnomah County Drug Court program (by reason of arrest or charges of Possession of Controlled Substance I or II) whose cases had closed during the years 1992-1993 or 1997-1998). Sampling was stratified by year in order to obtain roughly equal numbers per year. All of the year 1992 cases (423), every other year 1993 case (645), and a random selection of cases (roughly 25%) from 1997 (540) and 1998 (545) were extracted (total of 2,153).

The most feasible datum for identifying cases is the date on which the case was closed. As noted, closed case records were pulled from two time periods, 1992-93 and 1997-98. The intention in choosing those years was to have one study group that came before the implementation of Medicaid managed care and one that came after its implementation.

However, the most useful "index" date for analyses was not the close date, but rather the date of the court hearing ("petition hearing") at which the eligible person announced whether or not he/she would try drug court. Index and closing dates were not uniformly 12 months apart. Drug court eligibles selected on closing date had index dates distributed over several years (Table 3). However, the time periods between index and closing dates for FFS subjects were within the FFS era. Similarly, time periods between index and closing dates for MC subjects were within the MC era.

The petition hearing index date was also used to denote Medicaid eligibility. Subjects were categorized based on state Medicaid data as being (a) "yes" Medicaid eligible, (b) "no", i.e. not Medicaid eligible, or (c) "unknown" with regard to Medicaid during the 180 day window extending from 90 days before to 90 days after the index date. This tabulation includes "unknown" cases who were without a match in the Medicaid database. Conversely, individuals in the "no" category had at one time been Medicaid clients, but not within the 90-day windows before or after the index date. A separate chapter discusses the challenges of linkage between Medicaid management and other administrative data systems.

District Attorney case number, name, date of arrest, and charge were obtained for the 2,153 cases selected from the MPD list. Then, the District Attorney case number was used to obtain information from the District Attorney's Computerized Tracking System (DACTS). Data on the incident leading to placement on the MPD's list was extracted from DACTS including charge; felony/misdemeanor; class of felony or misdemeanor (A, B, C); arrest date;

date of birth, gender; police-recorded ethnicity; criminal justice and law enforcement database identification numbers; and sentence including jail time, prison time, probation or parole, and conditions of probation.

Of the 2,153 cases originally selected from the list of persons eligible for drug court; 214 were discarded, leaving 1,939. Of the 214 cases discarded, 62 were removed because they spanned eras, 34 because the charges against them had been dropped, 32 because they were still in the program (having been closed but later reopened), 24 because they had died during the program or within three years after the index date, 23 because of "merging cases" (cases that started out as separate were later determined to be the same case),19 because the "exit" was "miscellaneous disposition," seven because the District Attorney denied drug court program participation, seven because the case closing date came before the case opening date (bad data), three because the "exit" was "conditional discharge", and three for which a reason was not recorded.

Subjects were followed for at least three years forward from the index date. This follow-up period includes 12 months for the drug program and 24 more months for outcomes, as recommended by Belenko (1998) and Peters (1996). Fortunately (because the drug court length of stay was often longer than 12 calendar months), there were data for at least two years after closing and for two years before the index (*i.e.,* petition hearing date) for all subjects.

Regarding criminal justice data, arrests related to the index crime are <u>not</u> included in the post-index count of arrests. However, arrests related to the index crime *are* included in the pre-index counts.

Matching of records proved especially challenging. Indeed, a separate chapter is devoted to lessons learned about linkage (or lack thereof) among record systems pertinent to Medicaid clients being treated for substance abuse problems. In particular, as will be described, numerous subjects were assigned to an "unknown" condition with regard to Medicaid eligibility status.

Subjects with unknown Medicaid eligibility were included in many analyses. For some of these analyses, indicator variables were used to distinguish the three groups: Medicaid yes, Medicaid no, and unknown Medicaid. In other of these analyses, the subjects with "unknown" Medicaid status were, in effect, lumped together with people known to have "no" Medicaid eligibility status. Still other analyses focused just on subjects with known (either yes or no) Medicaid status.

As noted, information for this project was obtained from several criminal justice databases and Medicaid enrollment files while ensuring protection for human subjects. Law enforcement and criminal justice data are public records. Medicaid eligibility and substance abuse treatment administrative data pertained to a public benefits program (Code of Federal Regulations 45.56). Linkage of data was conducted under an agreement with the State of Oregon Department of Human Services. The researchers worked with a de-identified, linked data set. The research project was approved by the Oregon Health and Science University Institutional Review Board.

Suffice it to say here that it was not feasible to link all the available data. Nonetheless, the project was able to address its hypotheses as will be described.

RESULTS

Sample Demographics

As planned in the sampling strategy, about half the total sample (52%) was in the fee for service (FFS) era and half in the managed care (MC) era. While the sampling strategy did not control for choice of drug court versus trial, close to half (about 45%) did choose drug court. There was a decline in choice of drug court (from 48% to 41%) between the two eras (chi-squared test with continuity correction = 9.3, p = .002). Table 4 shows the distribution of the sample among the four cells in the two-by-two design. Roughly a quarter of the sample falls into each cell.

Women comprised from 20 percent to 28 percent of the subjects in each of the four cells. Overall, some 76% of subjects were male. The variation in representation of women among the four cells was not statistically significant.

Table 4. Frequencies for Medicaid era and court type

	Court		
Medicaid era	**Criminal**	**Drug court**	**Total**
Fee for service	524 (52%)	485 (48%)	1009
Managed care	548 (59%)	382 (41%)	930
Total	1072	867	1939

Fee for service = index year of 1991 through 1993
Managed care = index year of 1996 through 1998

The average age was 32 with median age also 32. The range of mean ages in the four cells of the research design was 30 to 33. The average ages (at the index date) did vary significantly among the cells. The youngest subjects (average age 30) were in the FFS era criminal court, the next youngest (average age 32) were in the FFS era drug court, and the oldest were in the MC era (both criminal and drug court average age was 33). The difference between Medicaid eras was statistically significant ($p < .001$ by analysis of variance) as was the overall difference between court types ($p = .007$). The interaction between era and court type was modestly significant ($p = .05$).

Over half the subjects (57%) were white, 23% were African-American, and 16% were Hispanic. The remaining 4% were American Indian, Asian-American, or unknown. Table 5 shows the distribution of the racial/ethnic groups in the four cells of the research design. There is a statistically significant increase in the proportion of whites in the criminal court (and a corresponding decrease in the drug court) in the MC era by comparison with the FFS era. For whites and African-Americans there was a shift from drug court to criminal court after managed care but the opposite for Hispanics. During the FFS era, the racial differences in court choice were highly statistically significant (chi-squared with two degrees of freedom = 24.1, p less than 0.0001). However, there was not such racial disparity in the MC era (chi-squared with two degrees of freedom = 2.3, p = not significant). Looking at whites versus non-whites, during the FFS era, some 48% of whites chose criminal court versus 57% of non-whites (chi-squared with continuity correction = 7.2, p = 0.007). Conversely, during MC some 59% of whites chose criminal court versus 60% of non-whites (chi-squared with continuity correction = 0.06, p = not significant). As it happens, these apparent racial differences between eras were not statistically significant (Mantel-Haenszel heterogeneity chi-squared with one degree of freedom = 2.48, p = not significant).

Table 5. Race and ethnicity by Medicaid era and court type

	Court	
Medicaid era	**Criminal**	**Drug court**
Fee for service		
White	237 (45%)	259 (53%)
African American	112 (21%)	125 (26%)
Hispanic	158 (30%)	82 (17%)
Other or unknown	17 (4%)	19 (4%)
Managed care		
White	362 (66%)	252 (66%)
African American	133 (24%)	74 (19%)
Hispanic	34 (6%)	27 (7%)
Other or unknown	19 (4%)	29 (8%)

There were additional differences among subjects in the four cells with regards to arrests prior to the index date. It was possible to identify some 1817 subjects in the various criminal justice databases. For the initial analysis of arrests prior to the index date, subjects who could not be found in the criminal justice databases were considered to be missing and were omitted. On this basis, subjects in the FFS era who chose criminal court had an average of 2.9 arrests in the two years prior to the index date versus 3.2 arrests for the drug court subjects. In the MC era, criminal court subjects had on average 3.6 arrests in the two years prior to the index date versus an average of 2.8 arrests for the drug court participants. The difference between eras is statistically significant ($p < .001$) as is the interaction term ($p < .001$). However the difference between criminal versus drug court is not different statistically.

It should be noted that (by virtue of arrest) subjects had assorted times "at risk" in the community prior to the index date. In other words, subjects could have been in jail or prison during the two years prior to the index date and, therefore, not at risk for arrest. However, the incarceration times were relatively brief. For example, 95 percent of subjects had at least 588 days in the community during the two years (730 days) prior to the index date. Most (55 percent) of subjects had at least 727 days in the community during those two years.

Subjects' cases were closed for several reasons including the following. Numerous individuals absconded prior to petitioning the court for either criminal court or drug court assignment. These absconders were put on "pre-petition bench warrant" status (N = 458). Other individuals either declined drug court or tried drug court for a short period of time (typically just a few days) but then withdrew (N = 607). Yet other subjects participated in drug court but failed to graduate and, therefore, underwent a stipulated facts trial (N = 508). Finally, subjects participated in and graduated from the drug court program (N = 359).

As expected, the days from index date to closing date varied markedly among these several groups. The pre-petition bench warrant subjects had a mean "open" case duration of 2.4 days (standard deviation 21.5 days), declined or withdrew subjects' open duration was 11.1 days (standard deviation 47.4 days), stipulated facts trial subjects had open duration of 274.0 days (standard deviation of 183. 1 days), and graduates had open duration of 425.1 days (standard deviation of 89.2 days). Interestingly enough, minimum open durations for the first three groups were all one day whereas the maximum open durations were 371 days (for pre-petition bench warrant), 506 days (for declined or withdrew), and 1439 days for stipulated facts trial subjects. For graduates, the minimum open duration was 247 days and the maximum was 1439 days.

TESTS OF THE HYPOTHESES

In the following analyses, subjects from the FFS era are compared to subjects from the MC care era in order to assess the impact of managed care on the drug court program.

Hypothesis 1: Proportion Eligible For Medicaid Increased Under Managed Care

The purpose of Medicaid managed care was to rationalize utilization, while increasing access for the working poor to Medicaid coverage. Table 6 is a cross-tabulation of (a) FFS versus MC, (b) Medicaid or not (within 90 days before or after the index date), and (c) drug court vs. criminal court. This tabulation includes "unknown" cases who were without a match in the Medicaid database. On the other hand, individuals in the "no" category had at one time been Medicaid clients, but not within the 90-day windows before or after the index date.

Table 6. Medicaid enrollment by Medicaid era and court type

	Court	
Medicaid era	**Criminal**	**Drug court**
Fee for service		
Medicaid within 90 days	66 (13%)	63 (13%)
No Medicaid within 90 days	116 (22%)	150 (31%)
Unknown	342 (65%)	272 (56%)
Managed care		
Medicaid within 90 days	194 (35%)	174 (46%)
No Medicaid within 90 days	170 (31%)	87 (23%)
Unknown	184 (34%)	121 (32%)

Within 90 days refers to the three months prior to and the three months following the index date.

Type of Medicaid coverage was known for many but by no means all subjects. The most common type (260 subjects) was the so-called "standard" coverage under the Oregon Medicaid program (known as the Oregon Health Plan). The standard coverage pertained chiefly to working poor individuals. Temporary Assistance to Needy Families or its predecessor Aid to Families with Dependent Children accounted for 93 subjects. There were 84 individuals with Medicaid due to Supplemental Security Income or other indication of disability. Finally, there were 60 people with Medicaid for other reasons.

As expected, the number with Medicaid eligibility within 90 days (before or after the index date) rose from about 13% to 40% after the introduction of MC. The number not eligible within 90 days stayed at about 27%. "Unknowns" dropped from about 61% to 33% with most of the aggregate difference — over 300 cases — apparently going into the Medicaid eligible category.

The change was especially dramatic among drug court participants. During FFS, individuals known to be current Medicaid clients (as of the index date) were under-represented in the drug court group. Conversely, during MC, current Medicaid clients were greatly over-represented among drug court participants. This change is highly significant statistically ($p = .003$ for the parameter corresponding to current Medicaid client status in a logistic regression model with dependent variable being criminal court versus drug court and predictors being Medicaid era and Medicaid client status including yes, no, and unknown).

Not surprisingly, there were marked differences between subjects who had known Medicaid eligibility status (*i.e.,* either eligible during the 90 days before or after index date or not eligible during that time period) versus those with unknown Medicaid eligibility. For example, as was just mentioned, Medicaid era powerfully predicted knowledge of Medicaid status (with marked drop in "unknown" status after introduction of managed care). In a multiple logistic regression model, era was a highly significant predictor ($p < .0001$) such that those in the managed care era were 61% less likely than those in fee for service to have unknown Medicaid eligibility status. Subjects with known (either yes or no) Medicaid eligibility status were also more likely than those with unknown status to be drug court participants ($p = .02$), female ($p < .0001$), older ($p = .001$), and non-Hispanic ($p < .0001$). It also turned out that persons with known Medicaid eligibility status (either yes or no) were more likely to be arrested during follow-up than subjects with unknown Medicaid status ($p < .0001$). Men were over twice as likely as women to have unknown Medicaid status and Hispanics were over seven times as likely as non-Hispanics to have unknown Medicaid status. Interestingly, arrests in the two years prior to index date did not predict known versus unknown Medicaid status nor did African-American race.

Hypothesis 2: Time in Treatment Will Decrease Under Managed Care

A mediating variable between drug treatment and outcome is *time in treatment* — the more treatment time, the better the outcome. Time in treatment is measured in months (counting only "good days" during which the patient is complying with and participating in the treatment program, as reported to the drug court). The drug court uses only good days to calculate time of graduation. Consequently, calendar time in the drug court often stretches well beyond 12 calendar months. As expected, time in treatment had a bi-modal distribution with numerous individuals clustered around zero days and another mode around 365 days in treatment.

In the FFS era, the 485 participants received 9.6 months of treatment (with standard deviation of 5.1 months). As expected in the MC era, the 382 participants received less treatment, 8.3 months (with standard deviation of 5.6 months). The difference was significant ($p < .001$).

In a multiple linear regression model, predictors of reduced time in treatment included Managed Care era ($p < .0001$), black race ($p = .04$), Hispanic ethnicity ($p < .0001$), and prior arrests ($p < .0001$). The reduction of treatment time due to Managed Care era was some 58 days while the reductions were 28 days for black race, 86 days for Hispanic ethnicity, and 15 days for each prior arrest. Each year of age increased treatment time by about two days ($p = .01$). Gender had no effect. Importantly, there was no effect for the Medicaid eligibility indicator nor for the interaction term (Medicaid eligibility times Managed Care era indicator).

Time in treatment, above, is for all the persons who chose to participate in drug court. Among these drug court participants, there was a group who graduated and a group who failed (and were given a stipulated facts trial). Time in treatment for the 210 drug court participants who graduated during FFS was 13.5 months (standard deviation of 2.7 months) versus 13.6 months (standard deviation 1.8 months) for the 149 subjects who graduated during MC. For graduates, the time in treatment during both eras was normally distributed and was about a month and a half longer than required for graduation. Among these graduated subjects, the numbers of months in treatment under fee-for-service versus managed care were not statistically significantly different. In a linear regression model for graduates with time in treatment as dependent variable, there were no statistically significant effects for age, gender, race, ethnicity, arrests in the two years prior to index date, Medicaid era, Medicaid eligibility, or the interaction of era times eligibility.

Turning now to drug court participants who failed, the 275 individuals who received stipulated facts trials during FFS averaged 6.5 months of treatment (standard deviation of 4.4 months) versus 4.9 months of treatment (standard deviation of 4.5 months) for the 233 treatment failures during MC. This difference was highly significant statistically ($p < .001$). Therefore, the overall decrease in time in treatment under MC seems to be due to those who failed. Even after adjustment for gender, age, race, ethnicity, arrests in the two years prior to index date, Medicaid eligibility, and the interaction of era times Medicaid eligibility, individuals who had stipulated facts trials during MC had about three months less treatment than did such individuals during FFS ($p < .001$ in a multiple linear regression model).

Because the distribution of treatment time was markedly skewed (with zero as the modal value), a generalized linear model was employed in which the days in treatment dependent variable was considered to have a Poisson distribution. Predictors again included age, gender, race, ethnicity, numbers of arrests in the two years prior to index date, Medicaid era, Medicaid eligibility, and the interaction term of era with eligibility. Again, the effect of era was highly statistically significant ($p < .001$).

Hypothesis 3: Treatment Failure Will not be Increased by Managed Care

The first outcome of treatment is graduation or failure (and a stipulated facts trial). As shown in Table 7, under FFS, about 57% of drug court participants failed (*i.e.,* exited with a stipulated facts trial rather than graduation). Conversely, under MC about 61% ended up with a stipulated facts trial rather than graduation. This direction is contrary to the hypothesis, but the difference is not statistically significant (chi-squared with continuity correction = 1.45, p = NS). In a logistic regression model including as predictors age, gender, race, ethnicity, numbers of arrests prior to index date, Medicaid era indicator, Medicaid eligibility indicator, and interaction of era times eligibility the only statistically significant predictors of graduation were age, prior arrests, race, and ethnicity (all with $p < .001$). Each year of age increased the adjusted odds to graduation by four percent whereas black race decreased chances of graduation by half and Hispanic ethnicity by 74%. Each prior arrest decreased adjusted odds of graduation by 36%.

Table 7. Treatment outcomes by Medicaid era

	Exit category	
Medicaid era	**Stipulated facts trial**	**Graduation**
Fee for service	275 (57%)	210 (43%)
Managed care	233 (61%)	149 (39%)

Hypothesis 4: Managed Care Will Not Increase Arrests

The outcome of concern in a drug court program is the impact on criminal activity (recidivism). There are several measures of criminal activity with arrests being a key indicator. The research design made comparisons feasible for the entire sample for about three years.

As the FFS and MC eras are sequential, other factors may have influenced criminal history. A simple historical confound would be reflected in differences in arrests between the two eras for the entire sample, regardless of treatment conditions. Therefore, analyses focused 1,818 cases who had arrest records in at least one of the state and sheriff databases. Some 121 cases with no arrest records were treated as "missing." The numbers of arrests among all persons eligible to participate in drug court (including those who did not) in the three years following their index dates averaged 5.17 (standard deviation 4.78) for the 912 FFS era individuals versus 5.83 (standard deviation of 6.39) for the 906 MC era subjects. In both FFS and MC eras some 15% of subjects had no arrests during follow-up. In both eras, the median number of arrests during the three years of follow-up was three.

Pre-index arrests (for the two years prior to index date) were then used as a covariate. Not surprisingly, the covariate was highly statistically significant ($p < .0001$). In this model there were more arrests in the MC era although the differences were slight, statistically insignificant, and the 95% confidence intervals (CIs) overlap. Specifically, the adjusted FFS adjusted mean was 5.28 (with 95% confidence interval 4.96 to 5.61) versus adjusted mean of 5.73 (5.40 to 6.05) in the MC era. This result is consistent with the hypothesis.

The outcome of MC is also seen in a comparison of arrests between those choosing drug court in the FFS versus MC eras. For the 445 drug court participants in the FFS era the mean arrests (within the three years after index date) was 5.56 (standard deviation 4.84) versus 5.23 (standard deviation 5.76) for the 367 drug court participants in the MC era. Again using prior arrests as covariate, the adjusted means become 5.44 (4.99 to 5.89) for FFS versus 5.37 (4.87 to 5.89) in MC. There were actually fewer arrests among drug court participants in the MC era, although the difference is small, not statistically significant and the 95% confidence intervals overlap. These data are consistent with the hypothesis.

Poisson regression models were then constructed with numbers of arrests (in three years following the index date) as dependent variable. The predictors included age, gender, race, ethnicity, prior arrests, Medicaid eligibility, era, drug court participation, as well as the two-way interaction terms (eligibility with era, eligibility with drug court participation, and participation with era) plus the triple interaction (era times eligibility times participation). The parameter of chief interest is the triple interaction term.

In a model that lumped "unknown" with "no" Medicaid status subjects the triple interaction term which was statistically significant (p = .02) and associated with increased arrests. Conversely, in a model that distinguished "no" from "unknown" Medicaid status subjects, the triple interaction term was not statistically significant. Age, race, ethnicity, and prior arrests were highly associated with numbers of arrests during follow-up. Also significant in this model were the indicators showing drug court participation, Medicaid "yes", and Medicaid "unknown" as well as the interaction terms for Medicaid (yes) times era and drug court participation times era. A model restricted to the 996 subjects with either "yes" or "no" (*i.e.,* known) Medicaid status had similar results. Namely, the triple interaction term was not statistically significant. In this model, the statistically significant predictors were age, race, ethnicity, prior arrests, and Medicaid status.

Also of interest is the effect of MC on those drug court participants who graduated from treatment. For the 185 FFS drug court graduates, the arrests averaged 2.17 (standard deviation of 2.78) versus 1.55 (standard deviation of 2.15) for the 140 MC graduates. The adjusted means (using prior arrests as covariate) were 2.15 (1.80 to 2.50) for FFS versus 1.57 (1.17 to 1.98) under MC. In other words, there were fewer arrests among graduated drug court participants in the MC era. The difference is significant (p = 0.034). These data are consistent with the hypothesis.

Conversely, there was no apparent effect of MC on the drug court participants who failed in treatment. The adjusted means were 7.82 (7.20 to 8.44) under FFS versus 7.66 (7.00 to 8.33) under MC. There were no statistically significant differences in number of arrests. These data are consistent with the hypothesis.

Hypothesis 5: Managed Care will not Decrease Time Until First Arrest / Booking

The number of months that subjects "survived" until their first arrest or booking (excluding the index arrests) is also an outcome. [Similarly, the proportion of subjects arrested by one year, by two years, etc., is such a measure.] Table 8 shows only those clients with arrest records in both state and sheriff databases. Some 83 clients with arrest records in only one of the databases were treated as "missing." First, Table 8 shows the effect of MC on survival for all drug court eligibles. It was expected that MC would not decrease that time. Table 8 shows the number of months (during the first three years after the index date) until the first arrest/booking for all eligible subjects (including arrests pursuant to bench warrants).

There were no significant differences in survival between the FFS and MC eras (by the log rank test), which is consistent with the hypothesis.

Cox regression models were employed to examine impact of gender, age, race, ethnicity, arrests in the two years prior to index date, Medicaid eligibility, era, drug court participation, the two-way interaction terms (eligibility by era, eligibility by participation, and era by participation) plus the three-way interaction term (eligibility by era by participation).

Table 8. Time until first arrest by Medicaid era

Medicaid era	Mean months (Std Error)	Median months (Std Error)
All drug court eligibles		
Fee for service	9.9 (.42)	4.0 (.24)
Managed care	9.9 (.41)	4.0 (.22)
Drug court participants		
Fee for service	9.3 (.57)	4.0 (.25)
Managed care	10.9 (.65)	5.0 (.39)

Models were constructed in which "no" Medicaid eligibility subjects were lumped with "unknown" Medicaid subjects as well as models that distinguished between those with "no" versus those with "unknown" Medicaid eligibility, respectively. There were also models focusing exclusively on subjects with known (either yes or no) Medicaid eligibility.

Here the three-way interaction term was not statistically significant in any model. For the model which lumped "no" with "unknown" Medicaid status subjects, increasing age was associated with longer survival ($p = .02$) whereas prior arrests ($p < .0001$), black race ($p < .0001$), and Hispanic ethnicity ($p = .02$) were associated with briefer survival. Gender was not associated with survival time. African-American subjects had adjusted hazard ratio roughly 44% higher than whites while Hispanic subjects had adjusted hazard ratio some 21% higher than whites. Each prior arrest increased the adjusted hazard ratio by about ten percent whereas each year of age decreased the adjusted hazard ratio by about one percent.

Interestingly enough, in the model that distinguished "no" from "unknown" Medicaid status, African-American subjects had increased survival (adjusted hazard ratio was reduced by 29%, $p < .0001$) as did Hispanic subjects (adjusted hazard ratio reduced by 28%, $p < .0001$). Prior arrests remained highly predictive of reduced survival in the community whereas increased age predicted longer survival free of arrest (both adjusted hazard ratios were similar to those in the previous model). In the model restricted to subjects with known Medicaid status, again black race was associated with 26% reduced adjusted hazard of re-arrest ($p < .001$) but ethnicity was not a statistically significant predictor. Prior arrests remained statistically significant ($p < .001$) as predictor of subsequent arrests (adjusted hazard ratio increased ten percent for each prior arrest).

The number of months that drug court participants "survived" until their first arrest or booking (excluding the index arrest) is also an outcome. [Similarly, the proportion of participants arrested by one year, by two years, etc., is such a measure.] It was expected that MC would not decrease that time. Table 8 shows the number of months (during the first three years after the index date) until the first arrest/booking for all drug court participants (including arrests pursuant to bench warrants). Drug court participants "survived" about a month longer in the MC era, which is consistent with the hypothesis. However, the differences are not significant.

A Cox regression analysis for drug court participants used pre-arrests as a covariate; controlled for age, gender, race, and ethnicity; and included indicators for Medicaid eligibility and era plus the interaction of era with eligibility. In this model the two-way interaction term (era times Medicaid eligibility) was statistically significant ($p = .04$) and indicated increase in survival until first arrest or booking. The adjusted hazard ratio was reduced by some 32%. Increasing age was associated with longer survival ($p = .009$) whereas prior arrests ($p < .0001$), black race ($p < .0001$), and Hispanic ethnicity ($p = .002$) were associated with briefer survival. Gender was not associated with survival times. African-American participants had adjusted hazard ratio roughly 48% higher than whites while Hispanic participants had adjusted hazard ratio elevated by 45%. Each prior arrest increased the adjusted hazard ratio by about 13% whereas each year of age decreased the adjusted hazard ratio by about one percent.

Hypothesis 6: Managed Care will Not Reduce Days in the Community

Days in the community represent another outcome. It was expected that MC would not reduce days in the community. Table 9 shows that the MC period yielded fewer days in the community for drug court eligibles (including those who chose criminal court). The difference is about 18 days, or less than two percent, but statistically significant ($p = .005$ in a model that adjusted for prior arrests). There was a 14 day decline in community days looking at the adjusted means.

Table 9. Days in the community by Medicaid era

Medicaid era	N	Mean (std dev)	Adjusted mean (95% CI)
All drug court eligibles			
Fee for service	884	1007 (93)	1005 (998 to 1012)
Managed care	901	989 (140)	991 (984 to 998)
Drug court participants			
Fee for service	427	1003 (95)	1005 (996 to 1014)
Managed care	364	1012 (112)	1009 (999 to 1019)

Std dev = Standard deviation
CI = confidence interval
Adjusted for arrests in two years prior to index date

However, it was not surprising to find that days in the community were markedly skewed. For example, about 14% of subjects (by far the largest group) had the maximum 1,095 days in the community. Roughly half the subjects had 1,035 days or more in the community. Therefore, logistic regression was conducted where the dependent variable was less versus more than 1,035 days in the community. The predictors included gender, age, race, ethnicity, arrests in the two years prior to index date, Medicaid eligibility, era, drug court participation, the two-way interaction terms (eligibility by era, eligibility by participation, and era by participation) plus the three-way interaction term (eligibility by era by participation). The three-way interaction term was not statistically significant in any model.

For the model that lumped "no" with "unknown" Medicaid eligibility, the two-way interaction of era by drug court participation was significant ($p = .01$) and associated with more days in the community (adjusted odds of 1.9). The other two-way interaction terms were not statistically significant nor were the indicators for era, drug court participation, or Medicaid eligibility. In the logistic regression model, the statistically significant predictors of more days in the community included age ($p = .01$). Each year of age increased the adjusted odds of greater days in the community by about two percent. Predictors of fewer days in the community included black race ($p < .001$), Hispanic ethnicity ($p = .006$), and prior arrests ($p < .001$). African-Americans were about half as likely as whites to have longer time in the community while Hispanics were about 35 percent less likely. Each prior arrest reduced the adjusted odds of more days in the community by about 27%. Gender did not predict more days in the community. Results were very similar from the logistic regression model that distinguish "no" from "unknown" Medicaid eligibility subjects. Medicaid "unknown" status was associated with doubled adjusted odds of longer community tenure ($p < .001$). Findings from the logistic regression model restricted to subjects with known (either "yes" or "no" Medicaid status) were also similar except that ethnicity was not a statistically significant predictor of community tenure.

Table 9 also reports more days in the community for drug court participants during the MC era. This finding is consistent with the hypothesis. However the difference is small (four days) and statistically insignificant in a model that adjusted for prior arrests. The same results were found for both graduates and treatment failures separately.

Interestingly enough, in the logistic regression approach for drug court participants, Managed Care era predicted decreased (by 43%) adjusted odds of more days in the community ($p = .004$). However, neither the interaction of Medicaid eligibility with era nor the Medicaid eligibility indicator were statistically significant. Age and gender were not statistically significant predictors but black race, Hispanic ethnicity, and prior arrests were all associated with increased adjusted odds of fewer days in the community. Among drug court participants, African- Americans ($p < .001$) and Hispanics ($p = .01$) both had about half the adjusted odds of increased days in the community. Each prior arrest reduced the adjusted odds of increased community days by about 25% ($p < .001$).

DISCUSSION

The distributions of cases, ages, genders, and the three major race/ethnic groups among the cells of the two-by-two design yield sufficient cases in each cell. There was a shift from drug court to criminal court under MC for whites and blacks but the opposite for Hispanics. The race distribution could have been a confounder in the hypothesis tests.

Hypothesis 1: Proportion Eligible for Medicaid Increased Under Managed Care

Thc introduction of managed care in Oregon had the intended result of increasing the numbers of people eligible for Medicaid. The percentage of known Medicaid eligibles went from about 13% to 40%, amounting to 305 cases.

Hypothesis 2: Time in Treatment Will Decrease Under Managed Care

Time in treatment received by drug court participants actually decreased under MC. The amount of treatment received by the drug court participants in the FFS era was 9.55 months (286.5 good days) of treatment. In the MC era, participants received less, 8.28 months (247.4 good days). The difference was significant. Drug court participants who succeeded in the treatment program and graduated received 13.50 months (405.0 days) under fee-for-service versus 13.55 (406.5 days) under MC. The difference was not significant. Drug court participants who failed in the treatment program and were given a stipulated facts trial received 6.54 months (196.2 days) in the FFS era but only 4.91 months (147.3 days) in the MC era. The difference was statistically significant. The 40 days reduced time in treatment for participants is mainly attributable to 49 fewer days received by treatment failures.

Hypothesis 3: Treatment Failure will not Be Increased by Managed Care

There was no significant difference between FFS and MC eras in the proportion of drug court participants finishing with a stipulated facts trial rather than a graduation.

Hypothesis 4: Managed care will not increase arrests (a measure of criminal recidivism)

There were more arrests in the MC era among persons eligible to participate in the drug court, although the differences were slight and insignificant. There does not appear to have been a historical confound affecting arrest rate. There were actually fewer arrests among drug court participants in the MC era, although the difference was small and insignificant. There were fewer arrests among graduates (significant) and treatment failures (not significant) both. Consistent with the hypothesis, MC did not increase arrest rates generally and, for graduates, arrests actually decreased.

Focusing on individuals known to be eligible for Medicaid, one statistical model did (barely) suggest that there might have been an increase in arrests among drug MC versus FFS drug court participants (who were Medicaid eligible). However, two other statistical models showed no impact of managed care on arrests among Medicaid eligible drug court participants. The most likely explanation is that the data do not indicate an increased arrest rate in this group.

Hypothesis 5: Managed Care will not Decrease Time Until First Arrest / Booking

There were no significant differences in survival until first arrest, which is consistent with the hypothesis. Moreover, statistical models focused on Medicaid eligible drug court participants showed no decrease in survival time under managed care for this group.

Hypothesis 6. Medicaid managed care will not reduce days in the community

The drug court eligibles spent fewer days in the community under MC. The difference was about 18 days, less than 2%, but statistically significant. This outcome appeared due to those who chose criminal court. Drug court participants actually spent 10 more days in the community under MC (not significant); graduates spent seven more days in the community under MC (not significant); and failures spent 13 more days in the community under MC (not significant). Apparently, criminal court participants spent fewer days in the community under MC, offsetting the direction of the drug court participants who spent more days in the community. Statistical models focused on Medicaid eligible drug court participants found no evidence that managed care decreased days in the community for this group.

Study Limitations

Of course, subjects were not assigned at random to the drug court program nor to Medicaid. Presumably, then, there were many differences between participants and comparison subjects and between those with versus without Medicaid. It is also possible that "pre" era subjects may have differed in many ways from "post" era subjects.

There were some data available (*e.g.,* prior arrests) that were used to adjust for differences between, say, drug court participants versus comparison subjects (within the several Medicaid categories). More troubling is the (likely) possibility that there may have been unobserved factors differentiating participants and comparison subjects (in any or all Medicaid categories). The problem of unobserved differences is particularly worrisome if the unobserved factors are correlated with the dependent variable (*e.g.,* with the re-arrest rate during follow-up). This problem of selection bias is common to observational studies and has been discussed by many authors (see, *e.g.,* Heckman, 1976, 1979; Heckman and Hotz, 1989; Lalonde, 1986; Manski, 1995; Rosenbaum, 1995).

Consideration was given to use of the propensity score (Rosenbaum and Rubin, 1983, 1984, 1985) to address selection bias. Conceptually, the propensity score method can match, say, drug court participants with comparison subjects who are as "similar" as possible (on the known variables). The drug court status (coded as participant equals one) is used as a binary dependent variable in a logistic regression where predictor variables would be items such as primary drug of abuse, employment, etc. The propensity score is the predicted value (from the estimated logistic regression model) for each subject. Individuals with high propensity scores "should be" drug court participants (if participation were to follow the logic of the logistic regression equation) and are therefore felt to be comparable. One then analyzes the data stratifying on the propensity score.

Obviously, the situation in this study was complicated because drug court participants and comparison subjects were also categorized based on Medicaid eligibility as well as managed care era. It is unclear whether, in these circumstances, one should use an overall logistic regression or a stratified approach to generate the propensity score(s). Given the project's inherent complexity, a simpler analytic approach was undertaken in which known confounders were included as predictors in assorted regression models. Consequently, conclusions need to be made with caution.

Statistical power is another potential limitation. Looking at the before versus after managed care comparisons, there were substantial numbers of subjects (at least one hundred) in each cell. Ignoring Medicaid eligibility, one can think of the before versus after comparison as two contrasting two-by-two tables. One dimension of each two-by-two table would be drug court participation versus criminal court. The other dimension would be the outcome (*e.g.*, arrests). For example, one could split the subjects on median follow-up arrests (namely three arrests) and show numbers of individuals with three or fewer arrests versus individuals with four or more arrests during follow-up. Then in the before era one has drug court participants versus criminal court defendants crossed with above versus below median arrests during follow-up. There is an analogous two-by-two table for the after managed care group. As noted, there should be at least a hundred subjects in each cell of each two-by-two table. In other words, there will be at least four hundred subjects in each two-by-two table.

Conceptually, one could think of each two-by-two table as, in effect, yielding a correlation coefficient. Then the statistical power question is, in effect, a comparison of two correlation coefficients. Cohen (1988) shows that for these sample sizes (at p-level of 0.05) there is 88% statistical power to detect a difference in correlation coefficients corresponding to an effect size of 0.2 which is in the small (0.1) to medium (0.3) range. Recalling that the standard deviation for arrests during follow-up was roughly five arrests, then an effect size of 0.2 is more or less equivalent to a difference (on average) of one arrest (over three years) between the groups. Given that the average follow-up arrests were about five (in each group) then there was adequate statistical power to detect a difference of approximately 20% from before to after managed care. This calculation is quite conservative because the total sample size is around 1,818 subjects. In other words, the sample size was (more than) adequate to detect a difference in arrests (from before to after managed care) that would be of interest to policy makers.

Of course, statistical power was reduced for sub-groups. In particular, there was interest in the Medicaid eligible subjects. Given the study's complexity, statistical power calculations were not straightforward. However, it is illuminating to examine confidence intervals in linear regression models. For example, consider a linear regression model with time in the community (during three years of follow-up) as the dependent variable and gender, age, race, ethnicity, arrests in the two years prior to index date, Medicaid eligibility, era, drug court participation, the two-way interaction terms (eligibility by era, eligibility by participation, and era by participation) plus the three-way interaction term (eligibility by era by participation) as predictors. In this model, the 95% confidence interval for the three-way interaction term was (- 88 days to +12 days). That is, the Medicaid eligible drug court participants in the managed care era could, at worst, have had 88 fewer days in the community than expected. Recall that mean and median community days during follow-up were roughly 1,000. Then, at worst,

Medicaid eligible drug court participants would have experienced roughly nine percent fewer community days than expected. Admittedly this computation is crude. To cite but one difficulty, as noted, days in the community were markedly skewed. Nonetheless, this computation suggests that the project had adequate sample size to address policy-makers' concerns about Medicaid managed care for drug court participants.

CONCLUSION

As expected, under managed care, less time was invested in treatment, especially for the drug court failures. Among the subgroups choosing the drug court, treatment failures got about a month and a half less treatment under managed care than they had under fee-for-service. Graduates, however, did not get less time in treatment.

It was expected that less time in treatment would, nonetheless, not worsen outcomes. There were no more failures in the managed care period, as reflected in the numbers of stipulated facts trials. There were actually fewer arrests under managed care, but only for graduates. Notably, treatment failures did not experience more arrests under managed care with its shorter treatment for treatment failures. As expected, managed care had no effect on other measures of recidivism, such as survival time to first arrest and days in the community for drug court participants.

Numerous analyses focused on Medicaid eligible drug court participants suggested, overall, that managed care had no impact on this group's numbers of arrests during follow-up, time to first follow-up arrest, or days in the community during follow-up. There appeared to be adequate sample sizes to detect meaningful impact of managed care.

As in previous studies using different populations, different interventions, and different measures, managed care seems have reduced services to drug court participants (primarily those who failed treatment) without affecting outcomes. Time in treatment may well be related to outcomes, but only when efficiency is comparable. This result suggests a higher degree of prudence in the allocation of resources which is, of course, one of the missions of managed care.

Of course, as was mentioned, the study had numerous challenges. The next chapter examines in detail one such challenge – namely the linkage of data from diverse administrative systems.

ACKNOWLEDGMENTS

Supported in part by National Institute on Drug Abuse grant number R01 DA 013091.

REFERENCES

Aaron, H. J. (2002). The unsurprising surprise of renewed health care cost inflation. *Health Affairs (Millwood), Web Supplement*, W85-87.

Alexander, J. A., and Lemak, C. H. (1997a). The effects of managed care on administrative burden in outpatient substance abuse treatment facilities. *Medical Care, 35*, 1060-1068.

Alexander, J. A., and Lemak, C. H. (1997b). Managed care penetration in outpatient substance abuse treatment units. *Medical Care Research and Review, 54*(4), 490-507.

Alterman, A. I., Snider, R. C., Cacciola, J. S., May, D. J., Parikh, G., Maany, I., et al. (1996). A quasi-experimental comparison of the effectiveness of 6- versus 12-hour per week outpatient treatments for cocaine dependence. *Journal of Nervous and Mental Disease, 184*, 54-65.

Altman, D. E., and Levitt, L. (2002). The sad history of health care cost containment as told in one chart. *Health Affairs (Millwood), Web Supplement*, W83-W84.

American Managed Behavioral Healthcare Association and the National Association of State Alcohol and Drug Abuse Directors (1999). Public substance abuse and managed behavioral healthcare. *Behavioral Healthcare Tomorrow*, 25-30.

American Society for Addiction Medicine (1996). *Patient placement criteria for the treatment of substance-related disorders, second edition* Chevy Chase, MD: American Society for Addiction Medicine.

Ashton, C. M., Petersen, N. J., Souchek, J., Menke, T. J., Yu, H. J., Pietz, K., et al. (1999). Geographic variations in utilization rates in Veterans Affairs hospitals and clinics. *New England Journal of Medicine, 340*, 32-39.

Belenko, S. (1998). Research on drug courts: A critical review. *National Drug Court Institute Review, 1*, 1-22.

Belenko, S. (Ed.). (1999). *Diverting drug offenders to treatment courts: The Portland experience*. Thousand Oaks, CA: Sage Publications.

Belenko, S., Patapis, N., and French, M. T. (2005). *Economic benefits of drug treatment: A critical review of the evidence for policy makers*. Philadelphia, PA: Treatment Research Institute.

Bergman, G. T. (1999). *A second generation of managed behavioral health programs emerge*. Rockville, MD: U.S. Department of Health and Human Services, Substance Abuse and Mental Health Services Administration, Managed Behavioral Healthcare Updates Series.

Bianconi, J. M., Mahler, J. M., and McFarland, B. H. (2006). Outcomes for rural Medicaid clients with severe mental illness in fee for service versus managed care. *Administration and Policy in Mental Health and Mental Health Services Research, 33*, 411-422.

Bien, T. H., Miller, W. R., and Tonigan, J. S. (1993). Brief interventions for alcohol problems: A review. *Addiction, 88*, 315-336.

Bigelow, D. A., McFarland, B. H., Gareau, M., and Young, D. J. (1991). Implementation and effectiveness of a bed reduction program. *Community Mental Health Journal, 27*, 125-133.

Bigelow, D. A., McFarland, B. H., McCamant, L. E., Deck, D. D., and Gabriel, R. M. (2004). Effect of managed care on access to mental health services among Medicaid enrollees receiving substance abuse treatment. *Psychiatric Services, 55*, 755-779.

Bodenheimer, T. (2002). The not-so-sad history of Medicare cost containment as told in one chart. *Health Affairs Web Supplement,* W88-90.

Bureau of Justice Assistance Drug Court Clearinghouse (2007). *Drug court activity update*. Washington, DC: American University.

Callahan, D. (1995). Once again reality: The lesson from the SUPPORT study Special Supplement. *Hastings Center Report, 24*, S33-S36.

Carey, S., and Finigan, M. (2003). *A Detailed Cost Analysis in a Mature Drug Court Setting: A Cost-Benefit Evaluation of the Multnomah County Drug Court*. Portland, OR: NPC Research, Inc.

Center for Substance Abuse Treatment (1997). *Substance abuse treatment planning guide and checklist for treatment-based drug courts (DHHS Publication Number SMA 97-3136).* Rockville, MD: Substance Abuse and Mental Health Services Administration.

Chandler, R., Fletcher, B.W., Volkow, N.D. (2009). Treating drug abuse and addiction in the criminal justice system: Improving public health and safety. *Journal of the American Medical Association,* 301, 183-190.

Cohen, J. (Ed.). (1988). *Statistical power analysis for the behavioral sciences, 2nd edition.* Hillsdale, NJ: Lawrence Erlbaum Associates.

Cutler, D. L., Bigelow, D., and McFarland, B. (1992). The cost of fragmented mental health financing: Is it worth it? *Community Mental Health Journal, 28,* 121-135.

Cutler, D. L., McFarland, B. H., and Winthrop, K. (1998). Mental health in the Oregon Health Plan: Integration or fragmentation? *Administration and Policy in Mental Health, 25,* 361-386.

Deck, D. D., McFarland, B. H., Titus, J. M., Laws, K. E., and Gabriel, R. M. (2000). Access to substance abuse treatment services under the Oregon Health Plan. *Journal of the American Medical Association, 284*(16), 2093-2099.

Drug Court Clearinghouse and Technical Assistance Project (1998). *Looking at a decade of drug courts*. Washington, DC: American University and Drug Courts Program Office, Office of Justice Programs, U.S. Department of Justice.

Drug Courts Program Office (1998). *Drug court activity: Summary information*. Washington, DC: Drug Courts Program Office, Office of Justice Programs, U.S. Department of Justice.

Drug Strategies (1999). *Millenium Hangover: Keeping Score on Alcohol*. Washington, DC: Drug Strategies.

Finigan, M. (1998). *An outcome program evaluation of the Multnomah County S.T.O.P. drug diversion program*. Portland, Oregon: Northwest Professional Consortium.

Finigan, M. W., Carey, S. M., and Cox, A. (2007). *The Impact of a mature drug court over 10 years of operation: Recidivism and costs (Final Report)*. Portland, OR: NPC Research.

Finn, P., and Newlyn, A. K. (1993). Miami drug court gives drug defendants a second chance. *National Institute of Justice Journal, November*, 13-20.

Finney, J. W., and Monahan, S. C. (1996). The cost-effectiveness of treatment for alcoholism: A second approximation. *Journal of Studies on Alcohol, 57*, 229-243.

Flaherty, J., and Kim, K. (1997). Managed care for psychiatric and addictive disorders. In N. Miller (Ed.), *The principles and practice of addictions in psychiatry*. Philadelphia: W.B. Saunders.

Frank, R. G., and McGuire, T. G. (1997). Savings from a Medicaid carve-out for mental health and substance abuse services in Massachusetts. *Psychiatric Services, 48,* 1147-1152.

Frank, R. G., McGuire, T. G., Notman, E. H., and Woodward, R. M (1996). Developments in Medicaid managed behavioral health care. In: R. W. Manderscheid, and M. A.

Sonnenschein (Eds.), *Mental Health, United States, 1996*, DHHS Pub. No. (SMA) 96-3098. Washington, DC: Superintendent of Documents, U.S. Government Printing Office.

Galanter, M. (1998). ASAM study to address the impact of managed care on addiction treatment. *ASAM News, 13*, 1-6.

General Accounting Office (1997). *Drug courts: Overview of growth, characteristics, and results.* Washington, DC: General Accounting Office.

Gerstein, D., and Harwood, H. (1990). *Treating drug problems: A study of the evolution, effectiveness, and financing of public and private drug treatment systems: Vol. 1.* Washington, DC: National Academy Press.

Government Accountability Office (2005). *Adult drug courts: Evidence indicates recidivism reductions and mixed results for other outcomes*. Washington DC: United States Government Accountability Office.

Harrell, A., Cavanagh, S., and Roman, J. (1998). *Final report: Findings from the evaluation of the DC superior court drug intervention program.* Washington, DC: Urban Institute.

Heckman, J. (1976). The common structure of statistical models of truncation, sample selection and limited dependent variables and a simple estimator for such models. *Annals of Economic and Social Measurement, 5*, 475-492.

Heckman, J. (1979). Sample selection bias as a specification error. *Econometrica, 47*, 153-161.

Heckman, J., and Hotz, V. (1989). Choosing among alternative nonexperimental methods for estimating the impact of social programs: the case of manpower training. *Journal of the American Statistical Association, 84*, 862-874.

Holder, H. (1998). Cost benefits of substance abuse treatment: an overview of results from alcohol and drug abuse. *Journal of Mental Health Policy and Economics, 1*, 23-29.

Huddleston, C. W., Marlowe, D. B., and Casebolt, R. (2008). *Painting the current picture: A national report card on drug courts and other problem solving court programs in the United States*. Alexandria, VA: National Drug Court Institute.

Humphreys, K., and Moos, R. H. (1996). Reduced substance-abuse-related health care costs among voluntary participants in Alcoholics Anonymous. *Psychiatric Services, 47*, 709-713.

Iglehart, J. K. (1999). The American health care system: Medicaid. *New England Journal of Medicine, 340*, 403-408.

Institute of Medicine (1990). *Broadening the base of treatment for alcohol problems.* Washington, DC: National Academy Press.

Institute of Medicine (1996). *Managing managed care: Quality improvement in behavioral health*. Washington, DC: National Academy Press.

Kihlstrom, L. C. (1997). Characteristics and growth of managed behavioral health firms. *Health Affairs, 16,* 127-130.

Kunnes, R., Niven, R., Gustafson, T., Brooks, N., Levin, S. M., Edmunds, M., et al. (1993). Financing and payment reform for primary health care and substance abuse treatment. *Journal of Addictive Diseases, 12*, 23-42.

Lalonde, R. (1986). Evaluating the econometric evaluations of training programs with experimental data. *American Economic Review, 76*, 604-620.

Lo, A., and Woodward, A. (1993). An evaluation of freestanding alcoholism treatment for Medicare recipients. *Addiction, 88,* 53-67.

Manski, C. F. (1995). *Identification problems in the social sciences*. Cambridge: Harvard University Press.

Marlowe, D. B., Festinger, D. S., and Lee, P. A. (2004). The judge is a key component of drug court. *National Drug Court Institute Review, IV,* 1-34.

Marlowe, D. B., Festinger, D. S., Dugosh, K. L., and Lee, P. A. (2003). Are judicial status hearings a key component of drug court? During-treatment data from a randomized trial. *Criminal Justice and Behavior, 30,* 141-162.

McFarland, B. H., and Blair, G. (1995). Delivering comprehensive services to homeless mentally ill offenders. *Psychiatric Services, 46,* 179-181.

McFarland, B. H., and Minkoff, K. (1996). Utilization management. In K. Minkoff and D. Pollack (Eds.), *Managed mental health care in the public sector: A survival manual.* Amsterdam: Harwood Academic Publishers.

McFarland, B. H., Bigelow, D. A., Smith, J. C., Hornbrook, M. C., Mofidi, A., and Payton, P (1995): A capitated payment system for involuntary mental health clients. *Health Affairs, 14,* 185-196.

McFarland, B. H., Deck, D. D., McCamant, L. E., Gabriel, R. M., and Bigelow, D. A. (2005). Outcomes for Medicaid clients with substance abuse problems before and after managed care. *Journal of Behavioral Health Services and Research, 32*(4), 351-367.

McFarland, B. H., McCamant, L. E., and Barron, N. M. (2005). Outcomes for clients of public substance abuse treatment programs before and after Medicaid managed care. *Journal of Substance Abuse Treatment, 28*, 149-157.

McFarland, B. H., Winthrop, K., and Cutler, D. L. (1997). Integrating mental health into the Oregon Health Plan. *Psychiatric Services 48,* 191-193.

McFarland, B., and George, R. (1995). Ethics and managed care. *Child and Adolescent Psychiatric Clinics of North America, 4*, 885-901.

McKenzie, D. A., Mullooly, J. P., McFarland, B. H., Semradek, J., and McCamant, L. E. (1999). Changes in antipsychotic drug use following shifts in policy: A multilevel analysis. *Research on Aging, 21*, 304-337.

McLellan, A. T., Belding, M., McKay, J. R., Zanis, D., and Alterman, A. I. (1996). Can the outcomes research literature inform the search for quality indicators in substance abuse treatment? In Institute of Medicine (Ed.), *Managing managed care: Quality improvement in behavioral health*. Washington, DC: National Academy Press.

Mechanic, D., Schlesinger, M., and McAlpine, D. D. (1995). Management of mental health and substance abuse services: State of the art and early results. *Milbank Quarterly, 73,* 19-55.

Miller, S. I. (1994). Drugs and alcohol: The clinician's view. In R. K. Schreter, S. S. Sharfstein and C. A. Schreter (Eds.), *Allies and adversaries*. Washington, DC: American Psychiatric Press, Inc.

Miller, W. R., and Hester, R. K. (1986). Inpatient alcoholism treatment: Who benefits? *American Psychologist, 41*, 794-805.

Moos, R. H., Pettit, B., and Gruber, V. (1995). Longer episodes of community residential care reduce substance abuse patients' readmission rates. *Journal of Studies on Alcohol, 56*, 433-443.

National Association of Drug Court Professionals (1997). *Defining drug courts: The key components*. Washington, DC: U.S. Department of Justice, Office of Justice Programs, Drug Court Programs Office.

National Clearinghouse for Alcohol and Drug Information (1997). *Clients in treatment, 1992.* Washington, DC: National Clearinghouse for Alcohol and Drug Information.

National Institute of Justice (2006). *Drug courts: The second decade.* Washington, D.C. U.S. Department of Justice, Office of Justice Programs, National Institute of Justice.

National Institute on Drug Abuse (2006). *Principles of drug abuse treatment for criminal justic populations: A research-based guide.* Bethesda, MD: National Institute on Drug Abuse, National Institutes of Health Publication Number 06-5316.

O'Brien, C., and McLellan, A. (1996). Myths about the treatment of addiction. *Lancet, 347*, 237-240.

Onken, L. S., Blaine, J. D., and Boren, J. J. (1997). Treatment for drug addiction: It won't work if they don't receive it. In *Beyond the therapeutic alliance: Keeping the drug dependent individual in treatment.* NIDA Research Monograph number 165.

Peters, R. H. (1996). *Evaluating drug court programs: an overview of issues and alternative strategies.* Washington, DC: American University Justice Programs Office.

Peters, R.H ,. Pennington, B. A., Wells, J. D., Rosenthal, L., Meeks, J., Brown, A., Kambo, R., and Singleton, M. (undated). *Treatment-based Drug Courts -- A Guide.* Tallahassee, FL: Office of the State Courts Administrator, Florida Supreme Court.

Pollack, D. A., McFarland, B. H., George, R. A., and Angell, R. H. (1994). Prioritization of mental health services in Oregon. *Milbank Quarterly, 72,* 515-550.

Prendergast, M. L., Podus, D., and Chang, E. (2000). Program factors and treatment outcomes in drug dependence treatment: An examination using meta-analysis. *Substance Use and Misuse, 35,* 1931-1965.

Reilly, D. A., and Pierre-Lawson, A. (2008). *Ensuring sustainability for drug courts: An overview of funding strategies.* Alexandria, VA.

Rosenbaum, P. R. (1995). Observational studies. New York: Springer-Verlag.

Rosenbaum, P. R., and Rubin, D. B. (1983). The central role of the propensity score in observational studies for causal effects. *Biometrika, 70*, 41-55.

Rosenbaum, P. R., and Rubin, D. B. (1984). Reducing bias in observational studies using subclassification on the propensity score. *Journal of the American Statistical Association, 79*, 516-524.

Rosenbaum, P. R., and Rubin, D. B. (1985). Constructing a control using multivariate matched sampling methods that incorporate the propensity score. *American Statistician, 39*, 33-38.

Ross, K. V., and McFarland, B. H. (2000). The mental health organizations. In R. R. Goetz, B. H. McFarland and K. V. Ross (Eds.), *What the Oregon Health Plan can teach us about managed mental health care. New Directions for Mental Health Services, 85:57-64.* San Francisco: Jossey-Bass.

Rothbard, A. B., McFarland, B. H., Shern, D. L., Morrisey, J. P., Leff, S. H., and Wylie, M. A. (2002). Managed care for persons with serious mental illness. *Drug Benefit Trends, 14*, 6-14.

Rothbard, A., Kuno, E., Hadley, T., and Dogin, J. (2004). Psychiatric service utilization and cost for persons with schizophrenia in a Medicaid managed care program. *Journal of Behavioral Health Services and Research, 31*, 1-12.

Sanford, S. J., and Arrigo, B. A. (2005). Lifting the cover on drug courts: Evaluation findings and policy concerns. *International Journal of Offender Therapy and Comparative Criminology, 49*(3), 239-259.

Schwartz, J. R., and Schwartz, L. P. (1998). The drug court: A new strategy for drug use prevention. *Obstetrics and Gynecology Clinics of North America, 25*, 255-268.

Scott, J. E. (1996). Alcoholism and alcohol abuse services research. In: B. L. Levin, and J. Petrilla (Eds.), *Mental health services: A public health perspective.* New York: Oxford University Press.

Silverman, C. (1994). Drugs and alcohol: The managed care view. In R. K. Schreter, S. S. Sharfstein and C. A. Schreter (Eds.), *Allies and adversaries*. Washington, DC: American Psychiatric Press, Inc.

Simpson, D. D., Joe, G. W., Fletcher, B. W., Hubbard, R. L., and Anglin, M. D. (1999). A national evaluation of treatment outcomes for cocaine dependence. *Archives of General Psychiatry, 56*, 507-514.

Substance Abuse and Mental Health Services Administration. (1998). *State profiles on public sector managed behavioral health care and other reforms.* Rockville, MD: Substance Abuse and Mental Health Services Administration.

Tauber, J. S. (1994). *National strategy for the co-funding of coordinated drug court systems.* Alexandria, VA: National Association of Drug Court Professionals.

Terry, W. C. (1999). Judicial change and dedicated treatment courts: Case studies in innovation. In W. C. Terry (Ed.), *The early drug courts*. Thousand Oaks, CA: Sage Publications.

Timko, C., Finney, J. W., Moos, R. H., and Moos, B. S. (1995). Short-term treatment careers and outcomes of previously untreated alcoholics. *Journal of Studies on Alcohol, 56*, 597-610.

United States Bureau of the Census (1998). *Statistical abstract of the United States 1998, 118th edition*. Washington, DC: U.S. Government Printing Office.

Walsh, D. C., Hingson, R. W., Merrigan, D. M., Levenson, S. M., Cupples, L. A., Heeren, T., et al. (1991). A randomized trial of treatment options for alcohol-abusing workers. *New England Journal of Medicine, 325*, 775-782.

Wennberg, J. (1999). Understanding geographic variations in health care delivery. *New England Journal of Medicine, 340*, 52-53.

Wilson, C. (1993). Substance abuse and managed care. In F. S. Goldman W (Ed.), *Managed mental health care. New Directions for Mental Health Services, Number 59*. San Francisco: Jossey-Bass.

Wilson, D. B. (2007). *Effects of drug courts on criminal offending and drug use*. Manassas, VA: George Mason University.

Zwick, W. R., and Bermon, M. (1992). Spectrum of services for the alcohol abusing patient. In J. L. Feldman and R. J. Fitzpatrick (Eds.), *Managed mental health care*. Washington, DC: American Psychiatric Press, Inc.

In: Medicaid and Treatment for People... ISBN 978-1-61470-742-4
Editors: B.H. McFarland, D.McCarty, et al, pp.163-179 ©2011 Nova Science Publishers, Inc.

Chapter 7

Research and Evaluation Challenges Pertaining to Medicaid Clients with Substance Abuse: Indeterminacy in Data Linkage

Anton Cox[1] and Douglas A. Bigelow[2]
[1] Department of Psychiatry, Oregon Health and Science University, Portland, OR (former association) and NPC Research Corporation, Portland, OR (former association), USA
[2] Department of Psychiatry, Oregon Health and Science University, Portland, OR, USA

Abstract

Medicaid clients (and especially clients with substance abuse problems) are often served by multiple agencies. Research and evaluation can be challenged by the need to link data generated by numerous administrative systems. Medicaid clients involved with the criminal justice system may be especially difficult for data linkage owing to numerous identities. This chapter describes methods used to verify matches pertaining to individuals eligible for drug court. Subjects were identified for the drug court and Medicaid managed care research project described in a previous chapter. Especially helpful were flow charts showing (a) the routes of individuals as they made contact with several agencies and (b) the creation of data elements describing those individuals by the numerous organizations. Building on this background, the chapter discusses matching problems as well as the several uncertainties that can arise. Case examples are provided showing results of assorted decisions made about possible linkages. Of some 2,153 potential cases, automated matching software would have retained only about 1,500 matched cases and many of those retained would have lacked demographic and-or service utilization data. Conversely, using manual methods, 214 potential cases were deleted chiefly due to the research project's inclusion and exclusion criteria. Only about 30 potential cases were deleted because of irresolvable data problems. Ultimately, some 1,939 subjects were deemed valid unique cases along with much of their identifying, demographic, and service utilization data. The manual linkage procedures decreased sampling error substantially which increased precision of the research project's data analyses.

INTRODUCTION

Linking data on individuals across health, social, justice, and employment service agencies is vital to the evaluation of policy and service initiatives, but linking records for an individual across administrative data bases can be very complicated (Hser and Evans, 2008). Agencies use different identifiers for individuals, such as name, coded name, Social Security Number (SSN), Federal Bureau of Investigation (FBI) number, and agency-assigned identifiers. Agencies also use different methods for identifying an individual at each contact with the person. Methods include self-declaration (*e.g.,* "my name is..."), documentation (*e.g.,* driver's license), and bio-markers (*e.g.,* fingerprints). Because different agencies use different identifiers and different methods of determining identity, linking an individual's records across agencies can be challenging.

The accuracy and completeness of identifiers (and other data elements, *e.g.,* insurance policy, ethnicity, driver's license, or even name) vary both within and across databases because the motivations for capturing each data element vary (Hser and Evans, 2008).

Inaccurate and incomplete data can suggest false negative matches (multiple individuals when there is, in fact, one) or false positive matches (a single person when there are, in fact, multiple individuals). Even when a match is found with certainty, inconsistent and incomplete demographic data from all sources for a single individual can preclude a dependable description of the individual (*e.g.,* the ethnicity may be wrong).

There are three approaches to linking data across agencies. First is to create a shared or central case registration system. We have had experience with several such systems and they work very well, once established. However, establishing such a shared or central case registration is a major policy decision and technical task. We were able to use such a system (Multnomah County Decision Support System) for subsequent projects pertaining to drug court in Oregon. The second approach is to use linking software to identify matching cases across data bases not otherwise linked. We also had experience with this approach using the Link King (*www.the-link-king.com)* to link a number of state databases. However, computerized matching algorithms like the Link King depend upon obvious, concrete ("determinative") correspondence between elements of the two or more databases being linked. A third approach uses a case-by-case examination of possible matches by researchers to identify likely matches. This examination depends upon understanding how data are collected, processed, and stored in each database so that clues can be interpreted and evaluated.

Data matching was required for the study described in an earlier chapter on possible impact of conversion from fee-for-service to managed care Medicaid on the effectiveness of a drug court diversion program. We used a two-by-two research design to examine cohorts of offenders processed by the Multnomah County (greater Portland, Oregon) court as either criminal or drug court diversion cases during a period of fee-for-service Medicaid and, later, a period of Medicaid managed care. The chief outcome measure was the re-arrest rate. A research database was constructed of participants and their data elements drawn from databases of the District Attorney, the Public Defender, and eight other agencies involved in drug offender cases processed by the Multnomah County drug court.

The research design required linking records on each individual among financial, treatment, law enforcement, judicial, and correctional agencies processing drug court individuals as will now be described.

METHODS

Drug court participants were selected from drug court records maintained by the District Attorney and the Metropolitan Public Defender. Under agreements and limitations established by each agency, identifiers and demographic data on participants were sent to database managers in other agencies providing drug court-related services to these individuals. Because the searches were conducted by agency personnel, the integrity of each database and maximum confidentiality for persons documented therein were maintained for each database.

All data are public record (except Medicaid eligibility which is data on a public benefits program qualifying for exemption under Code of Federal Regulations 45.56). The project was approved by the Oregon Health and Science University Institutional Review Board (project number 5480). There were data sharing agreements with the Oregon State Department of Human Services and the Oregon State Police. There was cooperation with law enforcement agencies including the Oregon State Police; Multnomah County Sheriff; Multnomah County District Attorney; Multnomah Metropolitan Public Defender; the drug court's treatment provider, InAct; Oregon State Department of Corrections; and Oregon State Department of Transportation Division of Motor Vehicles. Data matching was performed by the Oregon State Department of Human Services with technical assistance from the researchers. Once linking had been accomplished, a de-identified research database was generated for the study.

Data Matching Approach

We set out to accomplish two goals – first to identify and remove false matches and second to determine "consensus" sex, race, and date of birth (DOB) for each subject. Linking individuals across administrative databases was complex and labor-intensive. Although agencies usually assign and maintain their own identifiers to represent unique individuals within their own databases, those identifiers were not always shared across agencies. To facilitate cross-agency linking, universal identifiers such as State Identification number (SID), Oregon driver's license (ODL) and Social Security Number (SSN) were used. In addition, name, DOB, sex, and ethnicity were used in combination.

Each individual on the list was identified by several agency identifiers, universal identifiers, and demographic variables, with whatever level of completeness, consistency, and accuracy that existed. This situation was simple in concept, but not in practice. Most individual records on the list had multiple missing and inconsistent values when records from one agency were compared to records from another agency. These blanks and inconsistencies resulted from the needs of a given agency and its personnel for identifying data, the intentions of the individual disclosing self-identifying information, and the conditions under which data are collected by service agencies.

The following examples illustrate these challenges. Individuals sometimes identify themselves with a full formal name, sometimes with a nickname, and sometimes with alternate spellings. Individuals attempting to gain access to benefits or to avoid detection of criminal offenses sometimes identify themselves with false names and-or with borrowed, stolen or forged identity documents. Some individuals have multiple ODL, SSN, and other identifying documents.

The method for collecting the data differs from agency to agency. For example, one agency may note the apparent race of an individual whereas another may be more interested in the race with which a person self-identifies. Some agencies rely upon the data collected by other agencies and attempt to maintain consistency, even if the data are obviously incorrect. Treatment agencies may require a correct and valid social security number (SSN) to obtain payment for services but other agencies may only want the SSN for their records.

Law enforcement officers may collect identifying information under dangerous and tumultuous circumstances. Booking officers may collect information from incapacitated, ill or uncooperative persons or from persons unable to communicate in English or other languages known to available translators.

There can also be simple data entry errors such as misreading a "1" as a "7" or transposing numbers when recording a DOB. Even errors in documenting the sex of an individual occurred in this way. In some instances, corrections are entered without deletion of the original, incorrect entry, resulting in internal inconsistencies (*e.g.,* male and female) or even multiple cases (where the error is part of the identifier).

The end result is that a single individual can be "documented" in different ways in different databases, and even within the same data base.

The agencies involved in our study used search strategies appropriate to their circumstances and sent us records that met their criteria for a likely match. In addition to service records, each agency sent back their identifiers for the case. The number and type of identifiers varied depending on agreements that were made with each agency, legal constraints, and, as noted, the policies of the agencies' leadership.

We needed a method to distinguish the true matches (*i.e.,* where the potential match from the agency data base is the same person as the individual in our sample) from the false matches (*i.e.,* the potential match from the agency data base is not the same person as the individual in our sample). In our initial examination of the potentially linked pairs, we looked for high levels of agreement in the variables available for comparison. We also sought logical reasons for inconsistencies such as matched SSN, first name, and sex, but non-matching last name and DOB.

There were some cases on our list with multiple potential matches in another agency's data base. When we put all the agencies' potential matches for a case together, we realized we could develop a better method for discriminating between true and false matches by taking into consideration how a match was made, which agencies shared information with other agencies, and the direction of flow for information (*i.e.,* a logic model for construction of a case record).

Processing of Offenders

To apply our method for interpreting and evaluating potential matches, we first needed to understand how and when data are collected. Offenders enter the process shown in Figure 1 when arrested by the police or Sheriff, and, then, booked into the county jail by the Sheriff. The case is then forwarded to the Multnomah County District Attorney who determines if the case is eligible for diversion to drug court (rather than proceeding directly to criminal court or being released). If eligible, the case is forwarded to the Multnomah Public Defender. The offender chooses either to go to criminal court, or to stipulate to the facts (admitting to having committed the offense) and proceed to drug court. Those choosing Criminal Court are tried and, if found guilty, sentenced. These convicted persons are the comparison group in our study. Those choosing drug court are directed into treatment with a number of requirements, including drug testing (with "clean" results), attendance, and compliance with treatment protocol. If the requirements are met and drug treatment completed, the case is dismissed. If requirements are not met and corrective action ordered by the judge fails, or the individual absconds, a bench warrant is issued. Having stipulated to the facts, the individual is likely to be convicted and sentenced in criminal court.

Compilation of Data on Offender Cases

As offenders are processed through this system, data on the case are created (Figure 2). Information is collected by the police and Sheriff on the original contact. Fingerprinting creates a bio-marker sent to the Oregon State Police which searches its Law Enforcement Data System (LEDS). Based on the bio-marker, LEDS returns a State Identification Number (SID) and criminal history associated with that SID, while adding alternate or false names, dates of birth, and other information from its relational data base. Each agency data base has some internal auditing, reconciling and validating of identifiers and demographics (especially, to reduce duplicate cases). However, this data cleansing capability is limited. There is little ability to test validity of names or dates of birth or even SSN. If the offender provides false information or documents when booked (*e.g.,* name, DOB, driver's license, SSN), those false bits of information remain in the case record and are passed on to agencies further down the line. This phenomenon poses challenges to establishing both identity and demographic descriptors of cases.

Assembling the Sample and Data Elements Collected

Cases were identified in 2002 in the Metropolitan Public Defender's listing of all drug offenders 18 or older deemed by the District Attorney to be eligible for the Multnomah County Sanction, Treatment, Opportunity, Progress (STOP) drug court program. This data set comprised a list of 2,153 entries which contained some duplicates and otherwise invalid cases. The list included the District Attorney case number, name of offender, and the charge, while the associated District Attorney's database included Portland Police Data System number, Oregon Driver's License number (ODL), State Identification number (SID), Federal Bureau of Investigation identifier (FBIID), and up to five Social Security Numbers (SSNs).

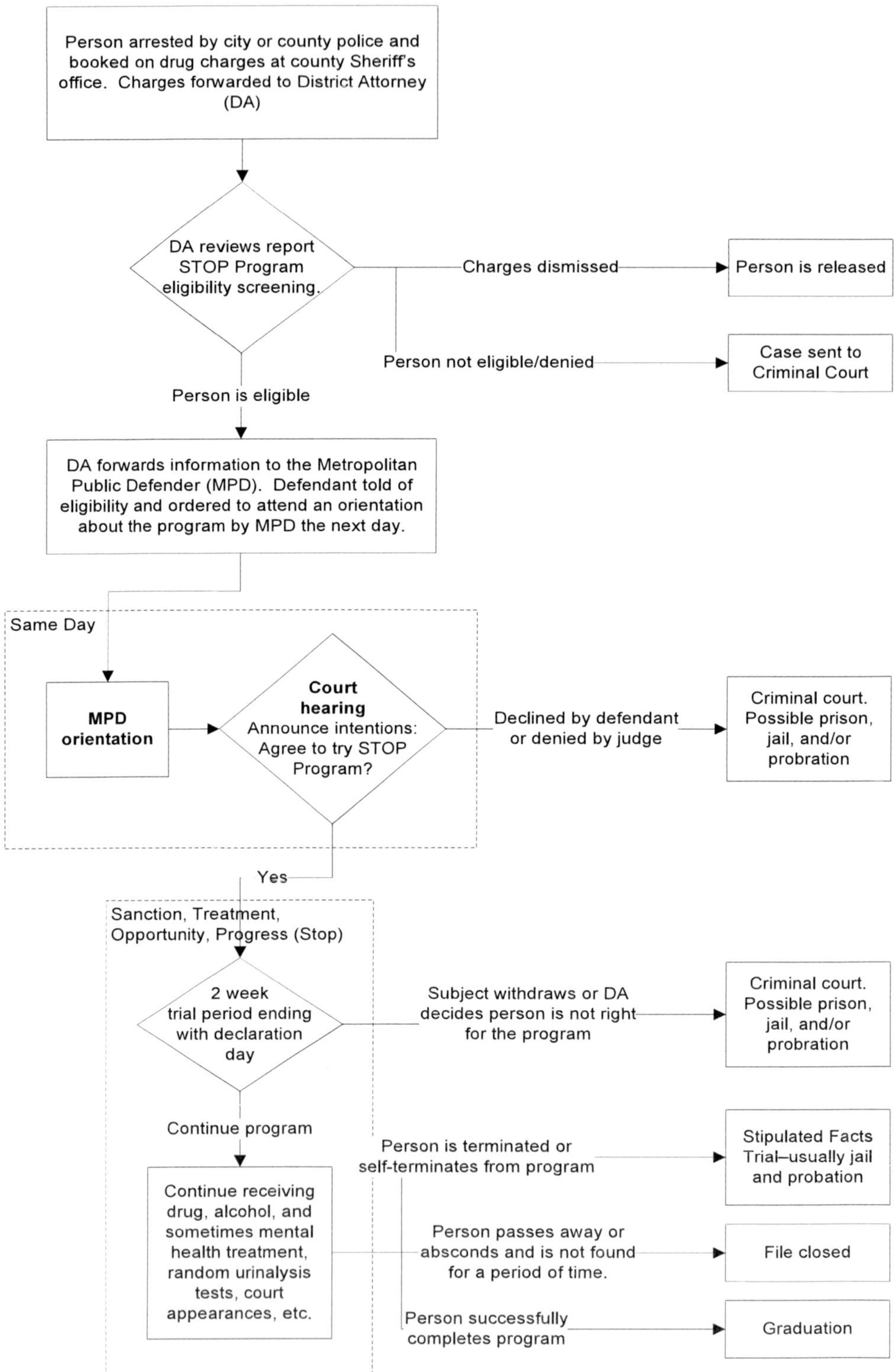

Figure 1. Processing of offenders.

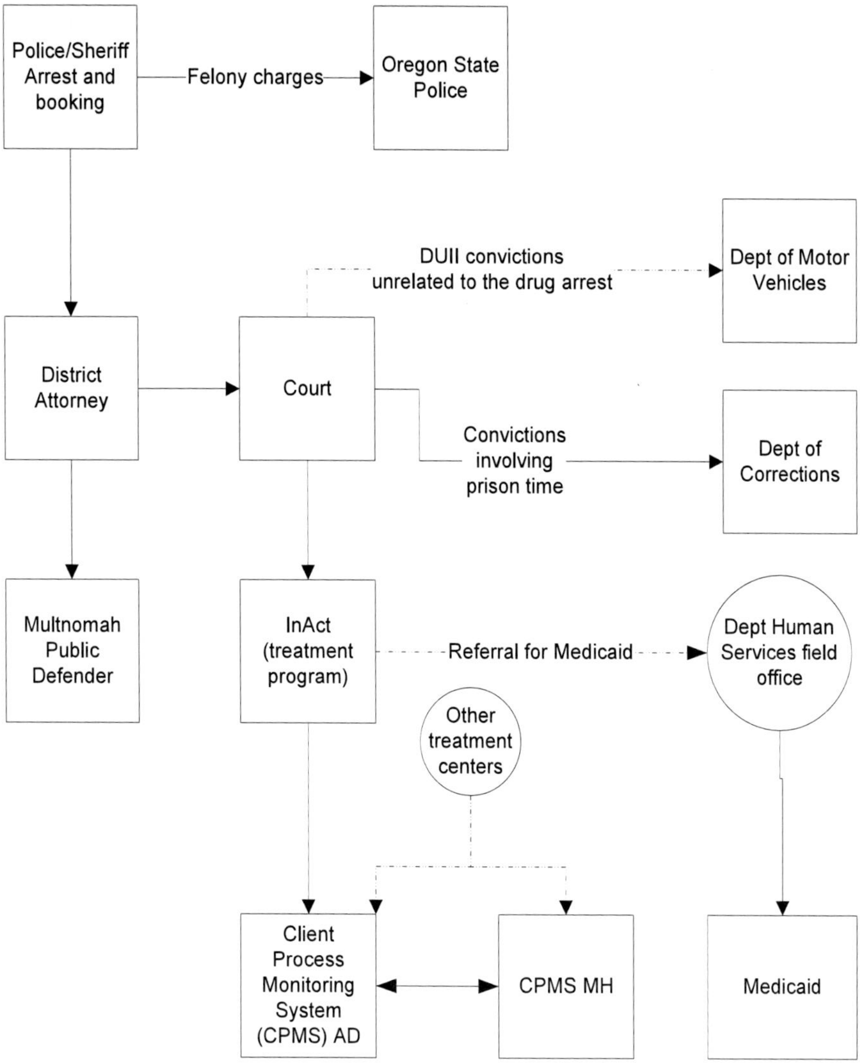

Figure 2. Compilation of data on offender cases.

We searched these data to find individuals who had more than one episode, finding close to 4% of such records. The demographic and identification data on cases were then sent to other agencies holding records on drug court offenders, under interagency agreements for matching cases across agencies. The sources of data were:

- *Multnomah County Public Defender:* District Attorney number; name; charge
- *Multnomah County District Attorney:* Incident charge details, arrest date, sentence, DOB, sex, police-recorded race, Portland Police Data System (PPDS) number, Oregon Driver's License (ODL) number, State Identification (SID) number, FBI ID, and up to five SSNs

- *Oregon State Police:* State Identification (SID) number associated with a fingerprint bio-marker, arrest incidents reported by Oregon county sheriffs, FBI ID, names, dates of birth, races, sexes, SSNs (note: in this relational data base, a SID points to all of the different identities and demographic values that the individual is known to have used)
- *Multnomah County Sheriff:* booking and release from county jail, SID (as provided to them by Oregon State Police)
- *Oregon State Department of Corrections:* SID, name, DOB, race, sex, convictions, admission and release from state prison
- *Oregon State Department of Transportation Driver and Motor Vehicles Services Division:* Oregon Driver's License (ODL), Driving Under Influence of Intoxicants (DUII) conviction dates; entry into diversion programs; license revocations (note: Driver and Motor Vehicles cannot by law provide name, although they can search on a name provided to them)
- *Oregon State Department of Human Services:* SSN, name, DOB, race, sex, dates of eligibility for Medicaid-paid drug and alcohol treatment episodes at hospital and outpatient facilities; admission and termination from publicly paid treatment episodes at community hospitals and state mental hospitals (with patient number), and community mental health and substance abuse treatment services (with Mental Health Information System number and coded name), especially those at drug court treatment provider InAct
- *InAct (the sole drug court treatment provider):* identifying and demographic data (as provided to them by drug court), admission date, "good days" (days in compliance with treatment regimen), termination date and status, and SSN

Agency Database Search and Matching Procedures

Each agency used its own searching and-or matching methods. Cases were returned with service data and additional demographic and identifiers (if available). Search and-or match procedures used by the agencies were as follows. Table 1 shows the numbers of the 1,939 study cases found in each agency's database.

Results

Multnomah County Public Defender and Multnomah County District Attorney

As was mentioned, we obtained a list of 2,153 cases potentially eligible for the research project from the Multnomah County Public Defender's (MPD) records and further identifying and demographic information from the District Attorney's (DA) Client Tracking database (DACT). We first found the State Identification (SID) number in the DACT where it was recorded in 1,465 of the 2,153 cases on that initial list.

Table 1. Agencies with matched cases

Agency with matched cases	Cases matched	Percent*
Multnomah County Sheriff	1782	91.9
Oregon State Police	1771	91.3
Driver and Motor Vehicles	1504	77.6
Medicaid	1020	52.6
Oregon Department of Corrections	891	46.0
Client Process Monitoring System (Substance Abuse)	787	40.6
Client Process Monitoring System (Mental Health)	377	19.4
State Mental Hospital	16	0.8

Percent of total study cases (N) = 1,939.

In other cases, individuals were not fingerprinted because (a) the officer processing the case expected the case to be non-reportable (to Oregon State Police), (b) the arrested individual was not able to be finger-printed (due to illness, for example) and was already known to booking officer, or (c) the individual was new to the system and a permanent SID was only assigned after the case has already been processed. For cases without SIDs, and which also have other incorrect identification, matching across databases is especially challenging.

Of the 2,153 cases originally selected from the list of persons eligible for drug court; 214 were discarded, leaving 1,939. Of the 214 cases discarded, 62 cases were removed because they spanned eras (before versus after Medicaid managed care) and therefore did not fit the study criteria, 34 because the charges against them had been dropped, 32 because they were still in the program (having been closed but later reopened, and open cases did not fit the study criteria), 24 because they had died during the program or within three years after the index date, 23 because of "merging cases" (cases that started out as separate were later determined to be the same case),19 because the "exit" was "miscellaneous disposition," seven because the District Attorney subsequently denied them program participation, seven because the case closing date came before the case opening date (bad data), three because the "exit" was "conditional discharge," and three for which a reason was not recorded.

Oregon State Police

The Oregon State Police (OSP) maintains a relational data base, the Law Enforcement Data System (LEDS) which uses as an identifier, the State Identification (SID) number that in turn is based on a bio-marker – namely fingerprints. In this system, fingerprints are converted to numeric bio-marker data at several levels of detail.

The SIDs are used in several ways. Local police use SIDs for known offenders already in their databases. Otherwise, local police assign temporary numbers and forward fingerprints to the OSP. The OSP searches LEDS for matching bio-markers, finds the SID and returns information to the local police. If a SID does not exist, the OSP forwards the fingerprints to a crime laboratory in San Francisco for matching against nation-wide records, returning the FBI ID number and data to the OSP where a new SID is created.

Matching on the SID became the gold standard for our study. It was the most reliable method in the state for identifying an individual. Most of the counties (approximately 20 of 36) use an automated system to check a person's identity against a fingerprint database. If the person has committed a crime in the past that led to the establishment of a SID, then the individual's identity can be established within a matter of hours at modernized facilities (such as Multnomah County).

OSP searched for records based on exact matches for SID, FBI ID, SSN (looking at each SSN digit individually) and also on first and last name, DOB, and sex considered together as a set. The OSP provided two tables that were extremely helpful in determining the weight of each potential match.

The first OSP table showed all the fields where OSP found matches in LEDS. This table also provided the SID the OSP had for that person.

The second OSP table showed all known alias and DOB combinations used by that person, an average of 7.8 name plus DOB combination for each case. Nine cases had more than 100 name plus DOB combinations with the highest being 162. The second OSP table aided the evaluation of matches made by all agencies, especially when the individual had used different identifying and demographic information in different agencies.

Of the ultimately valid 1,939 cases, the OSP found 1,771 valid matches (91.3%).

Multnomah County Sheriff

Potential matches were sought in two ways by the Sheriff. First, the Sheriff searched for matches using the SID (which is not their unique local ID, but is tracked by the Sheriff). Some 1,465 of the cases on our original list had a SID in the Public Defender / District Attorney databases. When no SID was available, the Sheriff searched by first and last name. When potential matches were found using this method, the Sheriff provided a SID for each (an additional 170 cases). Of the 1,939 ultimately valid cases, the Sheriff had found 1,782 valid matches (91.9%).

Oregon Department of Transportation Driver and Motor Vehicles Services Division

The Department of Transportation Driver and Motor Vehicles Services Division (DMV) searched their records in three ways and returned the results of each search in separate tables, which provided highly useful tools for evaluating each case. First, DMV looked for records based on the Oregon driver's license (ODL) number (when one was available). We had ODL for 1,221 of 2,153 on the original list. Next DMV searched using first name, last name, and year of birth considered together as a set. Finally, for 17 cases on our list that had neither an ODL nor a DOB listed, DMV searched on first and last name only. State law does not allow the DMV to give names to researchers, but we did receive sex, DOB, and the current county of residence for our cases to aid in match evaluation and assist in determining a consensus demographic picture. Keeping the possibility of identity theft and forged licenses in mind, we looked at the results in the following manner:

- When identical matches were found using ODL, name / year of birth, and the sex / DOB matched our sample, we gave the case the highest confidence in the match. We also placed more confidence in the sex / DOB when determining the consensus demographics because of the DMV's stringent proof of identity requirements. When a match was found using both methods, but these did not match each other, we looked to see if the sex and-or DOB matched our sample or the matches from other sources and made a decision based on the specifics of that case.
- When a match was made using ODL but not with name / year of birth, we compared the sex / DOB with the sample and the matches made by other sources. If they matched, we had high confidence whereas if they did not match, we kept the records but were less confident.
- When no match was found using the ODL (which we attributed to either a transcription error or to borrowed or forged license) or when no ODL was available, but one or more matches were found with the name / year of birth, we compared the sex and DOB with the sample and the matches made by other sources. If they matched, we had a medium to high confidence depending on how common the name in our sample was whereas if they did not match, we kept the records but were less confident.
- For the 17 cases where no ODL or DOB was recorded on the original list, we got some cases with no matches and some with many possible matches. Once again, we compared the sex with that listed in the sample and DOB with the matches made by other sources. Even when the demographics matched, our confidence was only medium.

Of the 1,939 ultimately valid cases, DMV found 1,504 valid matches (77.6%).

Oregon Department of Corrections

Potential matches were sought by the Department of Corrections (DOC) using a hierarchy that went from most reliable to least reliable basis for a match. If no match was found at one level (or if that variable was not available), DOC staff dropped down to the next level in the hierarchy. The hierarchy was, in descending order:

- SID (most reliable and most available)
- FBI ID (reliable but not available as often as SID)
- SSN
- Name and DOB, taken together

Of the 1,939 ultimately valid unique cases, DOC found 891 valid matches (46.0%).

Oregon Department of Human Services

The Department of Human Services (DHS) incorporates Medicaid as well as state-operated and publicly paid hospital and outpatient service episodes, including mental health and substance abuse services. Data are located in several different databases: Medicaid (using SSN), state mental hospital (using a patient identifier known as PTS), Mental Health (using an identifier from the Mental Health Information System or MHIS), and Substance Abuse (using MHIS). DHS searched for potential matches in three stages. First the DHS staff searched using a coded name (second, third, and fourth letters of the first and last name plus the DOB in MMDDYYYY format). If DHS staff found no match, they attempted exact matches using SSN. If that failed, staff looked up records by hand using the name and DOB. The DHS staff identified DOB, sex, race, and SSN (or PTS or MHIS) on file for each match they found.

Given the nature of the sample — as evidenced by so many aliases and SSNs being available for each person — our confidence in matches made with these data elements was not high unless the SSN and demographic data matched well with what was provided by other sources.

Of the 1,939 ultimately valid cases, DHS provided matches for 1,020 (52.6%) from Medicaid, 787 (40.6%) from substance abuse, 377 (19.4%) from mental health, and 16 (0.8%) from the state mental hospital.

InAct, Inc.

InAct, Inc. is the private outpatient substance abuse treatment facility subcontracted by the Oregon Department of Human Services substance abuse agency through Multnomah County and used by the Multnomah County drug court. InAct, Inc. records were matched using the District Attorney case number, which InAct staff obtained from a copy of the judge's docket. This approach enabled a one-to-one match of high confidence for any case where the person indicated he or she wanted to try the Multnomah County Department of Community Corrections Sanction, Treatment, Opportunity, Progress (STOP) drug court program. However, if the person indicated he or she did not want to try the program, the individual was not added to InAct's records. InAct provided name, DOB, sex, race and SSN (all of which were provided to InAct by the District Attorney and were on our list of cases).

Of the 1,939 ultimately valid cases, InAct found matches for the 867 who registered in the InAct program under the drug court.

When is a Match a Match?

We evaluated the validity of matches based on how a match was made, the number of agencies that found a match for a case, agreement of data elements across agencies for a case, and the flow of case information among agencies.

The State Identification number (SID) was our gold standard for identification, where available. The SID is a unique number assigned to a set of fingerprints and generated by the Oregon State Police. The SID indexes a relational database which includes many sets of information including names, arrests, convictions, and FBI ID. The SID is primarily used to track statewide arrest data ("criminal history"), but it is also a data element captured and used by other law enforcement agencies and some justice agencies. Many resources are used to determine if a set of fingerprints has been previously identified, both at the state level and with the FBI. Therefore the chance of two people sharing the same SID or of one person having two SIDs is extremely small.

The second highest level of confidence was generated by agencies searching once by a driver's license number and a second time by first and last name plus year of birth—and yielding with the same results both ways.

The third level of confidence was generated by agencies conducting a single search with a combination of identifiers.

The fourth level of confidence was obtained by agencies searching on a single variable, but finding other variables in agreement with those in the research data base.

Next, we did what computerized matching software cannot do. We looked at each case separately and made a judgment based on scenarios. For example, we saw matches when:

- There is only a slight difference in the spelling of the names and DOB or SSN are exact matches or close. "Sheryl" and "Cheryl" as likely first name matches and "Cooper" and "Copper" are likely to be last name matches if supported by agreement in other variables.
- One of the first names is a nickname for the other name such as "Cassie" and "Cassandra" or "Mike" and "Michael" and there is agreement in other variables.
- One name is included in or embedded in the other name such as last names of "Jenkins" and "Clark-Jenkins" and there is agreement in other variables.
- The last names differ but the first names match or are close, the subject is female, and DOB or SSN are exact matches or are similar.
- One name is an alternate spelling or homonym of the other such as "Bauers" and "Bowers" or "Louis" and "Lewis" and there is agreement in other variables.
- Sexes reported by agencies are different but the first name is strongly masculine or feminine and the majority of other variables were in agreement.
- The dates of birth are basically the same but a digit is missing from either the month or day and there is agreement in other variables, for example, 12/31/1969 and 2/31/1969 (a missing "1" in the month).
- Digits are transposed in the DOB, such as 12/31/1969 and 12/13/1969, and there is agreement in other variables.
- The month and day fields are transposed, such as 3/11/1969 and 11/3/1969, and there is agreement in other variables.
- The SSNs are basically the same except two numbers are transposed. We also treated transposed sections ("chunks") in the same way, but with some caution. For example, a match was declared if the first five digits matched and the last four digits were 4125 and 2541, and there is agreement in other variables.
- There is a difference in only one or two digits in the SSN and there is agreement in other variables, for example, 603-45-1111 and 603-45-1112.

(Note: although these examples represent actual cases, the identifiers have been fabricated for illustrative purposes.)

Table 2. Cases with matches in agency databases

Agencies	Cases	Percent of cases
0	79	4.07
1	44	2.27
2	174	8.97
3	373	19.24
4	394	20.32
5	352	18.15
6	365	18.82
7	153	7.89
8	5	0.26
Total	1,939	100.00

Agencies = number of agencies with matches for a given case (individual)
Cases = number of cases (individuals) with matches in the given number of agencies
Percent of cases = percent of study individuals (N = 1,939)

Race proved to be entirely undependable and was not used for matching. When age was less than 18 in all sources (*i.e.,* did not appear to be an erroneous DOB), we deleted the case because the study focused only on adults.

Most of the 1,939 cases were matched in several databases with an average of between three and four. Table 2 shows the agencies from which these matches came. About 600 of these matches included inconsistencies with the case identification and demographics found in the sample drawn from the Multnomah Public Defender and District Attorney databases. These inconsistencies led us to change sex in seven, race in 78, and age (DOB) in 126 of the ultimately valid cases.

In only 46 of the ultimately valid 1,939 cases did agencies other than Driver and Motor Vehicles find more than one possible match for a case we sent to them: nine in the Sheriff's database and 37 in the Oregon Department of Human Services data bases. However, there were 389 such cases in the Driver and Motor Vehicles database.

Case Examples

Following are examples showing approaches used to establish a case and the associated demographic descriptors.

Case 1. One example is a case (we concluded) for which the DOC, Sheriff, and OSP all found matches using the SID. The OSP had 24 different aliases using combinations of two first names, two last names, two middle names, and two dates of birth, and one of those combinations matched what was listed in the Public Defender - District Attorney list. These records also showed four SSNs, but no matches were found for medical services on those SSNs. When searching by name and year of birth, the DMV found a record that matched the sex and DOB exactly; when searching by ODL, they found a male with a completely different DOB that did not match any DOBs in the OSP database. This finding means there was a transcription error or that the driver's license was stolen or forged. The databases were consistent on race-ethnicity. Our conclusion was that this was a single case in which the individual is a male who was 41 years old on the index date.

Case 2. Another example is a case with exactly matched SID, SSN, name, DOB, sex, and services received across all databases. However, the race-ethnicity was white in some data bases and black in others and there was no logical way to determine which is correct. We concluded that this was a single case of unknown race.

Case 3. A case was matched on SID by OSP, Sheriff, and DOC. One of four aliases and a DOB from LEDS matched a record in the Sheriff's database. Two SSNs, differing by a single digit were found — one was used in the Medicaid database and the other in law enforcement databases. We concluded that these data represented a single male case.

Case 4. A case was matched on available data on all databases, except for two different Department of Human Services identification numbers on two identical sets of service records. Our conclusion was that a correction had been made to the database, but the original erroneous entries had not been deleted.

Case 5. A case was matched on SID but had different names and DOBs (mixed-and-matched) across agencies. The ODL matched DOB and some aliases in LEDS. All aliases were male names. We concluded that this was a single male case but of unknown name.

Case 6. We had only name, sex, and ODL. The name matched another in our database with a DOB but no ODL. The Portland Police database treated these entries as two different cases. The combined case matched another case in the Sheriff's database which matched one in the LEDS (on SID). The LEDS showed multiple arrests in multiple counties, including one arrest corresponding to the Sheriff's data on the incident arrest. A DMV search on ODL found the same name but different DOB from that found by the Sheriff. DMV also found two name-DOB matches. We concluded that these data represented one case, a white male of a certain age.

Case 7. This case also appeared twice in our sample. However, the case was matched on SID in LEDS, Sheriff, and DOC databases. The LEDS showed 16 different aliases, all with the same DOB, and three different SSNs. The second record in our sample had identical SID, FBI, Portland Police identifier, ODL, SSN, name and DOB. There was also another SSN which was used in accessing Medicaid coverage. We concluded this case was one person.

CONCLUSION

State and local databases are invaluable sources of information for program evaluation and policy research. However, goals and priorities of agencies maintaining databases, adversity of conditions under which data are collected, and shortage of database infrastructure (staff, equipment, and software) result in significant amounts of incomplete, inconsistent, and inaccurate information. Operational databases simply cannot achieve standards for resource-intensive research databases. Shared case registers improve data by necessitating reconciliation of information from the beginning. Matching software is useful for extracting a majority of linked data on a majority of cases. However, to obtain linked data on the remaining cases, a case-by-case examination is required—a labor-intensive and challenging task (Hser and Evans, 2008).

In this study we successfully undertook that linking task. In the course of this task, we discovered that the law enforcement system's identifier, based on a biomarker and containing all known variants of identifying and demographic data, was the gold standard.

While we received excellent cooperation and assistance from state and county agencies, we discovered that legal mandates (or lack thereof) are a barrier to the evaluation of state programs and policies. For example, one state agency refused to participate at all, despite requests from very high levels, despite easy and pre-tested logistics, despite having participated in similar research projects with other partners, and despite precedents in other states.

We found evidence that some clients of state programs access benefits and avoid detection of offenses by providing inaccurate identification and demographic information; some by obtaining multiple identification documents on false pretences, and some by borrowing, stealing, or forging them.

We also discovered that goals and priorities for data collection and maintenance differentially affect the completeness and accuracy of data. Case records at local providers do not always have corresponding records at state agencies, as mandated, in part because not all cases are cost-reimbursed by the state agency and, in part, because auditing does not take place.

Inadequate infrastructure for data-entry checking, auditing, and reconciliation makes it difficult to achieve and maintain data base completeness and accuracy. Beyond internal checking, comparison across databases would reveal conflicting dates of birth and sex for audit and reconciliation. Moreover, audit and reconciliation take place when required for agency operations, but not merely for the purpose of maintaining accurate data. For example, some databases accommodate multiple Social Security Numbers because they do, in fact, exist, but should not. Movement toward linked databases and state case registries may begin to resolve these reliability and validity problems.

We originally identified 2,153 potential cases. Had we used only an automated matching program, we may have identified roughly 1,500 matched cases, and we would have had many more missing demographic and service data. Of the 214 potential cases we deleted, most were because of the research project's inclusion and exclusion criteria. Only about 30 potential cases were deleted because of irresolvable data problems.

Ultimately, we identified 1,939 subjects we deemed valid unique cases, together with much of their identifying, demographic, and service data. The additional effort decreased sampling error substantially which increased precision of the research project's data analyses.

The following chapter is another example of research and evaluation pertaining to individuals who utilize services provided by multiple agencies – namely Medicaid clients involved with methadone maintenance treatment.

ACKNOWLEDGMENT

Supported in part by National Institute on Drug Abuse grant number R01 DA 013091.

REFERENCES

Hser, Y.-I., and Evans, E. (2008). Cross-system data linkage for treatment outcome evaluation: Lessons learned from the California Treatment Outcome Project. *Evaluation and Program Planning*, 31, 125-135

In: Medicaid and Treatment for People… ISBN 978-1-61470-742-4
Editor: B.H. McFarland, D.McCarty, et al, pp. 181-202

Chapter 8

MEDICAID AND METHADONE

Dennis Deck
RMC Research Corporation, Portland, OR, USA

ABSTRACT

This chapter describes a series of studies examining three facets of methadone maintenance treatment (MMT): access to care, retention in treatment, and outcomes. The work takes advantage of similarities and differences in MMT for the adjoining states of Oregon and Washington. Regarding access, much of the attention in prior research has focused on demonstrating the efficacy of methadone for treating opiate dependence. Very little, if any, research has been conducted on factors that influence access to care. This chapter addresses both systemic influences and client characteristics that predispose to use of services, reflect the need for services, or enable access to care. While MMT is usually considered a long-term form of substance abuse treatment, state systems differ in the typical duration of treatment. Although many previous studies have measured retention, few have examined the impact of Medicaid managed care. This chapter compares retention in a Medicaid managed care state with that in a fee for service state. Turning to outcomes, studies have shown a link between opiate use and crime and suggested that treatment for opiate addiction can reduce criminal activity. However, past studies have generally been short term. The project reported in this chapter followed the arrest history of clients for three years from an initial admission to MMT to take a unique look at the impact of treatment. In general, MMT access was strongly influenced by systemic factors such as geographic proximity to a treatment program as well as capacity. Medicaid coverage also predicted MMT access whereas Medicaid managed care *per se* had little or no impact. Retention in MMT was also strongly influenced by Medicaid coverage. Treatment duration (retention) was longer in Oregon (Medicaid managed care) than in Washington state (fee for service Medicaid). Provider practices (such as administrative discharges which were much less likely in Oregon versus Washington) also appeared to influence retention. Arrests were strongly related to time in MMT but especially so for clients with stable treatment patterns. Multi-level models suggested that long term (over 12 months) MMT retention led to greater than expected reduction in arrests.

Introduction

This chapter describes a series of studies that examine three facets of methadone maintenance treatment (MMT): access to care, retention in treatment, and outcomes. Here the importance of these concepts will be briefly reviewed. Trends over several years for publicly funded clients in the adjoining states of Oregon and Washington reveal similarities and differences in each component.

Access

Given the importance of MMT, it is surprising how little research has been conducted to examine individual and system characteristics influencing access to MMT. Indeed, much of the attention in prior research has focused on demonstrating the efficacy of methadone for treating opiate dependence. Very little, if any, research has been conducted on factors that influence access to care. There is interest both in systemic influences and in client characteristics that predispose to use of services, reflect the need for services, or enable access to care.

Among the most commonly cited explanations for the low access rates typically observed are financing, inaccessibility of methadone clinics, and stigma associated with heroin addiction (Lewis, 1999). Indeed, the majority of individuals admitted for opiate use (71%) are either unemployed or not in the labor force. Nevertheless, in 1999 only 25 states covered MMT in their Medicaid plans (McCarty et al., 1999). In those states that do offer treatment, limited capacity inhibits providers from meeting the high demand. Furthermore, individuals living in areas that lack treatment centers, especially rural areas, are less likely to receive treatment (Deck et al., 2000; Farabee et al., 1998; Greenfield et al. 1996).

To remedy this situation, government oversight has shifted toward accreditation standards similar to those in effect for other health care organizations. Provisions in government regulation should permit the development of new delivery models and changes in provider practice, such as take-home doses, which may help expand the availability of MMT, especially in rural and suburban settings (Substance Abuse and Mental Health Services Administration, 2002). Such changes may, however, take months or years to improve access to treatment.

Of those states that cover methadone treatment through Medicaid, 12 utilize managed care programs (McCarty et al., 1999). One of the primary concerns about managed care is that financial incentives associated with managed care will reduce access to substance abuse treatment (Zarkin and Dunlap, 1999). Appropriate care management could, however, improve access to mental health and substance abuse treatment while maintaining the quality of care. For example, analyses of Medicaid recipients enrolled in Massachusetts' behavioral health carve-out and Oregon's prepaid health plans suggest that access to substance abuse services overall increased under managed care (Deck et al, 2000; McCarty et al., 1999). However, even in Oregon, where the introduction of managed care was associated with expanded access to substance abuse treatment as a whole, access to methadone treatment decreased during the same period (Deck et al., 2000; Deck and Carlson, 2004). On the other hand, following the introduction of the Medicaid behavioral health carve-out in Massachusetts, methadone utilization increased by 20% (Steenrod et al., 2001). Examinations of the National Drug Abuse Treatment System Survey (NDATSS) suggest that the extent of penetration of managed care enrollment within the treatment facility influences the impact of managed care on access to substance abuse treatment. In the NDATSS, treatment providers with very high and very low managed care penetration demonstrated better access compared to organizations with more moderate penetration (Alexander et al., 2003). Therefore, the present project addressed managed care in the analyses pertaining to access. Following the access analyses, attention was also focused on retention in treatment.

Retention

Decades of research have provided abundant evidence that duration of substance abuse treatment, particularly MMT, is associated with improved outcomes (Cacciola et al., 1998; Hubbard et al., 1997; Maddux and Desmond, 1997; National Institutes of Health, 1998; Sees et al., 2000; Simpson, Joe, and Brown, 1997; Simpson, Joe, Chatham, et al, 1997; Simpson and Sells, 1982; Ward et al., 1999; Zhang et al., 2003). Based on the accumulation of evidence, the nation's leading substance abuse and health care providers, researchers, and policy makers issued a national consensus statement indicating that "continuity of treatment is crucial–patients who are treated for less than 3 months generally show little or no improvement, and most, if not all, patients require continuous treatment for many years, and perhaps for life." (National Institutes of Health, 1998, p. 1940).

Retention estimates for MMT from two large national studies, the National Treatment Improvement Evaluation Study (NTIES; Zhang et al., 2003) and the Drug Abuse Treatment Outcome Studies (DATOS; Simpson, Joe, Broome, et al., 1997) indicated that median retention ranged from nine months to 12 months, respectively. There was, however, wide variation across treatment providers. In DATOS, for example, the percentage of patients retained for 360 days ranged from 15% to 76%. Other studies that examine retention have reported average lengths of stay as low as four to six months and as high as 23 months (Friedmann et al., 2001; Greenfield et al. 1996; Hubbard et al., 1989; Magura et al., 1998) and one-year retention rates range from 25% to over 70% (Rowan-Szal et al., 2000; Simpson, Joe, Chatham, et al., 1997). Although there is little agreement about appropriate duration of treatment, which depends to a great extent on the individual and the goals of treatment, 12 months has been commonly suggested as the minimum necessary to achieve clinical benefit for most adult patients.

While the importance of retention in MMT has been well documented, there are still several gaps in thc literature. Few studies have examined treatment or system level characteristics including financing arrangements, treatment practices, and geographic considerations.

For example, it has been suggested that managed care may negatively influence retention in substance abuse services through utilization management practices including gate-keeping and concurrent review that may serve to shorten the duration of treatment (Simpson, Joe, and Brown, 1997). In many cases, the literature supports this concern (Steenrod et al., 2001). However, very few studies have examined the impact of managed care on retention in methadone maintenance and even fewer have examined whether predictors of retention differ in a managed care environment compared with non-managed care.

In addition, lack of insurance to cover treatment may influence treatment retention. For example, Garcia and colleagues (Garcia et al., 1999) found that uninsured clients enrolled in a nonprofit drug treatment program were 3.4 times less likely than others to complete treatment. These findings suggest that a majority of individuals seeking treatment must rely on either public funding or find a way to manage the fees on their own.

While the research literature suggests that improved retention should be associated with fewer arrests, less dependence on public assistance, less reliance on emergency health services, reduced Human Immuno-deficiency Virus (HIV) risk, and other important outcomes, this contention has not been verified in a naturalistic setting on a large scale. Such research would be particularly important in the current climate of state deficits and the pressure that has been put on Medicaid programs. To cite just one example, in March of 2003, the Oregon legislature removed the substance abuse and mental health benefit for a Medicaid expansion population in reaction to rising Medicaid costs that the state was experiencing due to an unprecedented budget deficit. The present project therefore examined MMT retention with emphases on managed care and financing. This work is important because it is believed that retention in MMT reduces crime and arrests.

Arrests

Addiction to heroin is often associated with criminal activity. Numerous studies have indicated that substance abuse treatment is effective in decreasing both substance use and criminal activities (Hubbard et al., 1997; Simpson, Joe, Broome, et al., 1997). National evaluations of treatment, including the Drug Abuse Reporting Program (Sells and Simpson, 1980), the Treatment Outcome Prospective Study (TOPS; Hubbard et al., 1989), the National Treatment Improvement Evaluation Study (NTIES; Center for Substance Abuse Treatment, 1995), and the Drug Abuse Treatment Outcome Study (DATOS; Hubbard et al., 1997) have documented decreases in opiate use and criminal involvement after treatment. Furthermore, longer retention in treatment is associated with more favorable outcomes (Hubbard et al., 1989; Sells and Simpson, 1980;Simpson and Sells, 1982). Compared to other modalities, MMT has been found to be an effective mode of treatment for reducing heroin use and criminal behaviors (Anglin et al., 1982; Anglin and McGlothlin, 1984; Marsch, 1998; Simpson and Sells, 1982). These findings are echoed in DATOS where follow-up measures indicated a 69% decline in the number of weekly heroin users and a 52% decline in illegal activity (Hubbard et al., 1997).

However, many opiate addicts do not receive methadone. A National Institutes of Health expert panel noted that less than 20% of the estimated 600,000 opiate addicts were participating in methadone maintenance treatment programs. Individuals with more severe substance abuse problems tend not to have either private or public insurance (Frank and McGuire, 1995; Oggins, 2003). In the DATOS study, for instance, only 10% of the clients admitted to methadone treatment had private insurance (Hubbard et al. 1997).

Researchers examining the consequences of terminating clients from methadone maintenance programs, either due to loss of funding for a clinic or loss of coverage for a client's treatment, have found that a majority of the clients are unable to pay out of pocket for methadone treatment (Rosenbaum et al., 1996). Most notably, when clients were forced to discontinue methadone treatment because of clinic closures, they were likely to return to heroin use and to be involved in criminal activities (Anglin et al., 1989; Rosenbaum et al., 1996; Rosenbaum et al., 1987). These studies suggested that financial concerns played a major role in a client's ability to continue treatment. For instance, Rosenbaum, Murphy, and Beck (1987) reported that implementing a client fee was associated with an increase in criminal activities, incarcerations, heroin use, and hospitalizations. Similarly, Anglin and colleagues (Anglin et al., 1989) found that among clients who were terminated from a publicly funded MMT program, only 43% were able to continue their treatment by transferring to a private methadone clinic. Another study examining the effects of closing publicly funded methadone clinics found that within 24 months 54% of the clients were using heroin and 73% had been rearrested (McGlothlin and Anglin, 1991). Therefore, the present project examined arrests in detail. The work was guided by a conceptual model.

Conceptual Model

The behavioral model of utilization described by Andersen (Andersen, 1995; see also Aday and Andersen, 1974; Gelberg et al., 2000) provides a useful organizer for the study of treatment process and outcomes. According to this model, individuals' health care utilization is a function of their predisposition to use services, their need for care, and factors that enable or impede the use of services. Furthermore, systemic factors are thought to influence the final placement decision.

The behavioral model has evolved over time, and the choice of factors to measure and their placement in the model may differ depending on the population studied. The model served as a guide in selecting and organizing predictors. It also served to call attention to important provider and systemic factors that should be considered in interpreting the results even though only proxy empirical measures were available. Figure 1 illustrates a reformulation of the behavioral model for methadone services. The work took place in the adjacent states of Oregon and Washington.

Oregon and Washington

Oregon and Washington have long covered methadone services under Medicaid. These neighboring states were similar in many ways—geography, client demographics, and treatment systems. Both states had similar data systems for documenting both Medicaid eligibility and use of substance abuse treatment services. The data sets included suitable measures of all three categories of individual characteristics: predisposing factors including demographic characteristics and Medicaid eligibility category; need characteristics including years of drug use, polydrug use, history of substance abuse treatment, and mental illness; and enabling characteristics including income, stability of Medicaid enrollment, geographic proximity to a methadone clinic, marital status, living situation, employment status, and criminal behavior history.

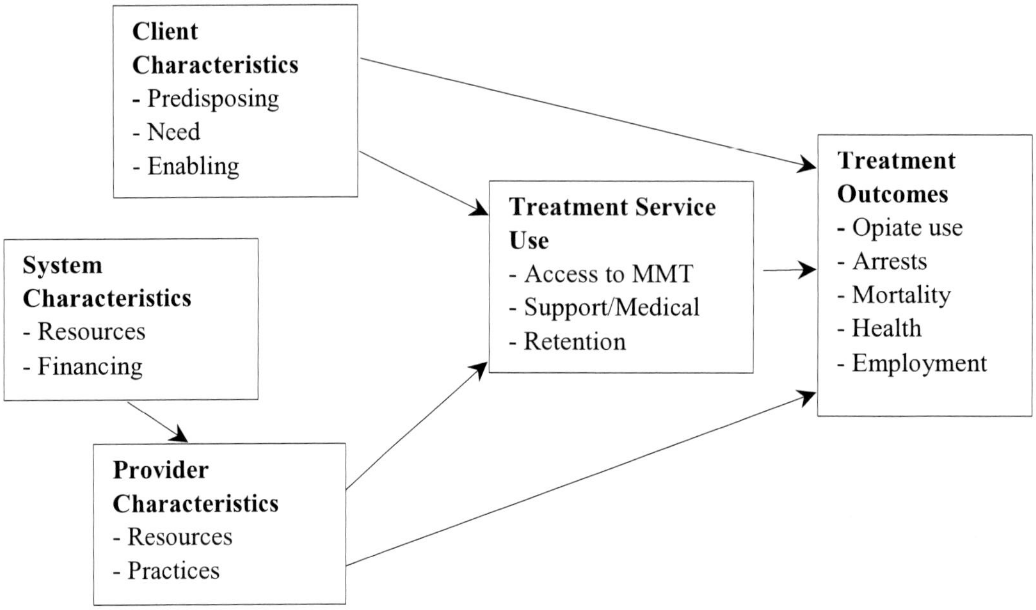

Figure 1. Conceptual model describing characteristics that affect service use and outcomes of methadone treatment.

State Practices in Oregon and Washington

As noted, Oregon and Washington were two of the 25 states that covered MMT as a Medicaid benefit. In both states, methadone clinics were geographically limited to the four most populous counties. However, there were some notable differences as well. One key difference was that Oregon shifted to managed care for Medicaid (Deck et al., 2000) while Washington retained a fee for service model. At the same time, there were anecdotal reports that MMT services in Washington were difficult to obtain with long waiting lists while there was no such issue apparent in Oregon.

Oregon provided full coverage for methadone under Medicaid managed care and administered the benefit through prepaid health plans. Enrollment in a prepaid health plan was mandated in most counties. In May 1995 the Oregon Health Plan (OHP) integrated the chemical dependency benefit with physical health care and took measures to prevent problems encountered in other demonstration projects. For example, patient placement criteria ensure that placement decisions are based on patient needs rather than financial considerations (Deck et al., 2003). A Section 1115 waiver, obtained from the Centers for Medicaid and Medicare Services, allowed Oregon to expand Medicaid coverage to all adults and their dependents who fell below the federal poverty level. (Deck et al., 2000)

While the neighboring state of Washington is geographically and demographically similar, substance abuse services were state administered and providers were reimbursed for treatment services to Medicaid recipients on a fee-for-service basis. Although Washington provided full coverage for MMT, matching funds are scarce and legislation limits the size and location of methadone clinics.

METHODS

To prepare data from the two states to follow the logic model, it was necessary to obtain and link client records from multiple state databases. Medicaid eligibility files identified the population of interest in each state. Client characteristics and treatment service use were available from the state treatment databases, Oregon's Client Process Monitoring System (CPMS) and Washington's Treatment and Report Generation Tool (TARGET), that track admissions and discharges to publicly funded treatment. Arrest data were obtained from the state police in each state. To link client records within each state from multiple data files, both deterministic and probabilistic algorithms were applied. A sophisticated data linkage package was adapted for this project (Campbell et al., 2006; Campbell et al., 2008).

RESULTS

Access

The number of eligible clients changed dramatically over the years in question in both states. To minimize the impact of this change, MMT access rates (admissions per 1,000 eligible clients) were calculated.

Figure 2 shows the MMT access rates in Oregon and Washington for the nine-year period from 1992 through 2000. The total unduplicated number of individuals admitted for treatment of opiate use in each year is included for context. As the number of individuals admitted increased to about 2000 in each state, access rates declined by 15 to 20 percentage points to a rate that was about two thirds of the previous rate. The change in access between the 1992 and 1996 cohorts was significant for both Oregon ($\chi^2 = 80.9$, $p < .001$) and Washington ($\chi^2 = 62.9$, $p < .001$). Access to MMT remained higher among opiate admissions in Oregon in all years.

The study also included logistic regression equations to predict access to MMT. Predictors were selected to represent predisposing, need, and enabling characteristics. While those results are not discussed here, one finding provides some insight for readers not particularly familiar with these two states. Proximity to methadone clinics was a strong predictor of access to MMT in both states. Individuals living in rural counties not adjacent to a county with a methadone clinic were about one fifth as likely to gain access to methadone compared to those living in counties with a methadone clinic in Oregon and only one tenth as likely in Washington (see Figure 3). The farther a client lives from the nearest methadone clinic the lower the probability of being placed in methadone maintenance treatment (MMT).

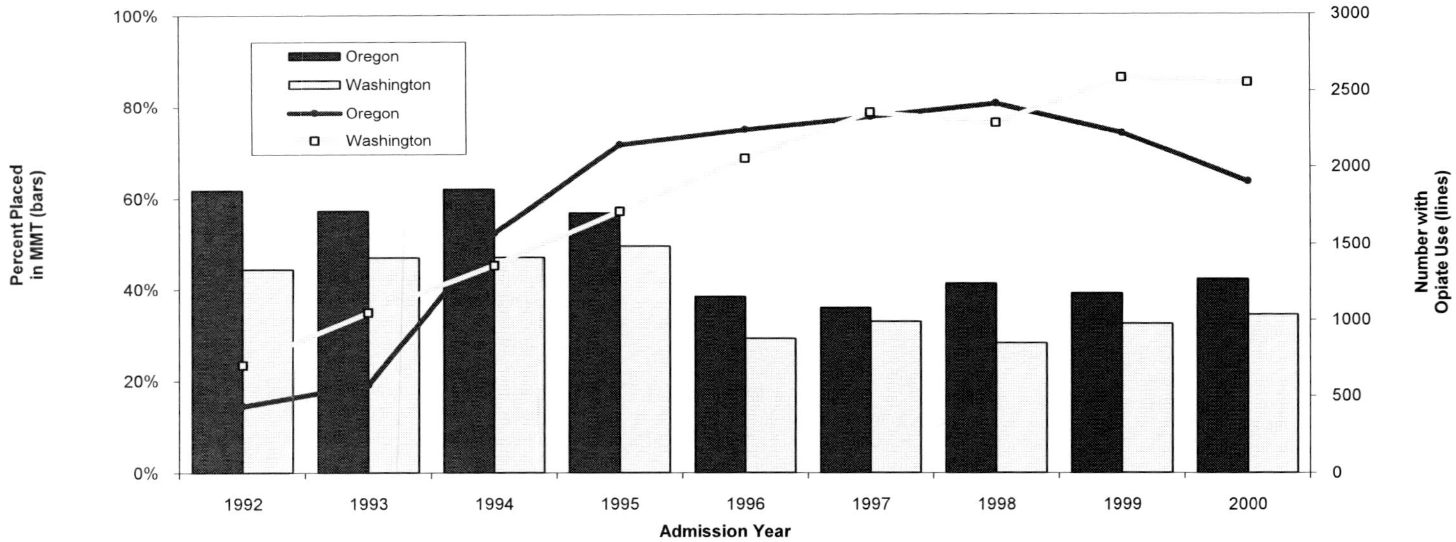

Figure 2. Methadone maintenance treatment (MMT) access rates by state and year.

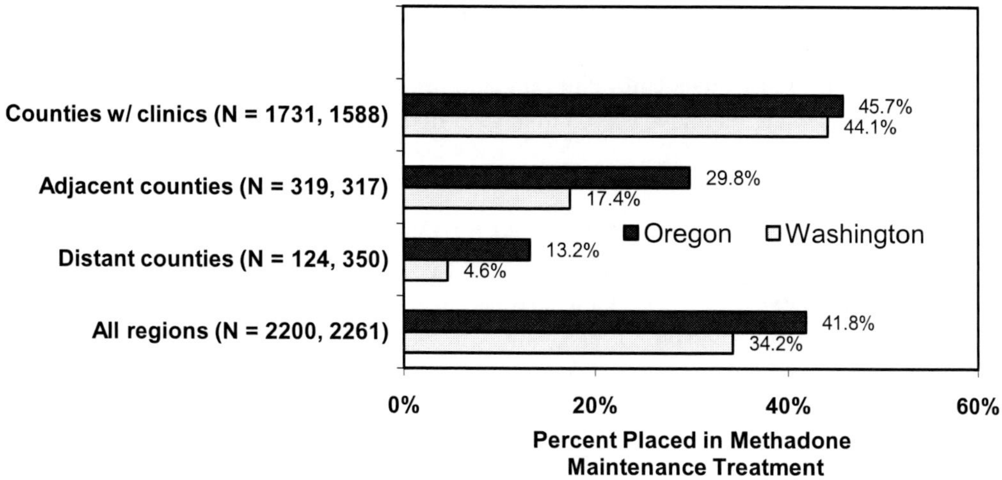

Figure 3. Methadone maintenance placements as a function of proximity to methadone clinics.

FINANCING AND CAPACITY

As the number of Medicaid-eligible adults admitted for treatment of opiate use increased in both Oregon and Washington, access rates declined sharply before leveling off. While shifts in the characteristics of these adults accounted for some of the change in access, the primary mechanism is probably due to constraints on funding and capacity. A focus group of methadone providers, state officials, managed care representatives, and researchers from both states helped the research team interpret these findings.

In Washington, a scarcity of matching funds and limits on the size and location of methadone clinics have conspired to restrict the availability of MMT. Fortunately, some of these barriers were removed during the 2001 legislative session. The state also puts an emphasis on residential services, especially for the indigent. In Oregon, expanded eligibility provided coverage to a large group of previously uninsured adults with a relatively high prevalence of opiate use, resulting in a dramatic increase in the number of MMT admissions between 1992 and 1995. After 1995 access to MMT in Oregon appears, however, also to have been limited by capacity despite evidence that access to substance abuse treatment in general increased (Deck et al., 2000; Deck and McFarland, 2002).

Despite concerns that the shift to managed care in Oregon might result in reduced use of substance abuse treatment services, in general access increased subsequent to the integration of the chemical dependency benefit with physical health care under the OHP (Deck et al., 2000; Deck and McFarland, 2002). The results for MMT services are, however, mixed. Expanded Medicaid eligibility resulted in a dramatic increase in the number of admissions for opiate use and the number of individuals placed in methadone programs, but the percentage of MMT placements dropped. Some health plan officials reported that opiate dependence was treated like other chronic illnesses—that is, treatment was essentially an entitlement—and MMT access rates were relatively high for these health plans. Some anecdotal evidence did, however, suggest that although prepaid health plans adopted a generally open policy toward MMT and did not deny services, they did exert some control over access. Examples of control mechanisms include establishing contracts with only a single methadone provider and temporarily freezing new admissions to MMT. Methadone providers typically received discounted rates for individuals enrolled in prepaid health plans (typically 75% to 85% of the state rate). The discount may have served to deter providers from expanding capacity.

Factors Influencing Access

As expected, demographic characteristics were not good predictors of access. Furthermore, no evidence in the current study suggests racial disparities in MMT in either state. Modest differences were observed for Washington whites, males, and the disabled as well as expansion category adults in Oregon.

In contrast, most need characteristics were significant predictors of access. Years of opiate use and needle use promoted access in both states. Prior use of MMT services was also a strong predictor of a methadone placement. Polydrug use, at least in the case of alcohol and amphetamines, hindered access in both states, perhaps because other modalities were viewed as effective in treating at least the secondary drug.

After controlling for predisposing and need client characteristics, adding enabling factors dramatically improved the prediction of access in both states. Thus a client's means of accessing care are particularly important determinants of access to MMT. This finding has systemic implications because these factors are more a function of state policies and provider practices than the predisposing or need characteristics.

Access to MMT has remained extremely limited in Oregon counties with no methadone clinic, especially in the rural portions of the state. Compared to Oregon, MMT services were more limited in Washington. Several factors, including the limited availability of treatment slots, appear to have acted as service delivery constraints that in turn have resulted in lower access.

Loss of Coverage

Late in 2002, news broke that the legislative finance committee in Oregon had taken a dramatic step to address a major budget shortfall in the state. As will be described in detail in later chapters, the legislature adopted premiums and co-payments for sub-groups of Medicaid clients (Mann and Artiga, 2004). Moreover, a large group of Medicaid clients (who are often not covered in other states) would lose coverage for substance abuse treatment, mental health treatment, or dental services starting March 2003. Although eventually coverage was partially restored for these clients in August 2004, the change created an unprecedented opportunity to examine MMT access rates before and after the removal of coverage.

Opiate Admission Rates

A descriptive study was conducted to document the effects of the benefit cut (Deck et al., 2006). By extending the time frames for the prior data extracts to cover this change, the study team was able to examine treatment and Medicaid eligibility records over a longer period. It was possible to compare methadone access rates for the year following the cut to rates during the year before the cuts for two large Medicaid eligibility groups, one which sustained the loss of coverage and another that retained coverage.

The loss of coverage affected a Medicaid expansion program for single adults and childless couples known as OHP Standard. There was no change in coverage for clients in mandatory categories, know collectively as OHP Plus. An extract of Oregon eligibility and treatment data covering 2002 and 2003 was prepared. This extract included 1,689 clients admitted to treatment for opiate dependence before the benefit cut and 555 adults admitted after the cut. Propensity scores were calculated to adjust for any differences between the two groups.

Analysis revealed that the 2003 cohort was heavily weighted by clients who had a prior treatment history. This finding suggested that the change had ended the normal influx of new clients addicted to opiates who had not previously been served by the substance abuse treatment system. Propensity scores were used to adjust for this change.

Figure 4 summarizes the number of new admissions for opiate addiction by month among OHP Standard adults as a rate per 1,000 eligible. Transfers between clinics or treatment modalities were excluded. The total count of adults addicted to opiates presenting for the first time for publicly funded treatment decreased by 84% for the last 3 quarters of 2003 compared to the same months in 2002. That drop represents a 59% decrease when expressed as a rate to control for the overall reduction in OHP Standard enrollments.

For comparison, Figure 4 also traces the monthly admission rates for opiate use among OHP Plus adults, again expressed as a rate. This group includes those eligible under the federally mandated programs and thus represents the traditional Medicaid population. This group showed no change in coverage and no disenrollment from Medicaid. Even for this group an unexpected 16% decrease in opiate admissions was observed in 2003 after the changes took effect in March, compared to 2002 for the same group.

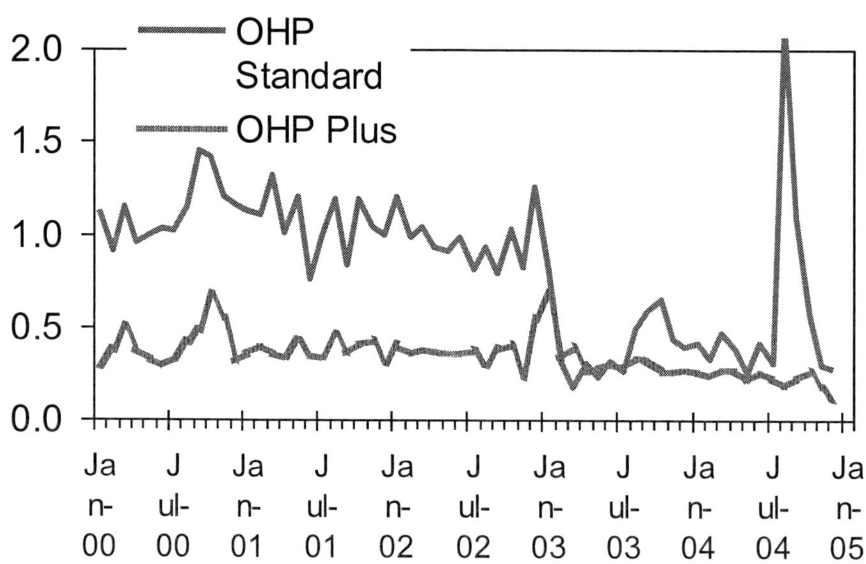

Figure 4. Oregon adult substance abuse treatment admissions for opiate addiction per thousand Medicaid clients enrolled by eligibility category before and after coverage was dropped.

The figure also shows a strong spike in admissions following the partial restoration of the benefit in August 2004. Only clients who had maintained their Medicaid eligibility could take advantage of the restored substance abuse treatment benefit so the rate was not sustained.

PROVIDER EXPERIENCE

Interviews with methadone providers confirmed that the apparent impact of the benefit cut was immediate and strongly felt (Laws et al., 2005–2007). For most providers, OHP Standard clients represented a substantial portion of their Medicaid caseload and thus a significant portion of their income. Two clinics closed their doors. The remaining ten clinics reported clinical staff lay offs, reductions in their staff's work week, elimination of staff health benefits, and other cost saving measures such as less individual contact with patients, increased treatment group size, and less urine analysis monitoring. Both treatment providers and patients began preparing for the loss of coverage even before the cut took effect.

A surprising number of patients elected to pay out of pocket after losing the benefit. Usually only those who had some source of income (from a job, family or friends or criminal activity) were able to do so. Treatment providers reported that as early as two months prior to the benefit cut, many patients were requesting methadone detoxification, as this approach provided a longer window of time than the minimum of 21 days required by the state if they waited until March 1. According to treatment providers, patients are reluctant to restart treatment even with restored benefits because providers could not assure them benefits would not be cut again, and the thought of going through another painful detoxification is something they did not want to endure.

There were, however, isolated instances of collaborative action to mitigate the impact of the benefit cut. In one area, the county, the hospital and the health plan split the costs of continuing to treat methadone patients who lost their benefit. A large urban county paid for some substance abuse treatment services through a special referendum that provided temporary (up to three years) funding for a variety of educational and social services.

RETENTION

A retention study was conducted to examine the impact of individual, treatment, and system-level characteristics on 12-month retention rates (Deck and Carlson, 2005). Administrative data collected over a nine-year period from the state substance abuse treatment agencies of the two states were analyzed to identify trends in utilization of MMT. In addition to examining individual and treatment characteristics, this study assessed the impact of system characteristics, including the introduction of managed care in Oregon, and the geographic distribution of methadone clinics in both states.

Retention was defined as continuous enrollment in an index treatment episode without discharge for at least 12 months following the admission date. The retention rates were calculated as the number of individuals retained in MMT for 12 months divided by the number of individuals admitted to MMT during the same period. The rates were expressed as percentages. The dependent variable for the logistic regressions was a binary variable coded as 1 if the patient was still enrolled in the index episode after 12 months and 0 if discharged prior to 12 months.

Figure 5 shows the percentage of Medicaid-eligible adults enrolled in methadone maintenance programs who were retained in treatment at least one year. The retention rates are presented by admission year cohort for each state. In Oregon, the retention rates doubled, from a low of 25% in 1994 to 50% in 1998 ($\chi^2 = 306.55$, $p < .001$, $N = 6{,}863$). In contrast, the retention rates in Washington increased only slightly, from 28% to 33%, during the same period ($\chi^2 = 8.6$, $p < .01$, $N = 5{,}308$).

To confirm that those results were not affected by the changes in the makeup of the sample, a second set of analyses was conducted. Only adults eligible under the disabled and welfare categories were included because the characteristics of these two groups were relatively stable during the study period. In Oregon, the retention rates for the stable subgroup paralleled those for the entire sample, ranging from 23% in 1994 to a high of 57% in 1998 ($\chi^2 = 113.8$, $p < .001$, $N = 1{,}840$). In Washington, the subgroup retention rates ranged from 27% to 36% during the same period ($\chi^2 = 12.6$, $p < .001$, $N = 3{,}756$).

The work also included a logistic regression predicting retention in each state. The most important enabling characteristic was stable Medicaid eligibility (defined as eligible at least 22 out of the first 24 weeks following admission). In Oregon, where a high proportion of the sample was in the expansion eligibility category and known to have difficulty staying eligible and enrolled, those with stable eligibility were about two and a half times as likely to be retained. In Washington, those with stable eligibility were about two thirds more likely to be retained.

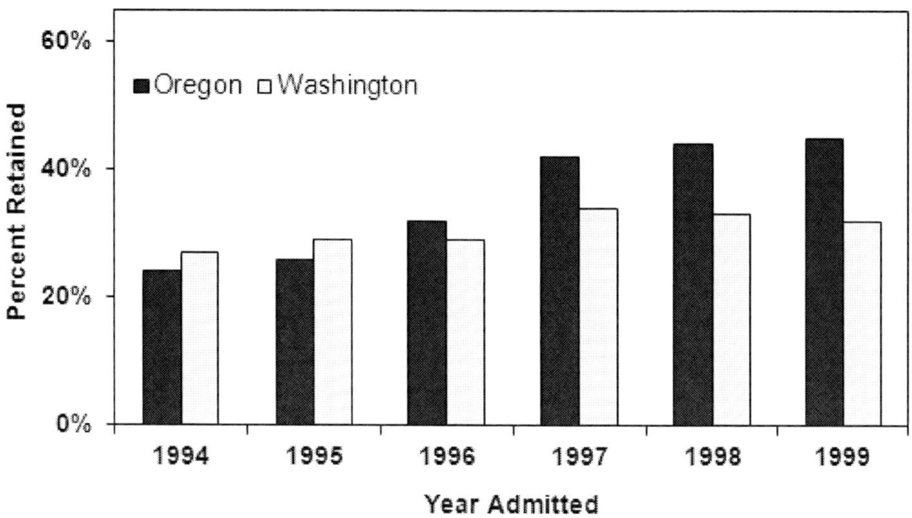

Figure 5. Retention rates by admission cohort for adults (ages 18–64) entering methadone maintenance programs in Oregon (N = 6,863) and Washington (N = 5,308).

There was also a time effect. Each successive admission year cohort was compared to 1994, the last year that treatment services were reimbursed on a fee-for-service basis under the OHP. In Oregon, the 1997, 1998, and 1999 cohorts were more likely retained, even after controlling for the comprehensive set of individual characteristics. The odds of retention for the 1998 cohort were about 3.5 times that of the 1994 cohort. In Washington, the odds of retention were marginally significant for the 1997 cohort but the overall test for the admission cohort factor was not significant.

Each of the largest agencies providing publicly funded methadone services within each state was compared to the average across providers for that state. In Oregon, two agencies achieved better than average retention controlling for patient characteristics, while another agency reported below average retention. One of these was well known for its emphasis on retention as well as its selective admission practices. A low retention agency was forced to close during the study period. In Washington, two small agencies differed in retention after controlling for patient differences. Both were Oregon providers serving individuals from nearby Clark County in Washington State under a special contract. The differences observed may be partly confounded with contracting issues.

FACTORS INFLUENCING RETENTION

Despite concerns that the shift to managed care in Oregon might result in reduced use of substance abuse treatment services, utilization of MMT increased noticeably under the OHP. Our study of access (Deck and Carlson, 2004) showed that although the number of patients entering MMT increased dramatically, the proportion of opiate dependent adults admitted to MMT actually decreased. This outcome occurred despite an overall improvement in access to substance abuse services for the general Medicaid population (Deck et al., 2000), thus ruling access out as the mechanism driving utilization rates.

The retention study suggested that the percentage retained dramatically increased subsequent to the integration of the chemical dependency benefit with physical health care under the OHP. No such increase was observed in Washington State, controlling for the same patient factors. While state differences in financing for MMT seemed the most plausible causal factor, a more systematic approach for considering alternative explanations seemed desirable. The research team convened an advisory panel of methadone providers, state officials, managed care representatives, and researchers from both states to identify and evaluate alternative hypotheses. The general conclusion of the panel was that at the provider level there were shifts in philosophy and changes in dosing practices in both states. However, state differences in financing influenced system capacity and provider practices differentially in the two states, and probably accounted for the more pronounced increase in utilization in Oregon.

Providers from both states reported that emerging findings from research on dosing practices led them to use higher methadone doses for many of their patients starting around 1997. Dosing level is one of the few methadone practices that has received much attention in the literature and has consistently been associated with better retention or other outcomes. At the same time, the prevailing philosophy about the role of methadone treatment shifted to focus on long-term maintenance and away from one that promoted a long-term abstinence goal. However, these changes were gradual, somewhat variable across providers, and subject to the realities of available funding and other constraints. Moreover, because providers in both states reported shifting to higher doses during the study period, dosing level did not appear to explain the differential retention patterns observed.

Washington providers reported that a scarcity of matching funds and limits on the size and location of methadone clinics conspired to restrict the availability of MMT. Fortunately, some of these barriers were removed during the 2001 legislative session, but during the study period providers reported long waiting lists. Two consequences of limited capacity were pressure to move patients out of treatment and a low tolerance for rule violations. In the words of one provider, clinicians "faced a moral dilemma"—to keep serving chronic rule violators or administratively discharge them to take on a new patient from the waiting list (Jackson, 2002). The treatment data appear to confirm this proposition. For 1994–1995 admissions, administrative discharges accounted for only 22% of the Oregon sample but 45% of the Washington sample. For 1998–1999 admissions, administrative discharges were down to 14% in Oregon but 37% in Washington.

In Oregon, expanded eligibility in 1994 provided coverage to a large group of previously uninsured adults with a relatively high prevalence of opiate use, resulting in a dramatic increase in the number of patients with coverage for substance abuse treatment, including methadone. The state imposed few limits on the services covered by the benefit. Consequently, provider capacity increased statewide during the early part of the study period. When prepaid health plans took over responsibility for the chemical dependency benefit in 1995, most adopted a generous posture toward substance abuse services, including methadone, often citing expected long term reductions in overall health costs. Most plans quickly moved away from managing care for individual patients but did implement quality assurance procedures during the latter part of the study period.

In contrast to Washington, Oregon providers reported no significant waiting lists and suggested that they had become more focused on retaining patients, even in light of rule violations. Subsequent analyses confirmed that of those not retained after 12 months, nearly 60% of the Washington patients were administratively discharged while 20% or less of the Oregon patients were discharged for rule violations. While this finding is consistent with the reported state differences in provider practices, more work is needed to determine whether this result adequately explains the differential trends in retention rates.

ARRESTS

A final study was conducted to examine the impact of sustained MMT on the likelihood of arrests. The hypothesis was that Medicaid coverage significantly improves access to MMT and that months in MMT significantly reduces the likelihood of felony arrests (Deck et al., 2009).

To examine arrests over time, each data set was converted into a set of monthly records covering a span of up to three years for each client. Both probabilistic and deterministic algorithms were applied to link records for a given client across data sets. Propensity score analysis was used to control for differences in client characteristics over time. Hierarchical linear models were used to estimate the effects of treatment over time. Parallel analyses were conducted with the Oregon and Washington samples.

Figure 6 shows the observed probability of felony or gross misdemeanor arrests in a given month for Oregon clients by treatment status for individuals with or without a prior history of arrest. Clients with at least one arrest in the year prior to the target treatment admission were about twice as likely to be arrested in a given month during the observation period. The probability of arrests was much lower during months in methadone maintenance treatment (solid line) compared to months untreated (dashed line). The red lines show results for individuals with a prior history of arrest (arrested at least once in the year prior to the initial opiate admission) and the blue lines show results for individuals with no arrests in the prior year. Arrests are much less likely as long as there is stable methadone enrollment.

The Washington model produced very similar results. Figure 7 shows a similar pattern in arrest rates. The probability of arrest was much lower during months in MMT than in months untreated, but again this relationship held only for clients with relatively stable MMT enrollment. As with Oregon, arrests were much less likely when enrolled in MMT as long as there is stable enrollment over time. A prior paper with a different sample and different methodology in Washington also showed similar patterns (Campbell et al. 2007).

There were, however, a few minor differences in the two models. For example, in Oregon a higher proportion of months in MMT was associated with a lower probability of arrest. Outpatient clients with prior arrests had a smaller decline in arrests than their counterparts with no prior arrests. In Washington, MMT clients with a prior arrest history had a higher arrest rate than their counterparts with no prior arrest. These reflect some minor differences between the states, but do not change the overall findings.

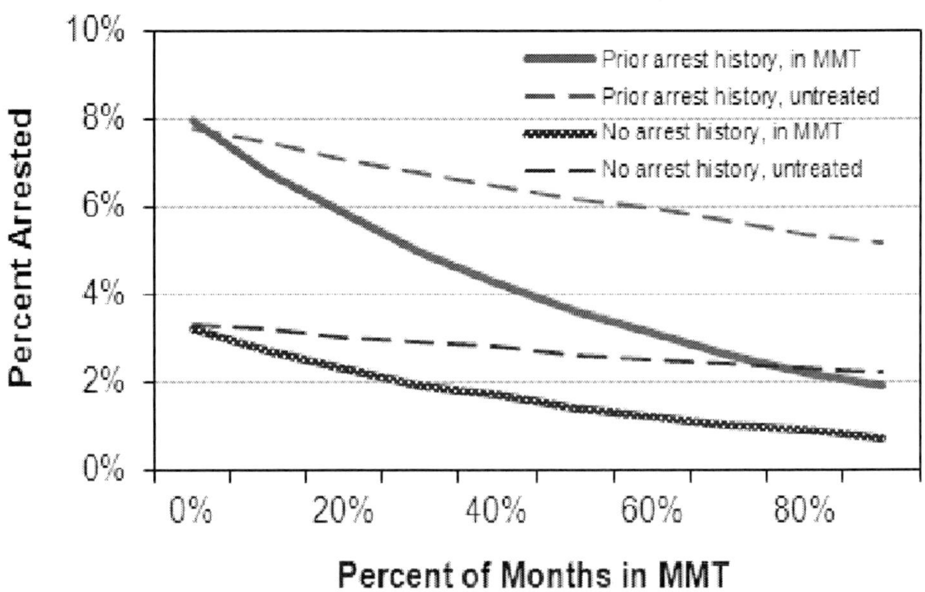

Figure 6. Predicted probability of a felony arrest in Oregon during months in methadone maintenance treatment (MMT; solid lines) compared to months untreated (dashed lines) by prior arrest history (red lines) or no prior arrest history (blue lines).

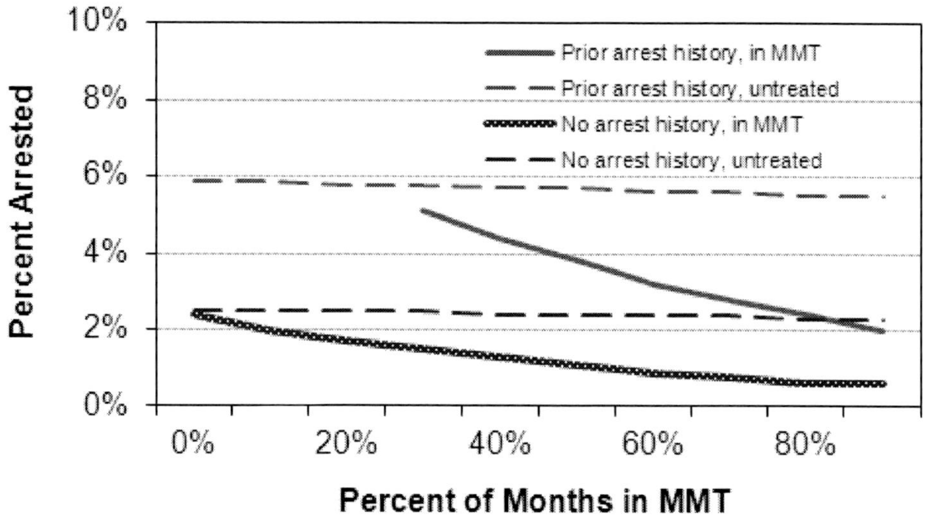

Figure 7. Predicted probability of a felony arrest in Washington during months in methadone maintenance treatment (MMT; solid line) compared to months untreated (dashed line) for clients with a prior arrest history (red lines) or no prior arrest history (blue lines).

Impact on Arrest Rates

As expected, during months in which individuals were enrolled in treatment, the odds of a felony arrest was much lower than in months when untreated. While clinical trials have suggested that methadone treatment should result in a reduction in arrests, this observational study was the first to confirm this hypothesis across two large statewide populations over a 10-year period. Such similar results from two different states after merging multiple administrative data sets (treatment, Medicaid, and state police) over extended time periods lend greater confidence to these findings.

The interaction with the proportion of months in treatment was an unexpected finding. The *a priori* hypothesis was that there would be a simple additive effect. Instead, the findings suggest that long-term retention leads to a greater reduction in arrests than originally expected while short-term retention is associated with little or no observable impact. Stable enrollment in methadone treatment was a critical factor in achieving the expected effect on arrests. There was little difference in arrest rates by treatment status for clients who were enrolled in methadone only a few months. Thus long-term retention is important, yet many prior studies have focused on rather brief and fixed lengths of stay. This finding lends support to the often-cited guideline that more than 12 months of MMT should be provided.

Overall, the arrest results from Oregon and Washington were quite similar. This finding was reassuring given that the analysis employed multiple administrative data sets from parallel, but not identical data systems, in both states. Furthermore, the findings were robust despite state differences in the financing of substance abuse services.

Conclusion

This chapter covered the results from several studies concerning Medicaid eligible adults in two states who accessed MMT services over a period of more than 10 years. While these observations are, of course, specific to those states, they shed light on issues that other states have likely faced or may face in the future.

Policy Implications

Reduction in the number of arrests is but one of the expected outcomes of methadone maintenance therapy. But it is a particularly important outcome because opiate addiction is highly associated with criminal activity and arrests account for a significant portion of the costs generated by untreated addiction. However, long term treatment raises issues about costs, though methadone is not expensive. The cost of opiate related crime has been estimated at about three times the cost of treatment (Center for Substance Abuse Treatment, 1995). In general, studies have found that long term MMT is quite cost effective. For example, an unpublished study (Norland et al., 2004) showed lower costs among MMT patients in Washington due primarily to reduced medical costs, especially among those in treatment longer than a year. A New York study (New York State Committee of Methadone Program Administrators, 1997) reported a $4 benefit for every $1 spent on MMT. In our sample, nearly every untreated client was arrested at least once during the observation period and some had many arrests.

Opiate addiction is considered a chronic condition like diabetes and enrollment in methadone maintenance is considered a long-term investment. Moreover, studies have shown that treatment is a relative bargain. The annual cost of treating a client in a methadone maintenance program was approximately $4,600 (Substance Abuse and Mental Health Services Administration, 2004), though unpublished studies in Washington state suggest the cost may be as low as $3,500 in some areas.

In summary, methadone maintenance treatment appears to be a worthwhile investment for state substance abuse and Medicaid agencies. Stable Medicaid coverage is an important predictor of access to and retention in methadone maintenance. In turn, methadone maintenance leads to positive outcomes such as minimization of arrests. Interestingly enough, managed care appeared not be detrimental for the population of Medicaid clients involved in methadone maintenance. The next chapter addresses Medicaid managed care impact for another special population – namely clients with co-occurring substance abuse and severe mental illness.

References

Aday, L. A., and Andersen, R. M. (1974). A framework for the study of access to medical care. *Health Services Research*, *9,* 208-220.

Alexander, J. A., Nahra, T. A., and Wheeler J. R. (2003). Managed care and access to substance abuse treatment services. *Journal of Behavioral Health Services and Research*, *30*, 161-175.

Andersen, R. M. (1995). Revisiting the behavioral model and access to medical care: Does it matter? *Journal of Health and Social Behavior, 36*, 1-10.

Anglin, M. D., and McGlothlin, W. H. (1984). Outcome of narcotic addict treatment in California. In F. M. Tims, and J. P. Ludford (Eds), *Drug abuse treatment evaluation: Strategies, progress, and prospects*. Rockville, MD: National Institute on Drug Abuse, NIDA Research Monograph Series, No. 5, 106-128.

Anglin, M. D., McGlothlin, W. H., Speckart, G. R., and Ryan, T. M. (1982). *Shutting off methadone: The closure of the San Diego Methadone Maintenance Program* (Final Report). Rockville, MD: National Institute on Drug Abuse.

Anglin, M. D., Speckart, G. R., Booth, M. W., and Ryan, T. M. (1989). Consequences and costs of shutting off methadone. *Addictive Behaviors*, *14*, 307-326.

Cacciola, J. S., Alterman, A. I., Rutherford, M. J., Mckay, J. R., and McLellan, A. T. (1998). The early course of change in methadone maintenance. *Addiction*, *93*, 41-49.

Campbell, K .M., Deck, D. D., Cox, A., and Broderick, C. (2006). *The Link King user manual Version 5.2.* Olympia, WA: Division of Alcohol and Substance Abuse. http://www.the-link-king.com/user_manual.zip

Campbell, K., Deck, D. D., and Krupski, A. (2007). Impact of substance abuse treatment on arrests among opiate users in Washington State. *American Journal on Addictions, 16*, 510-520.

Campbell, K., Deck, D. D., and Krupski, A. (2008). Record linkage software in the public domain: A comparison of Link Plus, The Link King, and a "basic" deterministic algorithm. *Healthy Informatics Journal, 14*, 5-15.

Center for Substance Abuse Treatment. (1995). *Methadone treatment outcomes in the National Treatment Improvement Studies (NTIES)*. Rockville, MD: Center for Substance Abuse Treatment, Department of Health and Human Services.

Deck, D. D. and Carlson, M. J. (2004). Access to publicly funded methadone maintenance treatment in two western states. *Journal of Behavioral Health Services Research*, *31*, 164-177.

Deck, D. D. and Carlson, M. J. (2005). Retention in publicly funded methadone maintenance treatment in two western states. *Journal of Behavioral Health Services and Research*, *32*, 43-60.

Deck, D. D., Gabriel, R. M., Knudsen, J. R. W., and Grams, G. (2003). Impact of client placement criteria on substance abuse treatment under the Oregon Health Plan. In D. R. Gastfriend (Ed.), *Addiction treatment matching: Research foundations of the American Society of Addiction Medicine (ASAM) criteria. New York: Haworth Medical Press.*

Deck, D. D. and McFarland, B. H. (2002). Use of substance abuse treatment services before and after Medicaid managed care. *Psychiatric Services, 53*, 802.

Deck, D. D., McFarland, B. H., Titus, J. M., Laws, K. E., and Gabriel, R. M. (2000). Access to substance abuse treatment services under the Oregon Health Plan. *Journal of the American Medical Association, 284*, 2093-2099.

Deck, D. D., Wiitala, W. L., and Laws, K. (2006) Medicaid coverage and access to publicly funded opiate treatment. *The Journal of Behavioral Health Services and Research, 33*, 324-334.

Deck, D. D., Wittala, W., McFarland, B., Campbell, K., Mulluly, J., Krupski, A., and McCarty, D. (2009). Medicaid coverage, methadone maintenance, and felony arrests: Outcomes of opiate treatment in two states. *Journal of Addictive Diseases, 28,* 89-102.

Farabee, D., Leukefeld, C. G., and Hays, L. (1998). Accessing drug abuse treatment: perceptions of out-of-treatment injectors. *Journal of Drug Issues*, *28*, 381-394.

Frank, R. G. and McGuire, T. G. (1995). Estimating costs of mental health and substance abuse coverage. *Health Affairs*, *14*, 102-115.

Friedmann, P. D., Lemon, S. C., and Stein, M. D. (2001). Transportation and retention in outpatient drug abuse treatment programs. *Journal of Substance Abuse Treatment*, *21*, 97-103.

Greenfield, L., Brady, J. V., Besteman, K. J., and De Smet, A. (1996). Patient retention in mobile and fixed-site methadone maintenance treatment. *Drug and Alcohol Dependence, 42*, 125-131.

Garcia, L. M., McGeary, K. A., Shultz, J. M., and McCoy, C. B. (1999). The impact of insurance status on drug abuse treatment completion. *Journal of Health Care Finance, 26*, 40-47.

Gelberg, L., Andersen, R. M., and Leake, B. D. (2000). The behavioral model for vulnerable populations: Application to medical care use and outcomes for homeless people. *Health Services Research*, *34*, 1273-1302.

Hubbard, R. L., Craddock, S. G., Flynn, P. M., Anderson, J., and Etheridge, R. M. (1997). Overview of 1-year follow-up outcomes in the drug abuse treatment outcome study (DATOS). *Psychology of Addictive Behaviors*, *11*, 261-278.

Hubbard, R. L., Marsden, M. E., Rachal, J. V., Harwood, H. J., Cavanaugh, E. R., and Ginzburg, H. M. (1989). *Drug abuse treatment: A national study of effectiveness.* Chapel Hill: University of North Carolina Press.

Laws, K. E., D'Ambrosio, R., and Deck, D. D. (2005-2007). Impact of changes in financing on publicly funded methadone maintenance treatment: A comparison between Oregon and Washington. *Journal of Maintenance in the Addictions* 3, 65-78.

Lewis, D. C. (1999). Access to narcotic addiction treatment and medical care: Prospects for the expansion of methadone maintenance treatment. *Journal of Addictive Diseases*, *18*, 5-21.

Maddux, J. F. and Desmond, D. P. (1997). Outcomes of methadone maintenance one year after admission. *Journal of Drug Issues*, *27*, 225-238.

Magura, S., Nwakeze, P. C., and Demsky, S. (1998). Pre- and in-treatment predictors of retention in methadone treatment using survival analysis. *Addiction*, *93*, 51-60.

Mann, C. and Artiga, S. (2004). *The impact of recent changes in health care coverage for low-income people: A first look at the research following changes in Oregon's Medicaid program.* Washington, DC: Kaiser Commission on Medicaid and the Uninsured.

Marsch, L. A. (1998). The efficacy of methadone maintenance interventions in reducing illicit opiate use, HIV risk behavior and criminality: A meta-analysis. *Addiction*, *93*, 515-532.

McCarty, D., Frank, R. G., and Denmead, G. C. (1999). Methadone maintenance and state Medicaid managed care programs. *The Milbank Quarterly, 77*, 341-362.

McGlothlin, W. H. and Anglin, M. D. (1991). Shutting off methadone. Costs and benefits. *Archives of General Psychiatry*, *38*, 885-892.

National Institutes of Health, National Consensus Development Panel on Effective Medical Treatment of Opiate Addiction. (1998). Effective medical treatment of opiate addiction. *Journal of the American Medical Association*, *280*, 1936-1943.

New York State Committee of Methadone Program Administrators. (1997). Regarding Methadone Treatment: A review. New York: Author.

Nordlund, D. J., Estee, S., Mancuso, D., and Felver, B. (2004). Methadone treatment for opiate addiction lowers health care costs and reduces arrests and convictions. Washington State Department of Social and Health Services, Research and Data Analysis Division. http://www1.dshs.wa.gov/pdf/ms/rda/research/4/49.pdf

Oggins, J. (2003). Changes in health insurance and payment for substance use treatment. *American Journal of Drug and Alcohol Abuse*, *9*, 55-74.

Rosenbaum, M., Murphy, S., and Beck, J. (1987). Money for methadone: Preliminary findings from a study of Alameda County's new maintenance policy. *Journal of Psychoactive Drugs*, *19*, 13-19.

Rosenbaum, M., Washburn, A., Knight, K., Kelley, M, and Irwin, J. (1996). Treatment as harm reduction, defunding as harm maximization: The case of methadone maintenance. *Journal of Psychoactive Drugs*, *28*, 241-249.

Rowan-Szal, G. A., Chatham, L. R., and Simpson, D. D. (2000). Importance of identifying cocaine and alcohol dependent methadone clients. *The American Journal on Addictions*, *9*, 38-50.

Sees, K. L., Delucchi, K. L., Masson, C., Rosen, A.; Clark, H. W., Robillard, H., Banys, P., and Hall, S. M. (2000) Methadone maintenance vs. 180-day psychosocially enriched detoxification for treatment of opioid dependence: A randomized controlled trial. *Journal of the American Medical Association*, *283*, 1303-1310.

Sells, S. B. and Simpson, D. D. (1980). A case for drug abuse treatment effectiveness based on the DARP research program. *British Journal of Addiction*, *75,* 117-132.

Simpson, D. D., Joe, G. W., Broome, K. M., Hiller, M. L., Knight, K., and Rowan-Szal, G. A. (1997). Program diversity and treatment retention rates in the drug abuse treatment outcome study (DATOS). *Psychology of Addictive Behaviors*, *11*, 279-293.

Simpson, D. D., Joe, G. W., and Brown, B. S. (1997). Treatment retention and follow-up outcomes in the drug abuse treatment outcomes study (DATOS). *Psychology of Addictive Behaviors*, *11*, 294-307.

Simpson, D. D., Joe, G. W., Chatham, L. R., and Dansereau, D. F. (1997). Strategies for improving methadone treatment process and outcomes. *Journal of Drug Issues*, *27*:239-260.

Simpson, D. D. and Sells, S. B. (1982). Effectiveness of treatment for drug abuse: An overview of the DARP research program. *Advances in Alcohol and Substance Abuse*, *2*, 7-29.

Steenrod, S., Brisson, A., McCarty, D., and Hodgkin, D. (2001). Effects of managed care on programs and practices for the treatment of alcohol and drug dependence. In Galanter M, (Ed.), *Recent Developments in Alcoholism, Volume 15: Services Research in the Era of Managed Care*. New York: Kluwer Academic/Plenum Publishers, 51-71.

Substance Abuse and Mental Health Services Administration. (2002). SAMHSA approves accrediting organizations for methadone treatment programs. Accessed May 16, 2002, from www.health.org/newsroom/releases/2002/Jan02/3.htm

Substance Abuse and Mental Health Services Administration. (2004). *Alcohol and Services Study (ADSS): The National Treatment System: Outpatient Methadone Facilities.* Rockville, MD: SAMSHA, Office of Applied Studies. Available at *http://www.oas.samhsa.gov/ADSS/methadone.pdf*

Ward, J., Hall, W., and Mattick, R. P. (1999). Role of maintenance treatment in opioid dependence. *The Lancet*, *353*, 221-226.

Zarkin, G. A. and Dunlap, L. J. (1999). Implication of managed care for methadone treatment: Findings from 5 case studies in New York State. *Journal of Substance Abuse Treatment*, *17*, 25-35.

Zhang, Z., Friedmann, P. D., and Gerstein, D. R. (2003). Does retention matter? Treatment duration and improvement in drug use. *Addiction*, *98*, 673-684.

In: Medicaid and Treatment for People… ISBN 978-1-61470-742-4
Editor: B.H. McFarland, D.McCarty, et al, pp. 203-222

Chapter 9

Concurrent Access to Mental Health and Substance Abuse Services for Medicaid Clients in Publicly Funded Treatment Systems

Roy M. Gabriel[1], Bentson H. McFarland[2], Brigid G. Zani[3], and Lynn E. McCamant[4]

[1] RMC Research Corporation, Portland, OR, USA
[2] Departments of Psychiatry and Public Health and Preventive Medicine, Oregon Health and Science University, Portland, OR, USA
[3] Early Assessment and Support Team, Mid-Valley Behavioral Care Network, Salem, OR (work performed while affiliated with the Department of Psychiatry, Oregon Health and Science University, Portland, OR), USA
[4] Department of Psychiatry, Oregon Health and Science University, Portland, OR (former affiliation), USA

Abstract

Medicaid clients with co-occurring mental health and substance abuse problems comprise substantial portions of the clienteles served by public sector mental health and chemical dependency treatment systems. However, little is known about implications of managed care for "dual diagnosis" Medicaid clients. This prospective study conducted in eight states used interviews to examine managed care impact on use of mental health services by adult Medicaid clients in treatment for substance abuse (N = 2,424) and on use of chemical dependency services by Medicaid clients with severe mental illness (N = 2,318). Compared with fee for service, managed care had no impact on use of mental health services by clients entering substance abuse treatment. Conversely, there was an apparent 26% reduction in substance abuse treatment ($p < .02$) among managed care (versus fee for service) Medicaid clients with severe mental illness. Managed care impact may vary among Medicaid sub-groups.

INTRODUCTION

Medicaid clients with co-occurring mental health and substance abuse problems comprise substantial portions of the clienteles served by the public mental health and chemical dependency treatment systems. Public behavioral health care programs have undergone marked change as Medicaid managed care has come to replace the previous fee for service arrangements (Buck et al., 2003; Coffey et al., 2001). Yet there has been little research into the implications of managed care for Medicaid clients with "dual diagnoses" pertaining to both mental health and substance abuse disorders. Important topics to be addressed include the impact of managed care (and the several managed care mechanisms) on recognition of co-occurring disorders, treatment planning for Medicaid clients with dual diagnoses, retention in care, and outcomes for these individuals. Information on these issues will be of considerable value to policy makers in state substance abuse, mental health, and Medicaid agencies who must devise optimal treatment programs for vulnerable populations while dealing with limited revenues and substantial caseloads (Smith et al., 2005). Specifically, state Medicaid, mental health and substance abuse agency policy makers need to decide whether clients with co-occurring mental health and substance abuse problems are best served by managed care systems or by fee for service programs.

CO-OCCURRING SUBSTANCE ABUSE AND MENTAL HEALTH DISORDERS

Individuals with primary substance abuse problems often have co-occurring mental health disorders (Babor et al., 1992; Miller and Ries, 1991; Substance Abuse and Mental Health Services Administration, 2002). Epidemiological studies show that primary chemical dependency problems are most closely related to anxiety and mood disorders (Grant et al., 2004; Regier et al., 1990; Samet and Hasin, 2008). Substance abuse treatment programs typically report 50% to 75% of their clients have a co-occurring mental health disorder (Sacks et al., 1997; Watkins et al., 2004).

Individuals with primary mental health disorders also have elevated rates of substance use (Menzes et al., 1996; Scott, 1993). Those with severe mental conditions such as schizophrenia or bipolar disorder have especially high rates of chemical dependency (Brunette and Mueser, 2006; Fowler et al., 1998; Green et al., 2007; Mueser et al., 1992) and the consequences of such co-morbidity include poorer overall health (cardiovascular problems, nutritional deficits and diabetes), worsened psychiatric symptoms, substantial days in the hospital, medication non-adherence, disruptive behavior, and poor social functioning (Buckley, 2006; Mueser et al., 1992; Owen et al., 1996). In addition, the prevalence of violence and victimization is higher among mentally ill people with substance use disorders than those without (Putkonen et al., 2004; Rasanen et al., 1998; Sells et al., 2003; Steadman et al., 1998).

Unsuccessfully treated elsewhere, persons with co-occurring disorders become disproportionately represented on the law enforcement, judicial, and correctional caseloads (Fzel et al., 2009). They are also more likely to be homeless (Reardon et al., 2003; Scott, 1993) and have family problems (Salyers and Meuser, 2001).

Long-term course and remission of symptoms (Brown et al., 1995) and the process of treatment are greatly affected by co-morbidity (Miller et al., 1997; Ouimette et al., 1998; Prince et al., 2009). There is evidence that individuals with co-occurring disorders typically do not receive adequate treatment to address all of their health and social needs (Calsyn et al., 2004; Drake and Mueser, 2000; Havassy et al., 2009; Timko and Moos, 2002). Chemical dependency clients who receive both substance abuse and mental health services fare better than those receiving only one type of treatment (Brunette and Mueser, 2006; Grella and Stein, 2006; Mueser et al., 1998; Ries, 1993; Ritsher et al., 2002). Conversely, without treatment for chemical dependency, substance use persists among mentally ill persons (Bartels et al., 1995; Cuffel and Chase, 1994; Kozarie-Kovacic et al., 1995; Morse et al., 1992; Okin et al., 1995).

Medicaid Managed Care and Behavioral Health Treatment

People with substance abuse and mental health problems depend heavily on the public sector for treatment (Substance Abuse and Mental Health Services Administration, 2002). In particular, Medicaid is a substantial payer for both chemical dependency and mental health services (Buck, 2001; Mark et al., 2005) and stability of coverage has been shown to be a strong influence on access to needed behavioral health services (Beinecke, 2005; Deck et al., 2006). Medicaid behavioral health care systems have undergone marked change (McFarland, 2000) as programs shifted away from fee for service and towards managed care approaches such as case rates or capitation (Institute of Medicine, 1998; Sosin and D'Aunno, 2001). Moreover, during the middle of the 1990s many states expanded Medicaid eligibility to include the "working poor".

Several studies have examined the impact of converting Medicaid from fee for service to managed care on clients with substance abuse problems (Deck and McFarland, 2002; Deck et al., 2000; Ettner et al., 2003; McCarty et al., 2003; McFarland et al., 2005). Similarly, there have also been studies on the switch from fee for service to managed care in programs for Medicaid clients with severe mental illness (Bianconi et al., 2006; Blank et al., 1996; Boothroyd et al., 2002; Christianson et al., 1992; Leff et al., 2005; Lurie and Belanger, 2002; Manning et al., 1999; McFarland et al., 2004; Morrissey et al., 2002; Rothbard et al., 2004; Stroup and Dorwart, 1995). While these shifts stimulated much concern within the policy community (Luft, 2003; Lurie et al., 1992; Mechanic, 2001), only a few studies have found empirical evidence of impact (see *e.g.*, Boothroyd et al., 2002; Deck et al., 2000; Manning et al., 1999; Stroup and Dorwart, 1995).

It is important to note that previous research focused on either substance abuse treatment or on mental health services for Medicaid clients. There have been few studies on concurrent use of substance abuse and mental health services in this population. Secondary analyses of a national dataset indicated marked variation across states in the availability of publicly-funded treatment services for persons with co-occurring conditions (McFarland and Gabriel, 2004). A small study from Oregon by Bigelow et al. (Bigelow et al., 2004) showed that use of mental health services did not differ between substance abuse treatment clients interviewed before versus after the change from fee for service to capitated (pre-paid) Medicaid managed care.

Challenges in serving so-called "dual diagnosis" clients in these rapidly changing environments have been well documented by researchers (see *e.g.,* Brunette and Mueser, 2006; Minkoff, 1998), practitioner associations (see *e.g.,* National Association of State Mental Health Program Directors and National Association of State Alcohol and Drug Abuse Directors, 1998), and federal agencies (Center for Substance Abuse Treatment, 2005; Substance Abuse and Mental Health Services Administration, 2002). Yet there has been little or no empirical research on the impact of these substantial changes in the organization and financing of services on Medicaid clients with co-occurring disorders.

Especially troubling is the possibility that managed care may reduce providers' interest in recognizing and addressing clients' concomitant substance abuse and mental health problems. The Substance Abuse and Mental Health Services Administration's (2002) Report to Congress concluded that conflicting rules, differing eligibility criteria, and duplication of required documentation and reporting to separate mental health and substance abuse funding and regulatory systems are substantial barriers. In other words, there are disincentives to clinician identification and procurement of treatment for clients' co-occurring conditions (Alexander et al., 2003).

Service provision for Medicaid clients with co-occurring mental health and substance abuse disorders is another area of concern. While the fee for service system rewards delivery of treatment, managed care financing mechanisms such as capitation may motivate providers to reduce services (Steenrod et al., 2001). Indeed, Etheridge et al. (1995) found nationwide a significant reduction over time in the number and range of services that substance abuse clients received. Because individuals with concurrent chemical dependency and mental health problems typically need volumes of services greater than people with just one condition, "dual diagnosis" clients may be especially vulnerable to treatment restrictions. However, little information is available about the impact of Medicaid managed care on services to clients with concurrent mental health and substance abuse disorders.

Summarily, people with substance abuse or mental health problems often have co-occurring mental health or substance abuse disorders, are typically treated in the public sector, and depend heavily on Medicaid for financing their treatments. Although there have been dramatic changes in the organization and financing of Medicaid programs as managed care systems have replaced fee for service programs, there has been little if any research to date on the impact of these events on recognition and service provision for clients with co-occurring chemical dependency and mental health problems. This project provides such information.

METHODS

This chapter draws on secondary datasets from the Substance Abuse and Mental Health Services Administration (SAMHSA) Medicaid Managed Behavioral Health Care and Vulnerable Populations studies of adults with alcohol or other drug chemical dependency (SAMHSA AOD) and adults with severe mental illness (SAMHSA SMI). These multi-state studies were designed to determine the effects of managed care (MC) organization and financing systems on the use, cost and outcomes of substance abuse treatment services for

Medicaid adults (Carlson and Gabriel, 2001; Larson et al., 2005) and mental health services for Medicaid adults (Leff et al., 2005; McFarland et al., 2004).

Data from the SAMHSA AOD study came from five states (Oregon, Washington, Massachusetts, Pennsylvania, and New York) and featured a prospective study of adult Medicaid clients participating in substance abuse treatment. A total N=2,424 participated in the initial interview with N=1,531 (63%) of these participating in a six-month follow-up interview. The study assessed these individuals via face-to-face interviews at treatment entry and six months later using a highly structured, standardized interview protocol that featured the Addiction Severity Index (ASI) (McLellan et al., 1992) and the SF-12 (Ware et al., 1996) at each point in time. The interview protocol also included information on respondents' living conditions, employment and prior medical and behavioral health care. Demographics included age, gender, race/ethnicity, education level, employment and marital status.

Data from the SAMHSA SMI study came from five states (Oregon, Pennsylvania, Virginia, Florida and Hawaii) and featured a prospective study of adult Medicaid clients participating in mental health treatment. A total N=2,318 participated in the initial interview, with N=1,969 (85%) of these participating in a six-month follow-up interview. The study assessed these individuals primarily through face-to-face interviews using a structured, standardized interview protocol at both points in time. Psychiatric symptoms and health functioning were assessed using the Brief Symptom Inventory (BSI) (DeRogatis, 1993) and the SF-12 (Ware et al., 1996), respectively. Demographics included age, gender, race/ethnicity, education level, employment, and marital status. Information on substance use included the ASI scales for alcohol use and drug use.

The Medicaid managed care systems for clients with severe mental illness have been described elsewhere (see *e.g.,* Bianconi et al., 2006; Leff et al., 2005; Morrissey et al., 2002; Ridgely et al., 2002; Rothbard et al., 2002; Stroup and Dorwart, 1995). Briefly, fee for service (FFS) Medicaid was replaced by assorted approaches to managed care (MC). In the mental health area, the preponderant alternative to fee for service was capitation in which managed care entities were pre-paid on a per capita basis to assume responsibility for mental health services.

With regard to substance abuse services, the Medicaid managed care systems were more variable across study states. They included states in which substance abuse and mental health services were carved out in the same system, carved out separately, and integrated with medical care (Ridgely et al., 2002; SAMHSA, 1999).

Comparable variables from both study samples were extracted from these datasets to examine the relationships between client characteristics and (a) mental health service use for the AOD sample and (b) substance abuse service use for the SMI sample. Andersen's (Andersen, 1995) Behavioral Model of access to health care, refined for use with vulnerable populations by Gelberg et al. (Gelberg et al., 2000), was employed as a framework guiding the analysis of these characteristics and their influence on subsequent behavioral health care. Client characteristics in both SAMHSA AOD and SAMHSA SMI studies are classified as *Predisposing*, *Enabling* or *Need* as prescribed by the model and are summarized in Table 1.

Table 1. Client characteristics used in the prediction of subsequent substance abuse or mental health service use in alcohol and other drug use and severe mental illness samples

Sample	Predisposing	Enabling	Need
Alcohol and other drug use sample	Age[1]	Ever had AOD Tx	ASI Alcohol Use[1]
	Gender	Ever had MH Tx	ASI Drug Use[1]
	Race/Ethnicity	Source of Referral	ASI Psychiatric[1]
	Education Level	MC/FFS	Activity Limits
	Employed		SF-12[1]
	Marital Status		
Severe mental illness sample	Age[1]	Ever had AOD Tx	ASI Alcohol Use[1]
	Gender	AOD Tx past 3 Mos	ASI Drug Use[1]
	Race/Ethnicity	MC/FFS	BSI Global[1]
	Education Level		SF-12[1]
	Employed		
	Marital Status		

[1] Continuous variable. All others are dichotomous.
AOD = Alcohol and other drugs
ASI = Addiction Severity Index
BSI = Brief Symptom Inventory
FFS = Fee for service
MC = Managed care
MH = Mental health
SF-12 = Short Form Health Survey
SMI = Severe mental illness
Tx = Treatment

Dependent Measures

The outcomes examined here are dichotomous. Stated simply, the research questions were:

1. Did SMI clients receive substance abuse treatment between the initial and follow-up interview? What client characteristics differentiate those who received these services from those who did not?
2. Did AOD clients receive mental health treatment between the initial and follow-up interview? What client characteristics differentiate those who received these services from those who did not?

These questions were asked six months after the initial interview for SAMHSA SMI and AOD samples. The term "follow-up" refers to these time points.

Predictor Variables

As shown in Table 1, the Predisposing characteristics were consistent across both study samples. All but age of the client were converted to dichotomous measures. Male, White, Married, High School or more, Employed, and Living Independently at the time of the initial interview served as the indicated (= 1) categorical value in the coding for subsequent logistic regression analyses.

Enabling characteristics were conceptually parallel but measured somewhat differently in the two samples. All were dichotomous. For the AOD sample, the source of referral (criminal justice as reference) was included, along with whether the client had ever had substance abuse treatment, or ever had mental health treatment prior to the initial interview. For the SMI sample, enabling characteristics included whether the client had ever had substance abuse treatment, and whether they had received substance abuse treatment in the three months prior to the initial interview. Clients in both samples were coded as to whether they were enrolled in a managed care (reference) or fee for service system.

Need factors again were conceptually parallel but measured somewhat differently in the two samples. For the AOD sample, three ASI composites were used as continuous predictors: alcohol use, drug use and psychiatric problems. In addition, a question as to whether the respondent's daily activity was limited by emotional problems was employed as another indicator of mental health problems. For the SMI sample, only the ASI alcohol use and drug use composites were available. Mental health problems were indicated using the BSI Global score. Both samples used the SF-12 physical health and mental health measures of general health functioning.

Analysis

Simple comparisons between clients in the managed care and fee for service conditions in both AOD and SMI samples were conducted using statistical techniques appropriate to the measurement scale of the variables. Mantel-Haenszel Common Odds Ratios and Chi-Squared tests were computed across sites for all dichotomous client characteristics. To assess whether these cross-site results were similar or different within the five states in each SAMHSA study, the Breslow-Day Chi-Squared test of Homogeneity was conducted. For continuous variables, means and standard deviations were computed within MC/FFS conditions and two-way analyses of variance (Site by MC/FFS condition ANOVAs) were conducted to determine (a) whether managed care clients were significantly different from fee for service clients on these variables (*i.e.,* the MC/FFS condition main effect), and (b) whether these differences were consistent across the states (*i.e.,* the Site by MC/FFS condition interaction).

Regression analysis to assess the association of the Predisposing, Enabling and Need characteristics with the receipt of mental health services for the AOD sample and receipt of substance abuse services for the SMI sample were performed using the stratified (by state) logistic regression procedure.

All analyses were done using the SPSS statistical software package.

Results

Sample sizes for the initial and follow-up interviews for the SAMHSA AOD and SAMHSA SMI study samples are shown by state and managed care and fee for service study condition in Table 2. In the AOD target population, initial interview sample sizes per condition ranged from n=108 (Managed Care sample in New York) to n=570 (Fee for Service sample in New York). Fee for Service samples were larger than Managed Care samples in each state, and represented nearly two-thirds (66.3%) of the full AOD study sample across states. In the SMI target population, initial interview sample sizes per condition ranged from n=138 (Fee for Service sample in Pennsylvania) to n=501 (Managed Care sample in Florida). Fee for Service samples were larger than Managed Care samples in three of the five study states, and across all states the sample was nearly balanced across Managed Care and Fee for Service conditions.

Table 2. Initial and follow-up sample sizes for alcohol and other drug use and severe mental illness samples by state and managed care / fee for service condition

	Fee for Service		Managed Care	
	Initial	**Follow-up**	**Initial**	**Follow-up**
Alcohol and other drug use sample				
Oregon/Washington	282	191	220	168
Massachusetts	444	284	230	154
New York	570	323	108	61
Pennsylvania	310	184	260	166
Total	1606	982	818	549
Severe mental illness sample				
Oregon	166	164	139	130
Pennsylvania	138	135	140	123
Hawaii	356	309	207	166
Virginia	308	244	176	108
Florida	187	159	501	431
Total	1155	1011	1163	958

Descriptive statistics (means or percentages) are displayed for Managed Care and Fee for Service conditions across the states for SAMHSA AOD and SAMHSA SMI samples in Table 3. Odds ratios or ANOVA F statistics test the cross-site comparison of Managed Care and Fee for Service clients for all predictor and outcome variables. Tests of the consistency of these comparisons across participating states are conducted using the Breslow-Day chi-square for dichotomous variables and the ANOVA F for the interaction between state and MC/FFS condition.

Table 3. Summary of sample and odds ratios or Analysis of Variance F-statistics for managed care / fee for service condition comparisons

	Fee for Service Condition (Mean / Percent)	Managed Care Condition (Mean / Percent)	Total	Odds Ratio or ANOVA F	Homogeneity Chi Square or ANOVA F
Alcohol and other drugs sample					
Predisposing characteristics					
Age	37.7	38.2	37.9	3.50*	10.57***
Gender (male)	66%	47%	60%	.39***	67.30***
Race/Ethnicity (% White)	38%	48%	42%	.89	14.48**
Education level (% HS+)	56%	60%	58%	.98	3.60
Employed	13%	17%	14%	1.03	29.66***
Ever married	35%	43%	38%	1.30**	5.10
Living, Home or Family	59%	71%	63%	1.94	14.48***
Enabling characteristics					
Ever Had AOD Tx	81%	83%	82%	1.06	15.69***
Ever Had MH Tx	39%	56%	49%	1.77***	72.65***
Crim. Justice Referral	27%	25%	26%	.95	35.97***
Need characteristics					
ASI Alcohol Use	.213	.213	.213	2.76	3.88**
ASI Drug Use	.157	.145	.152	12.74***	6.50***
ASI Psychiatric	.247	.357	.286	42.29***	14.75***
Limited Activity	50%	60%	54%	1.34***	18.56***
SF-12 Physical Health	48.62	44.99	47.40	35.45***	16.92***
SF-12 Mental Health	36.57	33.32	35.47	9.98**	2.87*
Outcome					
Received MH Tx	13%	24%	17%	1.93***	14.30**
Severe mental illness sample					
Predisposing characteristics					
Age	43	42.5	42.8	2.52	8.87***
Gender (male)	48%	35%	42%	1.45***	2.68
Race/Ethnicity (% White)	42%	48%	45%	1.02	13.18
Education level (% HS+)	66%	60%	63%	.87	24.19***
Employed	15%	12%	14%	.99	13.12
Ever married	45%	57%	51%	1.35***	1.64
Living independently	78%	92%	85%	2.38***	72.44**
Enabling characteristics					
Ever had AOD Tx	43%	37%	40%	.98	33.28***
Had AOD Tx, 3 Mos	26%	20%	23%	.86	29.49
Need characteristics					
ASI Alcohol Use	.047	.044	.046	.36	4.33**
ASI Drug Use	.024	.034	.029	10.61**	3.77**
BSI Global	46.20	48.33	47.27	27.17***	3.96**
SF-12 Physical Health	43.34	40.35	41.84	14.33***	.62
SF-12 Mental Health	40.03	36.65	38.33	23.69***	2.40*
Outcome					
Received AOD Tx	15%	9%	12%	.66**	65.86***

* $p<0.05$; ** $p<0.01$; *** $p<0.001$

Alcohol or Other Drug Sample

The full AOD sample was predominantly male (60%), non-White (58%), never married (62%), unemployed (86%), had at least a high school education (58%), were living at home or with family (63%), and were nearly 38 years old (37.9) on average. Clients' age, gender and the proportion who had ever been married varied significantly between Managed Care and Fee for Service conditions. Specifically, the Managed Care sample was older and predominantly female (53%) while the Fee for Service sample was predominantly male (66%), and adults in the Managed Care sample were more likely to be or have been married (43%) than those in Fee for Service (35%). Among these predisposing characteristics the relationships between age, gender, race/ethnicity, employment and living at home or with family with MC/FFS status differed across the five states.

Among the Enabling factors, the vast majority of these adults entering AOD treatment had been in substance abuse treatment before (82%), nearly half had had mental health treatment before (49%) and about one-fourth had come to their current treatment episode from a criminal justice referral (26%). Clients in the Managed Care condition were significantly more likely to have had experience with mental health treatment (56%) than their Fee for Service counterparts (39%). Relationships between all three Enabling factors and MC/FFS status differed among the five states.

Among the Need factors, all measures addressing mental health problems evidenced significantly greater severity among Managed Care clients. For example, ASI Psychiatric scores were significantly higher (indicating greater problem severity) and SF-12 Mental Health scores were significantly lower (less healthy) in the Managed Care condition. Moreover, a higher proportion of adults in Managed Care (60%) than in the Fee for Service condition (50%) indicated their daily activities were limited due to emotional problems. However, Fee for Service clients reported more severe drug problems on the ASI.

Severe Mental Illness Sample

The full SMI sample was predominantly female (58%), non-White (55%), had been or were currently married (51%), unemployed (86%), had at least a high school education (63%), were living independently, *i.e.,* not institutionalized (85%) and were, on average, nearly 43 (42.8) years old. Clients' gender, marital history and living situation varied between Managed Care and Fee for Service samples. Specifically, females outnumbered males nearly two to one in the Managed Care sample (65%), while in Fee for Service, gender was nearly equally distributed (52% female). Managed Care clients were also more likely to be or have been married (57% vs. 45%) and living independently (92% vs. 78%) than their Fee for Service counterparts. These relationships were consistent across states. Only the relations between education level and age with MC/FFS (non-significant in the aggregate) varied across the five states.

Among the Enabling characteristics, about 40% of these adults in mental health treatment had had substance abuse treatment in their lifetimes, and about 23% of them had had it in the three months prior to the initial interview. Neither of the proportions was significantly different between MC and FFS conditions across states. The relationship between lifetime history of substance abuse treatment and MC/FFS condition did differ across states, however.

Among the indicators of Need, Managed Care samples evidenced significantly greater problems in all areas except alcohol use. Specifically, they reported more severe drug problems (on the ASI), a higher frequency of mental health symptoms (on the BSI) and poorer mental and physical health (on the SF-12) than did their Fee for Service counterparts.

In terms of outcomes, about one in six AOD treatment clients (17%) received mental health treatment within six months prior to the follow-up interview. Managed care clients (24%) were significantly more likely to receive mental health treatment than Fee for Service clients (13%). In the SMI sample, about one in eight clients (12%) received substance abuse treatment within three months prior to the follow-up interview, with no significant difference in access across MC/FFS condition.

Predicting Mental Health Service Access Among Substance Abuse Treatment Participants

The results of the multivariate logistic regression, predicting mental health treatment access within the six months prior to the follow-up interview, are shown in Table 4. Among the Predisposing conditions, adults in AOD treatment were more likely to receive mental health services if they were older, female, White and not homeless. Among the Enabling factors, those with a history of mental health treatment were significantly more likely to access mental health treatment during their current substance abuse treatment episode. Among the Need factors, clients with greater psychiatric problem severity were significantly more likely to receive mental health treatment. Controlling for all of these client characteristics, adults in the Managed Care condition were marginally more likely ($p < 0.057$) to receive mental health treatment than those in the Fee for Service condition.

Predicting Substance Abuse Treatment Access Among Mental Health Treatment Participants

The results of the multivariate logistic regression, predicting substance abuse treatment access within the three months prior to the six-month follow-up interview among clients in mental health treatment, are also shown in Table 4. Among the Predisposing characteristics, only age was significantly related to substance abuse treatment access, with younger clients more likely to receive substance abuse treatment services. Among Enabling characteristics, clients with a prior history of substance abuse treatment were more likely to access it in their current episode. In terms of Need characteristics, those reporting more severe problems with drug use were more likely to receive AOD treatment. Controlling for all of these characteristics, clients in the Fee for Service condition were significantly more likely to receive substance abuse treatment ($p < 0.019$).

Table 4. Logistic regression predicting mental health treatment access for the alcohol and other drug use sample and substance abuse treatment access for the severe mental illness sample

	Exp (B)	Significance
Alcohol and other drugs sample		
Predisposing characteristics		
Age	1.017*	.014
Gender (male)	.648***	.001
Race/Ethnicity (White)	1.316*	.030
Education level (HS+)	1.059	.599
Employed	.738	.103
Marital status (Ever married)	1.009	.934
Living condition: Homeless	.594*	.031
Living condition: Institution	.950	.699
Enabling characteristics		
Ever Had AOD Tx	.999	.992
Ever Had MH Tx	2.178***	.001
Criminal Justice Referral	.897	.440
Managed Care Condition	1.239	.057
Need characteristics		
ASI Alcohol Use	.983	.931
ASI Drug Use	1.490	.294
ASI Psychiatric	3.101***	.001
Limited Activity	.934	.679
SF-12 Physical Health	.997	.602
SF-12 Mental Health	.988	.098
Severe mental illness sample		
Predisposing characteristics		
Age	.982**	.006
Gender (male)	.862	.266
Race/Ethnicity (White)	.865	.285
Education Level (HS+)	1.204	.198
Employed	1.279	.101
Marital Status (Ever married)	.996	.976
Living independently	1.020	.925
Enabling characteristics		
Ever had AOD Tx	3.759***	.001
Managed care condition	.739*	.019
Need characteristics		
ASI Alcohol Use	1.599	.330
ASI Drug Use	7.797*	.020
BSI Global	.994	.554
SF-12 Physical Health	1.011	.088
SF-12 Mental Health	.990	.135

* $p<0.05$; ** $p<0.01$; *** $p<0.001$

CONCLUSION

In summary, these analyses suggest that the conversion from fee for service to managed care Medicaid had differential impact on use of substance abuse versus mental health services by clients with co-occurring conditions. In general, it appears that implementation of substance abuse treatment managed care was associated with no change or perhaps slightly increased use of mental health services by Medicaid clients. Conversely, managed care was associated with decreased use of substance abuse treatment programs by Medicaid clients with severe mental illness. It should not be surprising that the study found differential impact. In many if not most of the study states, Medicaid substance abuse and mental health services were administered by distinctly different systems that had widely varying organizational and financial arrangements. In Oregon, for example, Medicaid mental health services were assigned to carved-out "mental health managed care organizations" (Ross and McFarland, 2000) while Medicaid substance abuse treatment was, at least theoretically, integrated into the responsibilities of fully capitated physical health maintenance organizations in 1995 (Laws et al., 2002). In contrast, Massachusetts implemented a statewide behavioral health carve-out in 1992 (Larson et al., 2005). Consequently, it might be expected that the fee for service to managed care conversion would have had varying impacts on these different systems. It is important for decision-makers to appreciate that policy changes may be associated with beneficial effects for some sub-groups and detrimental impacts on other sub-groups within the overall Medicaid population. Ongoing program evaluation is crucial to understand the impacts of such large-scale policy changes.

Also noteworthy in the present project is the apparent connection between components of the Andersen behavioral model of health care utilization and use of either mental health or substance abuse treatment services. It was gratifying and not surprising to observe that Need factors (such as measures of mental health or substance abuse problems) were powerful predictors of concurrent treatment access in both AOD and SMI samples. On the other hand, it is concerning and worthy of further investigation that Predisposing factors (independent of need for services) such as gender and race / ethnicity were also associated with access to services. In general, women were more likely than men to receive mental health services but less likely to receive substance abuse treatment. Racial/ethnic minority clients were less likely than whites to receive mental health services. These findings support current national concern for disparities in access to both substance abuse and mental health treatment.

Of course, there were many limitations to this observational study. Clients were not assigned at random to Fee for Service and Managed Care conditions. Regression approaches were employed to adjust for differences between the groups but there might well have been unobserved factors that may have confounded the results. On the other hand, in nearly all the study states, the managed care systems were implemented on the basis of geography (*e.g.*, county by county). In some sense, then, the study represented a "natural experiment." As was mentioned, there was substantial variation among (and within) states in the types of Medicaid managed care that replaced fee for service. It may well be the case that impacts of Medicaid managed care varied among the different types of programs that replaced fee for service systems. Nonetheless, from the policy perspective it is important to estimate the national impact of these substantial changes on different service populations within the Medicaid system.

Within these studies, the measures of some client characteristics, while conceptually parallel, were not always the same for AOD and SMI populations. For example, mental health service use after treatment entry in the AOD samples was asked with reference to the previous six months — essentially the entire period between baseline and follow-up interviews — while substance abuse treatment access in the SMI samples was asked with reference to the previous three months. This difference limits our ability to compare the overall likelihood of concurrent treatment access in AOD and SMI service samples, but it is unlikely that this discrepancy affects the predictive relationships exploring the association of client characteristics with mental health and substance abuse treatment access.

Finally, self-reported service use itself is another study limitation. It is conceivable, and perhaps likely, that clients did not always accurately distinguish between mental health and substance abuse treatment services. However, it is unlikely that there was differential misclassification among managed care and fee for service clients. Consequently, one could expect the misclassification measurement error to diminish the strength of the association between fee for service versus managed care and treatment utilization. Therefore, the estimates presented here are conservative.

In summary, Medicaid managed care appears to have had differential impact on clients with co-occurring substance abuse and mental health problems. For clients with primary substance abuse, use of mental health services seemed to remain unchanged or possibly increased under managed care. Conversely, for Medicaid clients with severe mental illness, there was decreased use of substance abuse treatment services. These findings show that large-scale changes in public policies can have widely varying impacts on sub-groups of the service population. The next chapters address impacts of unfortunate public policies – namely Medicaid cutbacks.

ACKNOWLEDGMENTS

This work was supported by a grant from the Robert Wood Johnson Substance Abuse Policy Research Program: No. 048278 (Bentson McFarland, Principal Investigator). In addition, the authors would like to thank the other principal investigators of the initial Substance Abuse and Mental Health Services Administration (SAMHSA)-funded studies from which the secondary analyses reported here drew data: Dr. Mary Jo Larson of New England Research Institute, Dr. Frank McCorry of the New York Office of Alcohol and Substance Abuse Services, Dr. Tom McLellan of the Treatment Research Institute, Dr. Joseph Morrissey of the University of North Carolina, Dr. Aileen Rothbard of the University of Pennsylvania, Dr. David Shern of the University of South Florida, and Dr. Michael Wylie of the University of Hawaii. These studies were ably coordinated by Dr. Virginia Mulkern, Dr. Stephen Leff and Mr. David Hughes of the Human Services Research Institute; and guided by SAMHSA project officers Dr. Mady Chalk and Ms. Frances Cotter of the Center for Substance Abuse Treatment and Dr. Jeffrey Buck of the Center for Mental Health Services.

REFERENCES

Alexander, J. A., Nahra, T. A., and Wheeler, J. R. C. (2003). Managed care and access to substance abuse treatment services. *Journal of Behavioral Health Services and Research, 30*, 161-175.

Andersen, R. (1995). Revisiting the Behavioral Model and access to medical care: Does it matter? *Journal of Health and Social Behavior, 36*(1), 1-10.

Babor, T. F., Dolinsky, Z. S., Meyer, R. E., Hesselbrock, M., Hofmann, M., and H, T. (1992). Types of alcoholics: Current and predictive validity of common classification schemes. *British Journal of Addiction, 87*, 1415-1431.

Bartels, S., Drake, R., and llach, M. (1995). Long-term course of substance use disorders among patients with severe mental illness. *Psychiatric Services, 46*, 248-251.

Beinecke, R. H. (2005). Stakeholder perspectives on public managed behavioral care in Massachusetts. *Administration and Policy in Mental Health and Mental Health Services Research, 32*(4), 427-438.

Bianconi, J. M., Mahler, J. M., and McFarland, B. H. (2006). Outcomes for rural Medicaid clients with severe mental illness in fee for service versus managed care. *Administration and Policy in Mental Health and Mental Health Services Research, 33*, 411-422.

Bigelow, D. A., McFarland, B. H., McCamant, L. E., Deck, D. D., and Gabriel, R. M. (2004). Effect of managed care on access to mental health services among Medicaid enrollees receiving substance abuse treatment. *Psychiatric Services, 55*, 755-779.

Blank, M. B., Eisenber, M. M., Hargrove, D. S., and Fox, J. C. (1996). Introduction to special issue: Health care reform and rural special populations. *Community Mental Health Journal, 32*, 427-429.

Boothroyd, R. A., Shern, D. L., and Bell, N. L. (2002). The effect of financial risk arrangements on service access and satisfaction among Medicaid beneficiaries. *Psychiatric Services, 53*, 299-303.

Brown, S., Inaba, B., Gillin, J., Schuckit, M., Stewart, M., and Irwin, M. (1995). Alcoholism and affective disorder: Clinical course of depressive symptoms. *American Journal of Psychiatry, 152*, 45-52.

Brunette, M. F., and Mueser, K. T. (2006). Psychosocial interventions for the long-term management of patients with severe mental illness and co-occurring substance use disorder. *Journal of Clinical Psychiatry, 67*(Suppl 7), 10-17.

Buck, J., Teich, J., and Miller, K. (2003). Use of mental health and substance abuse services among high-cost Medicaid enrollees. *Administration and Policy in Mental Health, 31*, 3-14.

Buck, J. A. (2001). Managed mental health care in Medicaid: Does the solution match the problem? *Administration and Policy in Mental Health, 29*(2), 177-180.

Buckley, P. F. (2006). Prevalence and consequences of the dual diagnosis of substance abuse and severe mental illness. *Journal of Clinical Psychiatry, 67*(Suppl 7), 5-9.

Calsyn, R. J., Klinkenberg, W. D., and Morse, G. A. (2004). Recruitment, engagement and retention of people living with HIV and co-occurring mental and substance use disorders. *AIDS Care, 16*(Suppl 1), S56-70.

Carlson, M. J., and Gabriel, R. M. (2001). Patient satisfaction, use of services, and one-year outcomes in publicly funded substance abuse treatment. *Psychiatric Services, 52*, 1230-1236.

Center for Substance Abuse Treatment (Ed.). (2005). *Substance abuse treatment for persons with co-occurring disorders: Treatment Improvement Protocol (TIP) Series 42. DHHS Publication No. (SMA) 05-3992*. Rockville, MD: U.S. Department of Health and Human Services, Substance Abuse and Mental Health Services Administration.

Christianson, J. B., Lurie, N., Finch, M., Moscovice, I. S., and Hartley, D. (1992). Use of community-based mental health programs by HMOs: Evidence from a Medicaid demonstration. *American Journal of Public Health, 82*(6), 790-796.

Coffey, R. M., Mark, T., King, E., Harwood, H., McKusick, D., Genuardi, J. et al. (2001). *National Estimates of Expenditures for Substance Abuse Treatment, 1997. SAMHSA Publication No. SMA-01-3511*. Rockville, MD: Center for Substance Abuse Treatment and Center for Mental Health Services, Substance Abuse and Mental Health Services Administration.

Cuffel, B., and Chase, P. (1994). Remission and relapse of substance use disorders in schizophrenia: Results from a one-year prospective study. *Journal of Nervous and Mental Disease, 182*, 342-348.

Deck, D. D., and McFarland, B. H. (2002). Medicaid managed care and substance abuse treatment. *Psychiatric Services, 53*, 802.

Deck, D. D., McFarland, B. H., Titus, J. M., Laws, K. E., and Gabriel, R. M. (2000). Access to substance abuse treatment services under the Oregon Health Plan. *Journal of the American Medical Association, 284*(16), 2093-2099.

Deck, D. D., Wiitala, W. L., and Laws, K. E. (2006). Medicaid coverage and access to publicly funded opiate treatment. *Journal of Behavioral Health Services and Research, 33*(3), 324-334.

DeRogatis, L. (Ed.). (1993). *Brief Symptom Inventory (BSI), 3rd edition. A brief form of the SCL-90-R, a self-report symptom inventory designed to measure psychological stress.* Minneapolis, MN: National Computer Systems.

Drake, R. E., and Mueser, K. T. (2000). Psychosocial approaches to dual diagnosis. *Schizophrenia Bulletin, 26*(1), 105-118.

Etheridge, R. M., Craddock, S. G., Dunteman, G. H., and Hubbard, R. L. (1995). Treatment services in two national studies of community-based drug abuse treatment programs. *Journal of Substance Abuse, 7*, 9-26.

Ettner, S. L., Argeriou, M., McCarty, D., Dilonardo, J., and Liu, H. (2003). How did the introduction of managed care for the uninsured in Iowa affect the use of substance abuse services? *Journal of Behavioral Health Services and Research, 30*, 26-40.

Fazel, S., Langstrom, N., Hjern, A., Grann, M., and Lichtenstein, P. (2009). Schizophrenia, substance abuse, and violent crime. *Journal of the American Medical Association*, 301, 2016-2023.

Fowler, I., Carr, V., Carter, N., and Lewin, T. J. (1998). Patterns of current and lifetime substance use in schizophrenia. *Schizophrenia Bulletin, 24*, 443-455.

Gelberg, L., Andersen, R. M., and Leaks, B. D. (2000). The Behavioral Model for vulnerable populations: Application to medical care use and outcomes for homeless people. *Health Services Research, 34*(6), 1273-1314.

Grant, B., Dawson, D., Stinson, F., Chou, S., Dufour, M., and Pickering, R. (2004). The 12-month prevalence and trends in DSM-IV alcohol abuse and dependence: United States, 1991-1992 and 2001-2002. *Drug and Alcohol Dependence, 74*, 223-234.

Green, A. I., Drake, R. E., Brunette, M. F., and Noordsy, D. L. (2007). Schizophrenia and co-occurring substance use disorder. *American Journal of Psychiatry,* 164, 408.402-

Grella, C. E. and Stein, J. A. (2006). Impact of program services on treatment outcomes of patients with comorbid mental and substance use disorders. *Psychiatric Services,* 57, 1007-1015.

Havassy, B. E., Alvidrez, J., and Mericle, A. A. (2009). Disparities in use of mental health and substance abuse services by persons with co-occurring disorders. *Psychiatric Services,* 60, 217-222.

Institute of Medicine (1998). *Summarizing population health: Directions for the development and application of population metrics*. Washington, DC: National Academy Press.

Kozarie-Kovacic, D., Folnegovic-Smalc, V., Folnegovic, Z., and Maruic, A. (1995). Influence of alcoholism on the prognosis of schizophrenic patients. *Journal of Studies on Alcohol, 56*, 622-627.

Larson, M. J., Zhang, A., Smith, K., and Kasten, L. (2005). Access to services: Multiple perspectives from adults with substance abuse disorders in Massachusetts. *Administration and Policy in Mental Health and Mental Health Services Research, 32*(4), 357-371.

Laws, K., Gabriel, R., and McFarland, B. H. (2002). Integration and its discontents: Substance abuse treatment in the Oregon Health Plan. *Health Affairs, 21*, 284-289.

Leff, H. S., Wieman, D. A., McFarland, B. H., Morrissey, J. P., Rothbard, A., Shern, D. L. et al. (2005). Assessment of Medicaid managed behavioral health care for persons with serious mental illness. *Psychiatric Services, 56*, 1245-1253.

Luft, H. (2003). Measuring quality in modern managed care. *Health Services Research, 38*, 1371-1384.

Lurie, J., and Belanger, R. J. (2002). The great debate: .Net vs. J2EE. *JavaWorld*, Retrieved March 23, 2005 from http://www.javaworld.com/javaworld/jw-2003-2002/jw-0308-j2002eenet.html.

Lurie, N., Moscovice, I. S., Finch, M., Christianson, J. B., and Popkin, M. K. (1992). Does capitation affect the health of the chronically mentally ill? Results from a randomized trial. *Journal of the American Medical Association, 267*(4), 3300-3303.

Manning, W. G., Liu, C., Stoner, T. J., Gray, D. Z., Lurie, N., Popkin, M. et al. (1999). Outcomes for Medicaid beneficiaries with schizophrenia under a prepaid mental health carve-out. *Journal of Behavioral Health Services and Research, 26*(4), 442-450.

Mark, T., Coffey, R. M., McKusick, D., Harwood, H., King, E., Bouchery, E. et al. (2005). *National expenditures for mental health services and substance abuse treatment: 1991-2001. SAMHSA Publication No. SMA 05-3999*. Rockville, MD: Substance Abuse and Mental Health Services Administration.

McCarty, D., Dilonardo, J., and Argeriou, M. (2003). State substance abuse and mental health managed care evaluation program. *Journal of Behavioral Health Services and Research, 30*, 7-17.

McFarland, B. H. (2000). Overview of Medicaid managed behavioral health care. In R. R. Goetz, B. H. McFarland and K. V. Ross (Eds.), *What the Oregon Health Plan can teach us about managed mental health care. New Directions for Mental Health Services, No. 85* (pp. 17-22). San Francisco: Jossey-Bass.

McFarland, B. H., Deck, D. D., McCamant, L. E., Gabriel, R. M., and Bigelow, D. A. (2005). Outcomes for Medicaid clients with substance abuse problems before and after managed care. *Journal of Behavioral Health Services and Research, 32*(4), 351-367.

McFarland, B. H., and Gabriel, R. M. (2004). Service availability for persons with co-occurring conditions. *Psychiatric Services, 55*, 978.

McFarland, B. H., Stroup, T. S., Rothbard, A. B., Rose, M. R., Stiles, P. G., Shern, D. L. et al. (2004). Antipsychotic medication use by Medicaid clients with severe mental illness. *Drug Benefit Trends, 16*, 204-208.

McLellan, A. T., Cacciola, J., Kushner, H., Peters, R., Smith, I., and Pettinati, H. (1992). The fifth edition of the Addiction Severity Index: Historical critique and normative data. *Journal of Substance Abuse Treatment, 9*, 199-213.

Mechanic, D. (2001). The managed care backlash: Perceptions and rhetoric in health care policy and the potential for health care reform. *Milbank Quarterly, 79*, 35-54.

Menzes, P., Johnson, S., Thornicraft, G., Marshall, J., Prosser, D., Bebbington, P. et al. (1996). Drug and alcohol problems among individuals with severe mental illness in South London. *British Journal of Psychiatry, 168*, 612-619.

Miller, N., and Ries, R. (1991). Drug and alcohol dependence and psychiatric populations: The need for diagnosis intervention and training. *Comprehensive Psychiatry, 32*, 268-276.

Miller, N. S., Ninonuevo, F. G., Klamen, D. L., Hoffmann, N. G., and Smith, D. E. (1997). Integration of treatment and posttreatment variables in predicting results of abstinence-based outpatient treatment after one year. *Journal of Psychoactive Drugs, 29*, 239-248.

Minkoff, K. (1998). *Co-occurring psychiatric and substance disorders in managed care systems: Standards of care practice guidelines workforce competencies and training curricula*. Rockville, MD: Center for Mental Health Services, SAMHSA.

Morrissey, J. P., Stroup, T. S., Ellis, A. R., and Merwin, E. (2002). Service use and health status of persons with severe mental illness in full-risk and non-risk Medicaid programs. *Psychiatric Services, 53*, 293-298.

Morse, G., Calsyn, R., Allen, G., Tempelhoff, B., and Smith, R. (1992). Experimental comparison of the effects of three treatment programs for homeless mentally ill people. *Hospital and Community Psychiatry, 43*, 1005-1010.

Mueser, K., Bellack, A., and Blanchard, J. (1992). Co-morbidity of schizophrenia and substance abuse: Implications for treatment. *Journal of Consulting and Clinical Psychology, 60*, 845-856.

Mueser, K., Drake, R., and Noordsy, D. (1998). Integrated mental health and substance abuse treatment for severe psychiatric disorders. *Journal of Practical Psychiatry and Behavioral Health, 4*, 129-139.

National Association of State Mental Health Program Directors (NASMHPD) and National Association of State Alcohol and Drug Abuse Directors (NASADAD) (Ed.). (1998). *National dialog on co-occurring mental health and substance abuse disorders (Conference, June 16-17 1998)*. Rockville, MD: Center for Substance Abuse Treatment and Center for Mental Health Services.

Okin, R., Borus, J., Baer, L., and Jones, A. L. (1995). Long-term outcome of state hospital patients discharged into structured community residential settings. *Psychiatric Services, 46*, 73-78.

Ouimette, P., Moos, R., and Finney, J. (1998). Influence of outpatient treatment and 12-step group involvement on one-year substance abuse treatment outcomes. *Journal on Studies of Alcohol, 59*, 513-522.

Owen, R., Rischer, E., Booth, B., and Cuffel, B. J. (1996). Medication noncompliance and substance abuse among patients with schizophrenia. *Psychiatric Services, 47*, 853-858.

Prince, J.D., Akincigil, A., Hoover, D.R., Walkup, J.T., Bilder, S., and Crystal, S. (2009). Substance abuse and hospitalization for mood disorder among Medicaid beneficiaries. *American Journal of Public Health,* 99, 160-167.

Putkonen, A., Kotilainen, I., and Joyal, C. C. (2004). Comorbid personality disorders and substance use disorders of mentally ill homicide offenders: A structured clinical study on dual and triple diagnoses. *Schizophrenia Bulletin, 30*(1), 59-72.

Rasanen, R., Tiihonen, J., Isohanni, M., Rantakallio, P., Lehtonen, J., and Moring, J. (1998). Schizophrenia alcohol abuse and violent behavior: A 26-year follow-up study of an unselected birth cohort. *Schizophrenia Bulletin, 24*, 437-441.

Reardon, M. L., Burns, A. B., Preist, R., Sachs-Ericsson, N., and Lang, A. (2003). Alcohol use and other psychiatric disorders in the formerly homeless and never homeless: Prevalence, age of onset, comorbidity, temporal sequencing, and service utilization. *Substance Use and Misuse, 38*, 601-644.

Regier, D., Farmer, M., Rae, D., Locke, B., Keith, S., Judd, L. et al. (1990). Comorbidity of mental disorders with alcohol and other drug abuse: Results from the Epidemiologic Catchment Area (ECA) study. *Journal of the American Medical Association, 264*, 2511-2518.

Ridgely, M. S., Giard, J., Shern, D., Mulkern, V., and Burnam, M. A. (2002). Managed behavioral health care: An instrument to characterize critical elements of public sector programs. *Health Services Research, 37*(4), 1105-1123.

Ridgely, M. S., Mulkern, V., Giard, J., and Shern, D. (2002). Critical elements of public-sector managed behavioral health programs for severe mental illness in five states. *Psychiatric Services, 53*, 397-399.

Ries, R. (1993). Clinical treatment matching models for co-occurring diagnosed patients. *Psychiatric Clinics of North America, 16*, 167-175.

Ritsher, J. B., Moos, R. H., and Finney, J. W. (2002). Relationship of treatment orientation and continuing care to remission among substance abuse patients. *Psychiatric Services, 53*, 595-601.

Ross, K. V., and McFarland, B. H. (2000). The mental health organizations. In R. R. Goetz, B. H. McFarland and K. V. Ross (Eds.), *What the Oregon Health Plan can teach us about managed mental health care. New Directions for Mental Health Services, 85:57-64*. San Francisco: Jossey-Bass.

Rothbard, A. B., Kuno, E., Hadley, T. R., and Dogin, J. (2004). Psychiatric service utilization and cost for persons with schizophrenia in a Medicaid managed care program. *Journal of Behavioral Health Services and Research, 31*, 1-12.

Rothbard, A. B., McFarland, B. H., Shern, D. L., Morrisey, J. P., Leff, S. H., and Wylie, M. A. (2002). Managed care for persons with serious mental illness. *Drug Benefit Trends, 14*, 6-14.

Sacks, S., Sacks, J., and DeLeon, G. (1997). Modified therapeutic community for mentally ill chemical abusers: Background, influences, program description; Preliminary findings. *Substance use and misuse, 32*(9), 1217-1259.

Salyers, M. P., and Meuser, K. T. (2001). Social functioning, psychopathology and medication side effects relation to substance use and abuse in schizophrenia. *Schizophrenia Research, 48*(1), 109-123.

Samet, S. and Hasin, D. (2008). Clinical implications of epidemiologic data for diagnosis and treatment of psychiatric comorbidity. *Psychiatric Annals,* 38, 709-715.

Scott, J. (1993). Homelessness and mental illness. *British Journal of Psychiatry, 162*, 314-324.

Sells, D. J., Rowe, M., and Fisk, D. (2003). Violent victimization of persons with co-occurring psychiatric and substance use disorders. *Psychiatric Services, 54*(9), 1253-1257.

Smith, V., Gifford, K., Ramesh, R., Ellis, E., and Wachino, V. (2005). *States respond to fiscal pressure: State Medicaid spending growth and cost containment in fiscal years 2003 and 2004: Results from a 50-state survey*. Washington, DC: Kaiser Commission on Medicaid and the Uninsured.

Sosin, M., and D'Aunno, T. (2001). The organization of substance abuse managed care. *Recent Developments in Alcoholism, 15*, 27-49.

Steadman, H., Mulvey, E., Monahan, J., Robbins, P., Appelbaum, P., Grisso, T. et al. (1998). Violence by people discharged from acute psychiatric facilities and by others in the same neighborhoods. *Archives of General Psychiatry, 55*, 393-401.

Steenrod, S., Brisson, A., McCarty, D., and Hodgkin, D. (2001). Effects of managed care on programs and practices for the treatment of alcohol and drug dependence. *Recent Developments in Alcoholism, 15*, 51-71.

Stroup, T. S., and Dorwart, R. A. (1995). Impact of a managed mental health program on Medicaid recipients with severe mental illness. *Psychiatric Services, 46*, 885-889.

Substance Abuse and Mental Health Services Administration (2002). *Report to Congress on the Prevention and Treatment of Co-occurring Substance Abuse Disorders and Mental Disorders*. Rockville, MD: Substance Abuse and Mental Health Services Administration Office of Applied Studies.

Substance Abuse and Mental Health Services Administration (Ed.). (1999). *Managed behavioral health care in the public sector: Interim report on baseline characteristics. Program report submitted by the project coordinating center, Human Services Research Institute*. Rockville, MD: U.S. Department of Health and Human Services.

Timko, C., and Moos, R. H. (2002). Symptom severity, amount of treatment, and one-year outcomes among dual diagnosis patients. *Administration and Policy in Mental Health, 30*, 33-54.

Ware, J., Kosinkski, M., and Keller, S. (1996). A 12-item short-form health survey: construction of scales and preliminary tests of reliability and validity. *Medical Care, 34*, 220-233.

Watkins, K., Hunter, S., and Wenzel, S. (2004). Prevalence and characteristics of clients with co-occurring disorders in outpatient substance abuse treatment. *American Journal of Drug and Alcohol Abuse, 30*(4), 749-764.

In: Medicaid and Treatment for People… ISBN 978-1-61470-742-4
Editor: B.H. McFarland, D.McCarty, et al, pp. 223-230

Chapter 10

Impact of Eliminating Medicaid Treatment Benefits

Dennis D. Deck and Roy M. Gabriel
RMC Research Corporation, Portland, OR, USA

Abstract

During the early 1990s Oregon dramatically expanded its Medicaid population through a series of federal waivers under a program known as the Oregon Health Plan (OHP). In 2002, the state split the Medicaid population into OHP Plus (traditional mandatory Medicaid-eligible persons), and OHP Standard (the expansion clients). Late in 2002 in response to a substantial budget shortfall, the Oregon legislature eliminated substance abuse, mental health, and dental benefits from OHP Standard coverage effective March 2003. Coverage for these services remained for the OHP Plus population. This chapter examines the impact of these Medicaid cutbacks. In brief, the benefit cutbacks led to dramatic reduction in the number of OHP Standard clients enrolled in Medicaid. Moreover, of those who remained enrolled, relatively few accessed substance abuse or mental health outpatient treatment while those services were not covered. Enrollment as well as use of mental health and substance abuse services by traditional Medicaid (OHP Plus) clients showed little change. Providers also felt the impact of cutbacks as agencies closed or dramatically reduced services. Medicaid cutbacks for substance abuse and mental health treatment can have substantial impact.

Introduction

During the early 1990s Oregon dramatically expanded its Medicaid population through a series of federal waivers. Together these changes came to be known as the Oregon Health Plan (OHP). Controlling costs through a prioritized list of covered treatments and other features, the plan included a significant expansion of the population covered by Medicaid. In 2002, the state split the OHP population into OHP Plus, consisting of the traditional mandatory Medicaid-eligible categories, and OHP Standard, a category that covered the expansion clients.

Late in 2002 the state faced a significant budget shortfall. Responding to the shortfall, the Oregon legislature instituted premiums and co-payments for OHP Standard clients (Mann and Artiga, 2004). In addition, the state eliminated substance abuse (SA), mental health (MH), and dental benefits from OHP Standard coverage effective March 2003. Coverage for these services remained for the OHP Plus population. The cutback of Medicaid benefits to deal with the budget shortfall came as a shock to many — especially Medicaid clients and treatment providers.

Some 17 months later, in August 2004, these benefits were finally re-instated. However enrollment in OHP Standard had been frozen so anyone who had dis-enrolled during the benefit elimination period was unable to re-enroll. While observers expected a reduction in access to treatment, no one was certain how dramatic the impact might be.

METHODS

Adults presenting for publicly funded treatment were identified using Oregon's Client Process Monitoring System (CPMS), a statewide treatment database. Medicaid eligibility at admission was verified by linking eligibility records from the state's Medicaid Management Information System (MMIS) to CPMS records. The sample consisted of adults (ages 18 to 64) accessing MH or SA treatment during 2000 through 2004 who were enrolled in Medicaid.

Table 1 shows the admission characteristics of the Medicaid-eligible adults presenting for MH or SA treatment in Oregon during the study period.

Table 1. Characteristics of Medicaid-eligible adults presenting for substance abuse and mental health treatment in Oregon between 2000 and 2004

Characteristic	Substance abuse (N = 35,153)	Mental health (N = 59,763)
Medicaid eligibility		
OHP Plus – Disabled	7%	16%
OHP Plus – Poverty	26%	30%
OHP Standard	63%	46%
Other Medicaid	4%	9%
Age		
18–25	26%	24%
26–35	32%	28%
36–45	30%	27%
46–64	12%	21%
Gender		
Female	46%	66%
Male	54%	35%
Ethnicity/Race		
White, not Hispanic	81%	88%
Black, not Hispanic	6%	4%
Hispanic	5%	4%
Native American	6%	1%
Other	2%	3%

Eligibility categories were mapped into OHP Standard, a Medicaid expansion program for single adults and childless couples, and OHP Plus, which included the mandatory Medicaid eligibility programs. For this study, OHP Plus was further divided into Disabled and Poverty since the latter group were most like OHP Standard enrollees. SA admissions associated with Driving Under the Influence of Intoxicants (DUII) were excluded for this study.

Three main categories of outpatient treatment services are covered under Medicaid in Oregon: Mental Health (MH), Substance Abuse (SA), and Methadone Maintenance Treatment (MMT). These will be covered separately.

RESULTS

First we examine the change in the Medicaid enrollments before and after the benefit cut. Next we look at the number of Medicaid-eligible adults entering each form of treatment each month. Finally we compute monthly access rates to show the net impact of the change.

Medicaid Enrollment

Figure 1 shows the number of adults enrolled in Medicaid from 2000 through 2004 for OHP Standard, OHP Plus-Poverty, and OHP Plus-Disabled. Vertical lines mark the beginning (March 2003) and end (August 2004) of the period during which MH, SA, and dental services were not covered.

The number of adults enrolled as OHP Standard dropped dramatically after the cutbacks to about half the prior enrollment. Although adults continuing their Medicaid enrollment retained coverage for medical problems, access to behavioral health services may have been a major factor in encouraging clients eligible for OHP standard to enroll and pay fees. As expected, enrollment for OHP Plus remained fairly stable during this period.

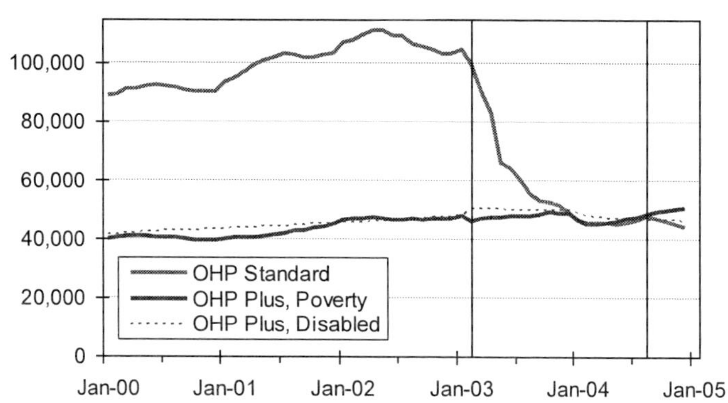

Figure 1. Monthly Medicaid enrollment: Number of Medicaid-eligible adults in Oregon from 2000 to 2004 by funding category.

Admissions to Treatment

Figures 2, 3, and 4 illustrate the monthly number of MH, SA, and MMT outpatient admissions in Oregon from 2000 through 2004 in each Medicaid eligibility category. As soon as treatment was no longer covered for OHP Standard clients, the number of admissions immediately dropped to a very low level for all three types of treatment.

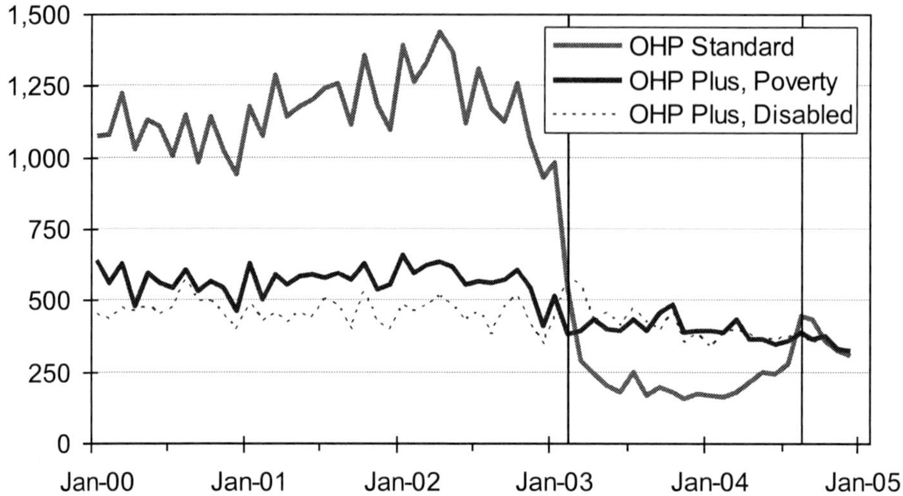

Figure 2. Outpatient mental health admissions: Number of adult outpatient mental health treatment admissions in Oregon from 2000 through 2004 by funding category

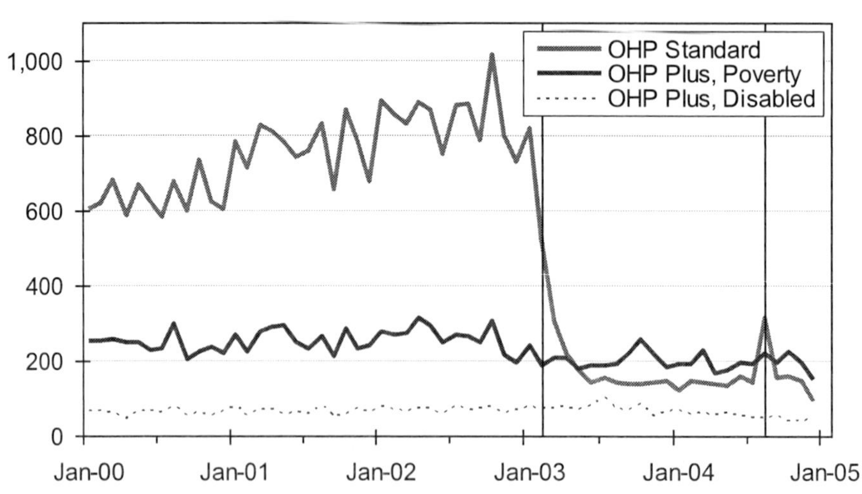

Figure 3. Outpatient substance abuse Admissions: Number of adult outpatient substance abuse treatment admissions in Oregon from 2000 through 2004 by funding category.

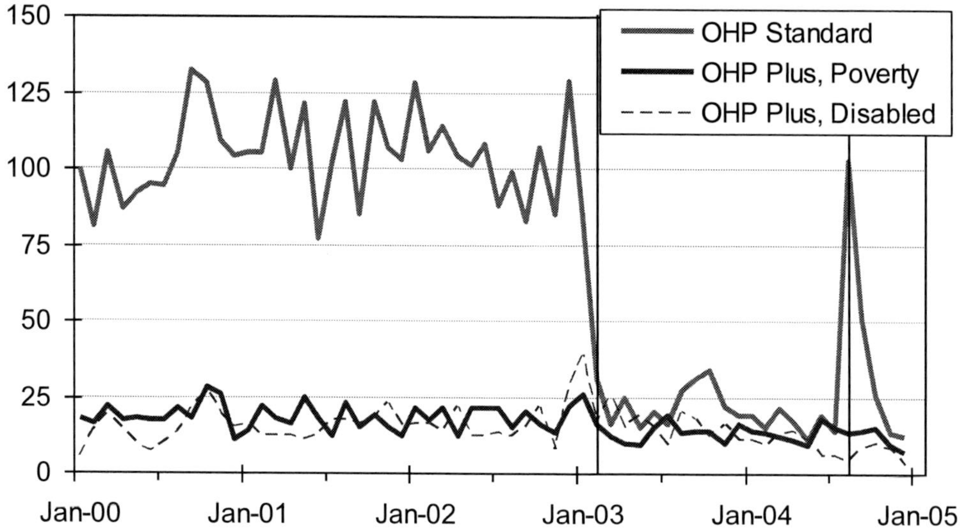

Figure 4. Methadone maintenance treatment admissions: Number of adult methadone maintenance admissions in Oregon from 2000 through 2004 by funding category.

The number of treatment admissions for OHP Plus Poverty dropped slightly over that same time period for each form of treatment as providers worked to rebalance caseloads with what they described as radically downsized staff.

Admission Rates

The number of adults presenting for treatment was converted to a rate to control for the large decline in OHP Standard enrollees under Medicaid. Figures 5, 6, and 7 display the outpatient treatment admission rates for each group, computed as the number of admissions per 1000 eligible members.

Rates declined dramatically among OHP Standard members—71% MH, 67% SA, and 57% MMT between 2002 and the last three quarters of 2003. The decline started slightly before the policy change took effect as providers were already cutting back services in anticipation of benefit elimination.

Somewhat surprisingly, there was also a decline in admissions for the Poverty group of OHP Plus members—28% MH, 25% SA, and 28% MMT. Qualitative inquiry among MMT providers suggested that anticipation of the dramatic loss of revenue for OHP Standard clients—much more than half of the served population—drove agency closures and staff turnover resulting in a decline in overall capacity.

Following reinstatement of treatment benefits for OHP Standard, there was an immediate but temporary increase in access, especially for methadone maintenance treatment. Although many clients had let eligibility lapse, those who continued paying the premium to cover their medical benefit immediately sought reinstatement into treatment. However the increase was not sustained without an influx of new OHP Standard clients.

Analysis revealed that those presenting for methadone maintenance treatment in 2003 often had a prior treatment history.

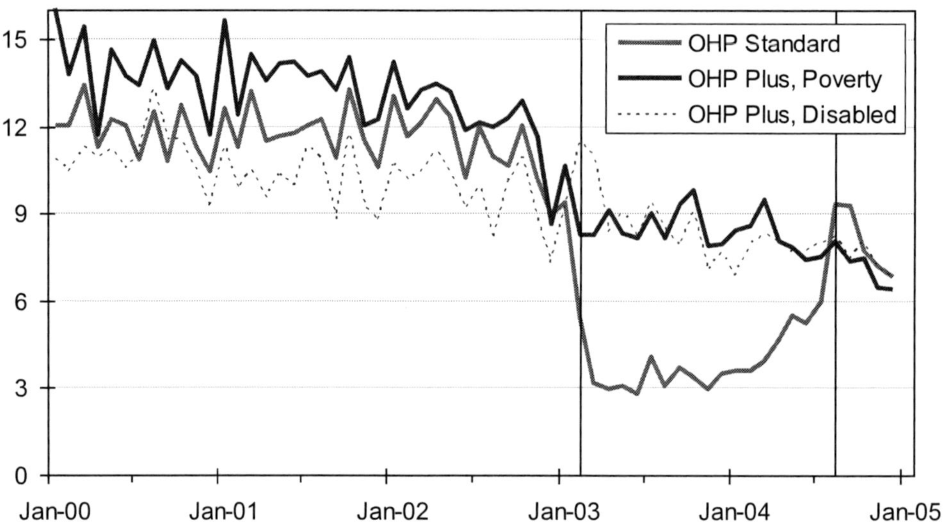

Figure 5. Outpatient mental health admissions rates: Admissions per 1,000 Medicaid-eligible adults to publicly funded outpatient mental health treatment in Oregon by funding category

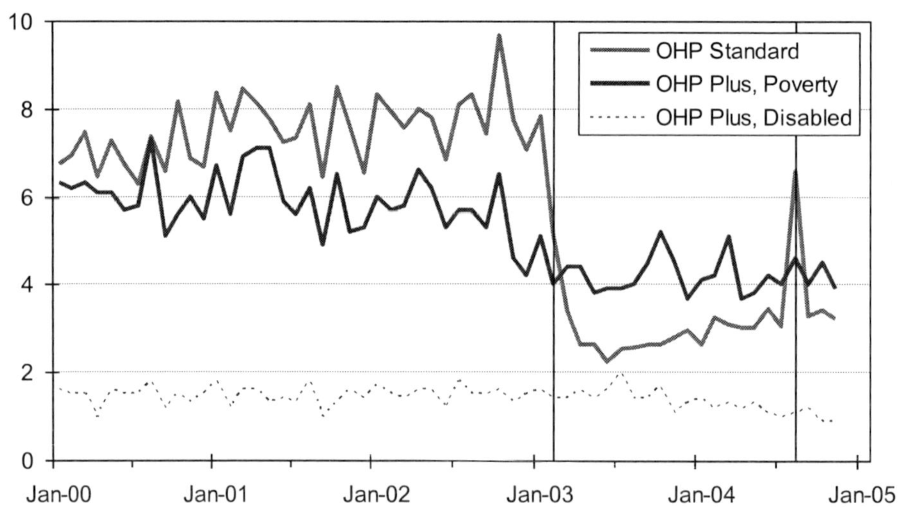

Figure 6. Outpatient substance abuse admission rates: Admissions per 1000 Medicaid-eligible adults to publicly funded outpatient substance abuse treatment in Oregon by funding category

This finding suggested that the cutbacks reduced the normal influx of new clients addicted to opiates who had not previously been served by the substance abuse treatment system. For further discussion see Deck et al. (2006).

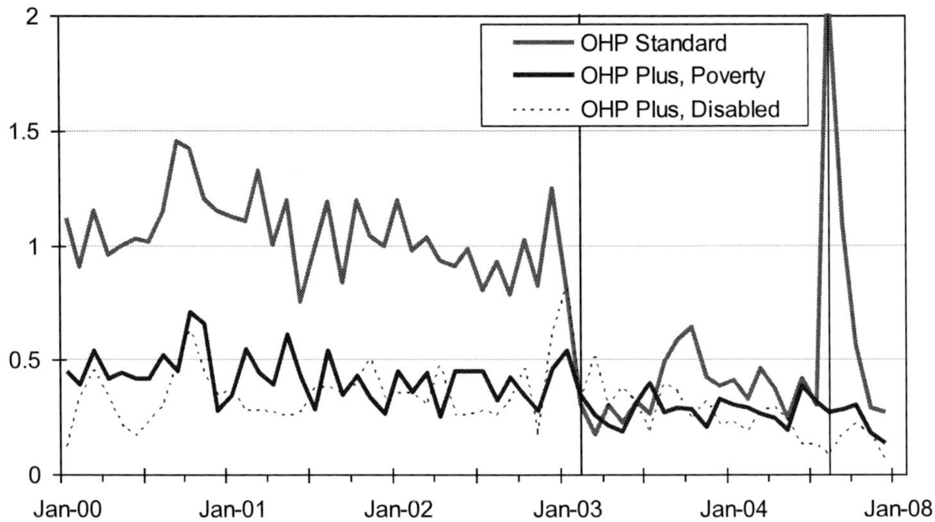

Figure 7. Methadone maintenance admission rates: Admissions per 1000 Medicaid-eligible adults to publicly funded methadone maintenance treatment in Oregon by funding category.

METHADONE MAINTENANCE TREATMENT PROVIDER EXPERIENCE

Interviews with methadone providers confirmed that the apparent impact of the benefit cut was immediate and strongly felt (Laws et al., 2008). For most providers, OHP Standard clients represented a substantial portion of their Medicaid caseload and thus a significant portion of their income. Two clinics closed their doors following loss of so many clients. The remaining clinics reported a number of changes: clinical staff lay offs, reductions in their staff's work week, elimination of staff health benefits, and other cost saving measures such as less individual contact with patients, increased treatment group size, and less urine analysis monitoring. Both treatment providers and patients began preparing for the loss of coverage even before the cut took effect.

A surprising number of patients elected to pay out of pocket after losing the benefit, though usually only those who had some source of income (from a job, family or friends or criminal activity) were able to do so. Treatment providers reported that as early as two months prior to the benefit cut, many patients were requesting methadone detoxification, as this approach provided a longer window of time than the minimum of 21 days required by the state if they waited until March 1. According to treatment providers, patients are reluctant to restart treatment even with restored benefits since providers could not reassure them that benefits would not be cut again, and the thought of going through another painful detoxification is something they did not want to endure.

There were also isolated instances of collaborative action to mitigate the impact of the benefit cut. In one area, the county, the hospital and the health plan split the costs of continuing to treat methadone patients who lost their benefit. A large urban county paid for some substance abuse treatment services through a special referendum that provided temporary (up to 3 years) funding for a variety of educational and social services.

While we suspect that outpatient MH and SA clinics had somewhat similar experiences, we only interviewed MMT providers so we can only speculate.

Conclusion

In conclusion, cutbacks led to a dramatic reduction in the number of OHP Standard clients enrolled in Medicaid. For those who remained enrolled, relatively few accessed SA or MH outpatient treatment while those services were not covered. When re-expressed as rates to control for the dramatic change in the number enrolled in Medicaid, the decreases are even more striking.

Although continued pressure eventually led the state to reinstate Medicaid coverage for these services, the impact was minimized by restricting this reinstatement to those who had retained their coverage. After a brief spike in admissions, especially for MMT, rates returned to a low level.

The next chapter addresses impact of these Medicaid cutbacks as assessed with survey data.

Acknowledgment

This research was supported by Robert Wood Johnson Substance Abuse Policy Research Program Grant number 51530 and National Institute on Drug Abuse (NIDA) Research Grant number R01 DA015060.

References

Deck, D. D., Wiitala, W., and Laws K. E. (2006). Medicaid coverage and access to publicly funded opiate treatment. *Journal of Behavioral Health Services and Research*, *33*, 324-334.

Laws, K. E., D'Ambrosio, R., and Deck, D. D. (2008). Impact of changes in financing on publicly funded methadone maintenance treatment: A comparison between Oregon and Washington. *Journal of Maintenance in the Addictions* 3, 65-78.

Mann, C. and Artiga, S. (2004). *The impact of recent changes in health care coverage for low-income people: A first look at the research following changes in Oregon's Medicaid program.* Washington, DC: Kaiser Commission on Medicaid and the Uninsured.

In: Medicaid and Treatment for People... ISBN 978-1-61470-742-4
Editor: B.H. McFarland, D.McCarty, et al, pp. 231-237

Chapter 11

ELIMINATING THEN (SORT OF) RESTORING SUBSTANCE ABUSE AND MENTAL HEALTH BENEFITS IN THE OREGON HEALTH PLAN: EFFECTS ON TREATMENT FOR THE MOST VULNERABLE MEDICAID CLIENTS

Roy M. Gabriel, Dennis D. Deck, Chandra K. Lewis, Kelly J. Vander Ley, and Katherine E. Laws
RMC Research Corporation, Portland, OR, USA

ABSTRACT

Cutbacks may differentially affect sub-groups within the Medicaid population. This chapter summarizes 2005 survey data from Oregon Health Plan members including both traditional Medicaid and expansion population clients. The statewide sample was augmented by clients currently in substance abuse treatment who had been Medicaid beneficiaries prior to the 2003 benefit cuts. Among those who had experienced or expressed need for substance abuse or mental health treatment there was no apparent decline in access to behavioral health care for either expansion or traditional Medicaid clients following benefit elimination in 2003. There was also no increase in access following restoration of the benefit in 2004. Clients who were receiving substance abuse or mental health treatment prior to the elimination of these benefits were significantly more likely to maintain access to care following the policy changes than were those who were in need but were not already in treatment prior to the policy change. These results are in marked contrast to the overall declines in behavioral health treatment shown by Oregon Medicaid population data as well as the decreases for Oregon methadone maintenance clients reported in previous chapters. On the other hand, the Oregon data reported here echo findings from California in an early chapter suggesting that at least some Medicaid clients in substance abuse treatment are able to continue care even in the absence of insurance coverage. An important message is that Medicaid policy changes can have assorted and widespread impacts.

Introduction

Oregon's progressive Medicaid expansion, known as the Oregon Health Plan (OHP), received national attention among health policy advocates and evidenced positive outcomes for its members through the 1990s (Deck et al., 2000). In 2003, dealing with what was then the state's worst fiscal recession since World War II, the Oregon legislature chose to cut health care costs by, among other things, eliminating substance abuse (SA) and mental health (MH) benefits from OHP for nearly half of its membership, the non-categorically eligible "expansion" population known as OHP Standard. The state also added premiums and co-payments for this group (Enos, 2006; Mann and Artiga, 2004). Within six months, over half the OHP Standard members dis-enrolled from OHP (McConnell and Wallace, 2004) and access to SA treatment declined dramatically for all OHP populations (Deck et al., 2005). In August 2004, as the state's fiscal outlook improved, SA and MH benefits were reinstated, although only for those OHP Standard members who retained their OHP coverage through the prior policy change period.

This chapter addresses the following research questions. For OHP members who reported experience with or need for SA or MH treatment, first, did access to SA and MH treatment decline following the elimination of these benefits? Second, did access to SA and MH treatment improve with the restoration of these benefits 17 months later? And third, did these policy changes affect the traditional Medicaid (OHP Plus) and "expansion" Medicaid (OHP Standard) populations differently? The policy change periods are shown in Table 1.

Table 1. Substance abuse and mental health benefit coverage by Oregon Health Plan eligibility group and policy change periods

	Oregon Health Plan benefit policy change periods		
Medicaid Population	Prior to Benefit Cuts (1/00–2/03)	Substance Abuse and Mental Health Benefits Eliminated (3/03–7/04)	Substance and Mental Health Benefits Restored (8/04–12/05)
OHP Standard	Covered	Not covered	Covered
OHP Plus	Covered	Covered	Covered

Notes:
OHP Standard = Oregon Health Plan non-categorically eligible Medicaid "expansion" population
OHP Plus = Oregon Health Plan traditional Medicaid population

Methods

Structured interviews, using Time Line Follow Back methodology (Sobell and Sobell, 1992) were conducted with 190 adults who were OHP members prior to benefit cuts in 2003. The sample was stratified by OHP Standard and OHP Plus membership.

The original sample was taken from a statewide survey of OHP membership (Wright et al., 2005) and included only those who had experience with or reported a need for SA or MH treatment. The small original sample size was later augmented by a sample of current SA treatment participants who had been OHP members prior to benefit cuts. Interviews were conducted from July to December of 2005.

The sample was predominantly White (72%), female (72%) and over 30 years old (73%), but differences existed between OHP Standard and Plus members in these and other demographic characteristics as shown in Table 2.

Table 2. Oregon Health Plan Standard and Plus demographics from survey and current treatment samples

	Oregon Health Plan survey sample (*n* = 100)		**Current treatment sample (*n* = 90)**		
	OHP Standard	**OHP Plus**	**OHP Standard**	**OHP Plus**	**Total Sample (*n* = 190)**
Characteristic [a]					
Female*	76%	82%	**57%**	81%	75%
White	78%	69%	71%	69%	72%
30 and younger**	16%	18%	**33%**	44%	27%
Married*	28%	16%	26%	29%	25%
High School or less	33%	51%	60%	58%	50%
Living independently	69%	67%	66%	58%	64%
Employed***	36%	**16%**	24%	**8%**	22%
Ever arrested***	15%	7%	43%	**31%**	23%

Notes.

[a] At time of Oregon Health Plan benefit policy change in March of 2003

OHP Standard = Oregon Health Plan non-categorically eligible Medicaid "expansion" population

OHP Plus = Oregon Health Plan traditional Medicaid population

Bolded percentages denote significant differences between Standard (expansion) and Plus (traditional Medicaid) groups

*$p < .05$; **$p < .01$; ***$p < .001$

Results

The prevalence of SA and MH problems prior to the policy changes differed slightly for OHP Standard and OHP Plus members, but dramatically for OHP survey and Current Treatment samples as shown in Table 3. Recent substance use prior to OHP policy changes was similar between OHP Standard and Plus populations, except for higher prevalence of heroin and opiate use among OHP Standard members. Lifetime mental health problems were also similar, except for higher rates of anxiety and schizophrenia among OHP Plus members. Adults from the current SA treatment sample reported significantly higher rates of prior substance use than those from the OHP survey sample for all substances but alcohol. Oregon Health Plan Standard members currently in SA treatment were less likely to report anxiety, depression and "other mental breakdowns" than all other groups. Oregon Health Plan Plus members in SA treatment were more likely to report post traumatic stress disorder (PTSD).

Table 3. Substance abuse and mental health problems for survey and current treatment samples

	Oregon Health Plan survey sample (n = 100)		Current treatment sample (n = 90)		
	OHP Standard	**OHP Plus**	**OHP Standard**	**OHP Plus**	**Total Sample (n = 190)**
Problem [a]					
Recent alcohol or illicit drug use					
Alcohol	71%	67%	79%	86%	76%
Marijuana*	42%	44%	**64%**	**73%**	55%
Methamphetamine***	16%	18%	**71%**	**65%**	41%
Heroin***	11%	2%	**33%**	**25%**	17%
Opiates***	20%	2%	**38%**	**25%**	21%
Crack/Cocaine***	13%	11%	**60%**	**44%**	31%
Other illicit drug**	9%	4%	**29%**	**19%**	15%
Lifetime mental health problem					
Anxiety**	53%	**76%**	38%	56%	56%
Sleep/eating disorder	53%	51%	33%	35%	44%
Major depression*	**54%**	**55%**	29%	**58%**	50%
PTSD*	40%	31%	43%	**63%**	44%
Depression**	**73%**	**67%**	38%	**65%**	62%
Schizophrenia***	7%	**31%**	7%	8%	13%
Other mental breakdown*	**55%**	**53%**	26%	**44%**	45%

Notes.

[a]At time of interview July to December 2005

OHP Standard = Oregon Health Plan non-categorically eligible Medicaid "expansion" population

OHP Plus = Oregon Health Plan traditional Medicaid population

PTSD = post-traumatic stress disorder

Bolded percentages denote groups significantly more severe than others.

$^{*}p < .05$; $^{**}p < .01$; $^{***}p < .001$.

Use of SA or MH treatment services differed markedly between OHP Standard and Plus members as shown in Table 4. OHP Standard members were more than twice as likely to access SA treatment than OHP Plus members in all three policy periods. OHP Plus members were more likely to access MH treatment than OHP Standard members prior to and after the benefit elimination, but not following the restoration of the benefits for OHP Standard members. For this sample—those who had experienced or expressed a need for SA or MH treatment—there was no apparent decline in access to SA or MH treatment following the elimination of the benefit in 2003 for either OHP Standard or Plus members. This result is in stark contrast to findings in the OHP population as a whole (Deck et al., 2005). There was also no increase in access following restoration of the benefit in 2004.

Those OHP members who were receiving SA or MH treatment prior to the elimination of these benefits were significantly more likely to maintain access to treatment following these policy changes than were those who were in need but were not already in treatment prior to the policy change as shown in Table 5.

Table 4. Treatment access prior to and after Oregon Health Plan policy changes

		OHP benefit policy change periods		
Group	Treatment Services	Prior to benefit cuts (1/02–2/03)	During benefit cuts (3/03–7/04)	After Treatment Benefits Restored (8/04–12/05)
OHP Standard (n = 97)	Substance Abuse	32%	32%	32%
	Mental Health	23%	30%	33%
OHP Plus (n = 93)	Substance Abuse	14%	16%	15%
	Mental Health	43%	43%	34%

OHP Standard = Oregon Health Plan non-categorically eligible Medicaid "expansion" population
OHP Plus = Oregon Health Plan traditional Medicaid population

Table 5. Treatment participation during benefit cut and restoration periods for prior treatment participants and non-participants

	OHP Standard		OHP Plus	
	During benefit cut period (3/03–7/04)	After restoration of benefit (8/04–12/05)	During benefit cut period (3/03–7/04)	After restoration of benefit (8/04–12/05)
Substance abuse treatment				
Prior treatment	65%	65%	85%	54%
No prior treatment	17%	17%	5%	9%
Mental health treatment				
Prior treatment	68%	64%	80%	68%
No prior treatment	19%	24%	15%	9%

OHP Standard = Oregon Health Plan non-categorically eligible Medicaid "expansion" population.
OHP Plus = Oregon Health Plan traditional Medicaid population.

DISCUSSION

The dramatic reduction in access to SA treatment for the OHP population as a whole (including those who maintained their enrollment through these periods of benefit changes) was not evident for that portion of the OHP population who was in (self-reported) need for treatment or had experienced treatment prior to these policy shifts.

Both OHP Standard and OHP Plus members who had participated in SA or MH treatment prior to the elimination of benefits were far more likely to access treatment through both benefit elimination and restoration periods than those who had not participated in treatment before the policy changes.

Qualitative evidence suggested that treatment agencies, both in anticipation of and during the benefit elimination period, found creative ways to finance current patients' care.

However, these findings do not account for the more than 60,000 OHP members who dis-enrolled or lost coverage during these policy shifting periods—generally the lowest income and most in need of medical and behavioral health care (Wright et al., 2005). Of the sample studied here, only 50% were able to maintain uninterrupted OHP coverage for the full study period (2002 through 2005).

CONCLUSION

At the population level, the sweeping policy changes mandated by the state legislature to eliminate SA and MH benefits for the expanded Medicaid population effected a dramatic decline in access to both SA and MH treatment.

Within the general population, however, those OHP Standard and Plus members who reported a need for, or prior experience with, SA or MH treatment did not exhibit this decline. More detailed analysis indicated this outcome was true only for OHP members who were already receiving SA or MH services prior to the elimination of benefits.

Because enrollment in OHP Standard was frozen when the SA and MH benefits were restored, any OHP members who had dis-enrolled during the benefit elimination period were unable to take advantage of restored SA and MH treatment coverage, leaving a substantial portion of the prior Medicaid population without coverage for SA and MH care. Therefore, the absence of dramatic increase in access to treatment following the restoration of benefits for OHP Standard is not surprising.

Policymakers are urged to consider the ramifications of sweeping (alleged) cost-saving measures in the health care arena. This study, and many others cited here, repeatedly show that individuals at lowest income levels and most in need of ongoing care are the ones who "slip through the cracks." While data presented here indicate that those treatment clients already receiving services often find ways (through a combination of self-pay and provider creativity) to maintain care even if they lose benefits, these solutions apply to only a small proportion of those affected by policy changes. An important message is that Medicaid policy changes can have assorted and widespread impacts. The next chapter focuses on another Medicaid sub-group potentially vulnerable to cutbacks – people who use emergency department services.

REFERENCES

Deck, D. D., Gabriel, R. M., Laws, K. E., McFarland, B. H., and McCarty, D. (2005). *Medicaid coverage and access to publicly funded substance abuse and mental health outpatient treatment.* Presentation at annual meeting of Addiction Health Services and Research, Santa Monica, CA, November 2005.

Deck, D. D., McFarland, B. H., Titus, J. M., Laws, K. E., and Gabriel, R. M. (2000). Access to substance abuse treatment services under the Oregon Health Plan. *Journal of the American Medical Association, 284,* 2093-2099.

Enos, G. (2006). *The Oregon Case. Special Report on Medicaid: Bridging the Gap between Care and Cost.* Washington, DC: Pew Center on the States, pages A18 and A19.

Mann, C. and Artiga, S. (2004). *The impact of recent changes in health care coverage for low-income people: A first look at the research following changes in Oregon's Medicaid program.* Washington, DC: Kaiser Commission on Medicaid and the Uninsured.

McConnell, K. J. and Wallace, N. (2004). *Impact of premium changes in the Oregon Health Plan.* Salem, OR: Office for Oregon Health Plan Policy and Research.

Sobell, L. C. and Sobell, M. B. (1992). Timeline follow-back: A technique for assessing self-reported alcohol consumption. In R. Litten and J. P. Allen (Eds.) *Measuring alcohol consumption: Psychosocial and biochemical methods.* Totowa, NJ: Human Press.

Wright, B. J., Carlson, M. J., Edlund, T., DeVoe, J., Gallia, C. and Smith, J. (2005). The impact of increased cost sharing on Medicaid enrollees. *Health Affairs, 24,* 1106-1116.

In: Medicaid and Treatment for People… ISBN 978-1-61470-742-4
Editor: B.H. McFarland, D.McCarty, et al, pp. 239-251 © 2011 Nova Science Publishers, Inc.

Chapter 12

THE IMPACT OF OREGON HEALTH PLAN CUTS ON SUBSTANCE ABUSE TREATMENT

Matthew J. Carlson[1], Bill J. Wright[2] and Robert A. Lowe[3]

[1] Department of Sociology, Portland State University, Portland, OR
[2] Providence Center for Health Outcomes Research Education, Portland, OR
[3] Department of Emergency Medicine, Oregon Health and Science University, Portland, OR, USA

ABSTRACT

This chapter describes cutbacks in the Oregon Health Plan and the effects of those Medicaid reductions at three distinct levels: individuals' access to substance abuse treatment, the substance abuse delivery system in Oregon, and Oregon's emergency departments. Data from several studies are examined to describe the impacts of major changes to the Oregon Health Plan's Standard (Medicaid expansion) program in early 2003 – particularly the increased cost sharing measures and coverage reduction including outpatient mental health and chemical dependency benefit cutbacks. The preponderance of evidence from these studies suggests that the impacts of program changes were felt profoundly by the individuals enrolled in OHP, by the clinics and treatment centers that form Oregon's substance abuse care delivery system, and in Oregon's emergency departments.

INTRODUCTION

Public financing plays a critical role in the delivery of substance abuse treatment services in the U.S. Approximately 77% of national expenditures for substance abuse treatment comes from public funds (Mark et al., 2007). State Medicaid programs, in particular, make up a substantial proportion of public funding, accounting for 18% of all spending on treatment services nationwide (Mark et al., 2005). In 2003, large state budget deficits caused nearly every state to implement cost saving strategies in their Medicaid programs including restricting eligibility and reducing benefits (Smith et al., 2004). Despite the important role that Medicaid plays in providing access to substance abuse treatment, there is very little information about the effects of restricted Medicaid eligibility and benefit reductions on substance abuse treatment.

This chapter describes cutbacks in the Oregon Health Plan and the effects of those cutbacks at three distinct levels: individuals' access to substance abuse treatment, the substance abuse delivery system in Oregon, and Oregon's emergency departments. Data from several studies are examined to describe the impacts of major changes to the Oregon Health Plan's Standard program in early 2003, particularly the increased cost sharing measures and reduction in key benefits, including outpatient mental health and chemical dependency benefits. The preponderance of evidence from these studies suggests that the impact of program changes were felt profoundly by the individuals enrolled in OHP, by the clinics and treatment centers that form Oregon's substance abuse care delivery system, and in Oregon's emergency departments.

Oregon Health Plan Cutbacks and Access to Substance Abuse Treatment

In February of 2003 Oregon responded to a large state budget shortfall by redesigning the Oregon Health Plan (OHP) to create OHP2. Based on the redesign, OHP2 consists of two distinct benefit packages: OHP Plus and OHP Standard. OHP Plus resembles the original OHP, and serves the traditional, categorically eligible Medicaid population (Temporary Aid to Needy Families, Old Age Assistance, and disabled populations). OHP Standard serves Oregon's expansion population (adults and couples with incomes under 100% of the federal poverty level). When OHP2 was launched in March 2003, nearly 90,000 OHP beneficiaries were transferred into the new OHP Standard program.

OHP Standard members experienced two basic types of program changes: cost sharing increases and benefit reductions (Mann and Artiga, 2004). Cost sharing changes included higher monthly premiums, added co-payments for services, and tightened administrative rules including elimination of premium exemptions and the imposition of a six-month lockout for missing a premium payment. These changes did not apply to OHP Plus members.

In addition to increased cost-sharing, OHP Standard members lost several benefits they had previously received. Most notably, coverage for outpatient mental health and chemical dependency treatment was eliminated, along with coverage for dental care, durable medical equipment (DME), and vision services. Prescription drug coverage was also briefly eliminated but was reinstated within a month of OHP2's launch. Due to a large outcry by patients, providers, and advocates, by August 2004 the state legislature restored behavioral health benefits for the entire OHP population (Mulligan, 2004, 2005).

IMPACTS ON INDIVIDUAL CLIENTS

The effects of these cutbacks on OHP enrollees were captured in the *OHP Panel Study*, a longitudinal study launched just after the OHP changes were implemented in early 2003. The study drew a representative sample of individuals who were enrolled before the cuts took effect and followed them over a three-year period, surveying them annually. One-half of the panel consisted of OHP Standard members (who were affected by the program cuts); the other half consisted of OHP Plus members (who did not experience program cuts). The purpose of the study was to estimate the relative effects over time of the OHP Standard program cuts on those enrolled when the changes were implemented (Wright et al., 2005).

Results showed a dramatic decline in OHP Standard enrollment in the months after the program cuts were implemented, driven heavily by the program changes themselves. The increased premiums, copayments, and "lock-out" for missed premium payments, along with benefit reductions, resulted in widespread disenrollment by OHP Standard beneficiaries: from 88,874 adults in February 2003 to 40,313 by August 2004, when mental health and chemical dependency benefits were reinstated (Oregon Division of Medical Assistance Programs, undated). This decline stands in stark contrast to the previous year, when enrollment decreased only slightly over a comparable time period, from 92,485 in January 2002 to 91,174 in December 2002 (Oregon Division of Medical Assistance Programs, undated).

Among OHP Standard beneficiaries who were enrolled prior to the OHP cuts, only 37% maintained their coverage over the subsequent 18 months; the remaining 63% lost coverage (Wright, Carlson, Smith, and Edlund, 2005). Figure 1 describes the coverage patterns in a cohort of OHP Standard and OHP Plus beneficiaries who were enrolled in February 2003, immediately prior to implementation of the OHP Changes. Compared with the Plus population, whose benefits did not change, the Standard population reported significantly higher levels of disenrollment and longer periods without insurance.

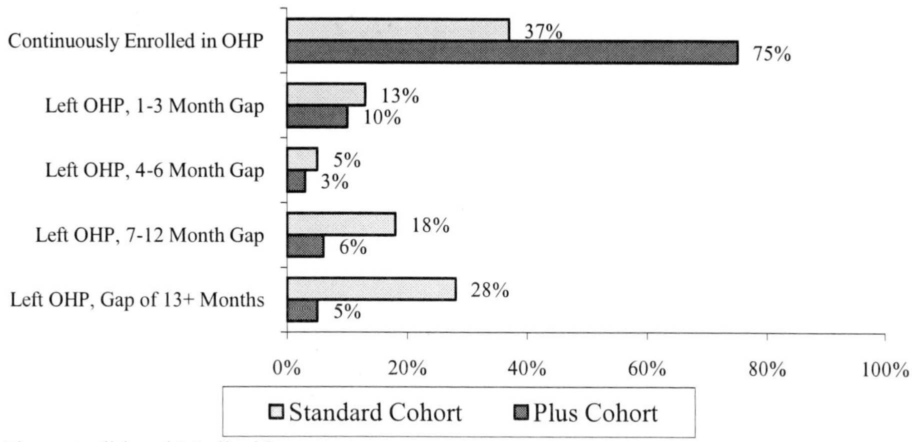

OHP Plus = traditional Medicaid

OHP Standard = Medicaid "expansion" population

Figure 1. 18-Month enrollment patterns of Oregon Health Plan Standard and Oregon Health Plan Plus.

Study results also showed that, for the most part, OHP Standard beneficiaries who lost coverage during this period were unable to regain any other type of health insurance coverage, and instead remained uninsured for substantial periods of time. Among those losing coverage, 29% were uninsured for seven to 12 months, and an additional 44% were uninsured for more than one year.

Taken together, this change meant that among all those who lost coverage, 73% were uninsured for a period of longer than six months. By the end of the study period, fewer than one-third of the former OHP Standard beneficiaries had regained coverage (Wright et al., 2005; Wright and Carlson, 2005).Compared to those who remained continuously insured, former OHP Standard members who had lost coverage after the 2003 OHP cuts reported significantly higher levels of unmet medical care, dental care, and medication needs, and substantially higher levels of financial strain related to unpaid medical bills across the remainder of the three-year study period (Carlson et al., 2006; Wright et al., 2005; Wright and Carlson, 2005).

The *OHP Panel Study* also found that the OHP cuts caused a substantial reduction in access to substance abuse treatment. As part of the surveys, respondents were asked whether they needed treatment for an alcohol or drug problem, and whether they were able to get that treatment. Just over 10% of the total study population, 234 individuals, reported a need for treatment. Among these, less than half of the OHP Standard population (42%) reported being able to receive needed treatment, a substantially smaller proportion than the 68% of OHP Plus members who reported receiving treatment (Carlson, 2007).

The OHP cohort study findings are strikingly similar to another study conducted during the same time period, in which OHP beneficiaries who were receiving methadone treatment in an urban clinic were prospectively followed for one year following elimination of benefits (Fuller et al., 2006). Of the 101 OHP Standard clients whose benefits were cut, only 45% were able to maintain their treatment for 12 months. Among OHP Plus clients, whose benefits were not cut, 82% were still in treatment one year later. This study also demonstrated that benefit cuts may have disproportionately harmed the most vulnerable clients; those who left treatment were more likely to use heroin and dirty needles, and reported greater drug, legal, and psychiatric problems both before and after the cuts. Moreover, loss of coverage for treatment disproportionately affected poor, homeless, and unemployed patients, and patients with little social support (Fuller et al., 2006).

Perhaps the most compelling evidence about the impacts of cutbacks comes from analysis of administrative data. As reported in another chapter, Deck and Gabriel used statewide administrative data to examine changes in the rates of new admissions to outpatient substance treatment for three years before and two years after the cuts. Between 2000 and the end of 2002, admission rates had consistently risen. However, between 2002 and 2003, OHP Standard admissions for substance abuse treatment declined by 67%. The decline in new admissions among the OHP Plus population during this period was still substantial, but much lower at 25% (Deck and Gabriel, this volume). Analyses of Oregon administrative data for new admissions to opiate treatment similarly indicated that new admission rates fell among OHP standard by 59% compared to 16% among the OHP Plus population during the same time period (Deck, this volume). A decline in admissions to treatment among OHP Standard enrollees who were no longer covered for these services was certainly not surprising. However, the decline in admissions among the OHP Plus enrollees, whose benefits did not change, was somewhat surprising – and probably attributable to the impacts on the service delivery system described in the next section.

IMPACTS ON THE SERVICE DELIVERY SYSTEM

Administrative data for OHP Standard clients show a dramatic decline in the number of chemical dependency claims just after the OHP benefit cuts, and a corresponding, but smaller, increase when benefits were restored (Figure 2) (Oregon Office of Mental Health and Addiction Services, 2007). Substance abuse treatment in Oregon, like many states, obtains a substantial portion of its funding from Medicaid. OHP Standard clients, for example, represented about 50% of all admissions to publicly funded community methadone clinics in 2003 (Deck et al., 2006). According to the Oregon Office of Mental Health and Addiction Services (2006), cuts in OHP Standard resulted in a loss in funding of over $10,000,000 per year in outpatient chemical dependency services. After these cuts, approximately 1,000 treatment staff lost their jobs and several clinics closed completely. These dramatic declines in service capacity led to extensive waiting lists in every Oregon county (Deck et al., 2006; Oregon OMHAS, 2006). As a result, even when benefits were restored in 2004, many clients were faced with the unpleasant experience of having coverage again, but having nowhere to go for care.

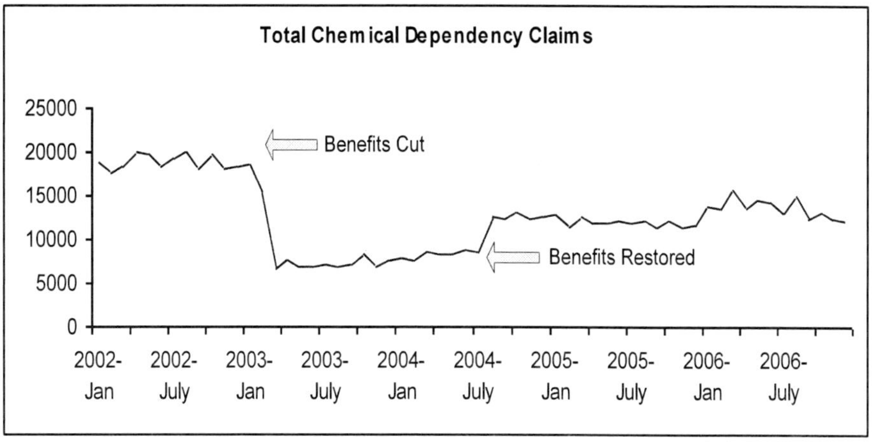

Source: OHP Claims Data Acquired December 2007.

Figure 2. Oregon Health Plan Standard chemical dependency claims, 2002–2006.

In summary, the turbulent period following the OHP redesign was characterized by a dramatic disenrollment of the OHP Standard population. Most of those who lost their health insurance coverage did not have access to an alternative and simply became uninsured. During this time, the elimination of OHP Standard's chemical dependency treatment benefits meant even those able to stay enrolled were no longer covered for many of the services they needed. Because the OHP Standard population represented a substantial proportion of substance abuse treatment clients around the state, the loss of revenue to treatment providers led to a substantially diminished service capacity. The result of these multiple trends was a highly unstable environment in which great need existed but there was a severe lack of access to outpatient services. The conditions created an intense new set of pressures on Oregon's emergency care system.

CHANGES IN EMERGENCY DEPARTMENT UTILIZATION

Hospital emergency departments (EDs) are a vital part of the medical care safety net. They disproportionately serve uninsured and under-insured patients who cannot reliably access care elsewhere, vulnerable populations such as minority groups, and – most important for this chapter – patients suffering from psychiatric disorders, alcoholism, and chemical dependency (Byrne et al., 2003; D'Onofrio et al., 1998a, 1998b; Mandelberg et al., 2000; Richardson and Hwang, 2001).

Although this situation may influence the U.S. health care delivery system adversely, interfering both with continuity of care and with coordination of the management of physical and behavioral health conditions, it also creates the opportunity to study chemical dependency by studying ED use for chemical dependency. ED utilization patterns have been shown to be sensitive indicators of access to care outside the ED (Christakis et al., 2001; Cunningham, 2006; Gill et al., 2000; Grumbach et al., 1993; Halfon et al., 1996; Li et al., 2003; Lombrail et al., 1997; Lowe et al., 2005; Mitchell and Remmel, 1992; O'Brien et al., 1997; Rask et al., 1994; Rosenblatt et al., 2000; Sarver et al., 2002; Wilson and Klein, 2000; Zuckerman and Shen, 2004), so EDs serve as a "canary in the coal mine" to understand problems with medical care delivery.

A statewide study of 22 Oregon EDs (Lowe et al., 2008) provides substantial insight into these new pressures. Administrative (billing) data were collected on all ED visits from August 2001 through February 2005, allowing comparison of ED utilization before versus after the OHP policy changes. These EDs account for approximately 55% of all ED visits statewide. They include 15 of Oregon's 20 urban EDs and seven of its 38 rural EDs. In this chapter, data are presented primarily for calendar years 2004 versus 2002, an approach that allows a pre-post comparison of ED trends before and after the 2003 OHP redesign, but that minimizes the effect of seasonal variation and avoids data from the period of instability closest to the date of the policy changes. Multivariable analyses presented elsewhere (Lowe et al., 2008) led to the same conclusions.

Emergency departments saw a substantial change in their traffic following the 2003 OHP redesign. Immediately following the OHP cutbacks, there was a substantial *decrease* in the number of OHP-sponsored ED visits for drug-related diagnoses and an increase in the number of uninsured ED visits for those conditions (Table 1). Drug-related visits by OHP-sponsored patients decreased from 3,365 in 2002 to 2,871 in 2004, while visits by uninsured patients increased from 1,235 to 3,364. The abrupt and sustained nature of these changes (Figure 3) suggests that they were due to the policy changes rather than other factors, which would likely have led to more gradual alterations.

One explanation for the rise in uninsured visits might be that frequent ED patients who may have had OHP coverage in 2002 continued to come to the ED in 2004, but were now uninsured. However, the combined number of drug-related visits by OHP-sponsored and uninsured patients rose 35%, from 4,600 in 2002 to 6,235 in 2004, (Table 1 and Figure 4) – an argument against a mere change in insurance status by ED patients with chemical dependency as the sole explanation.

Table 1. Drug-related Oregon Emergency Department visits, 2002 and 2004

Insurance category	2002	2004	% change
Commercial	1,274	1,551	+ 22%
Medicare	874	1,237	+ 41%
Oregon Health Plan (Medicaid)	3,365	2,871	- 15%
Uninsured	1,235	3,364	+ 172%
Other	472	749	+ 59%
Total	7,220	9,772	+ 35%

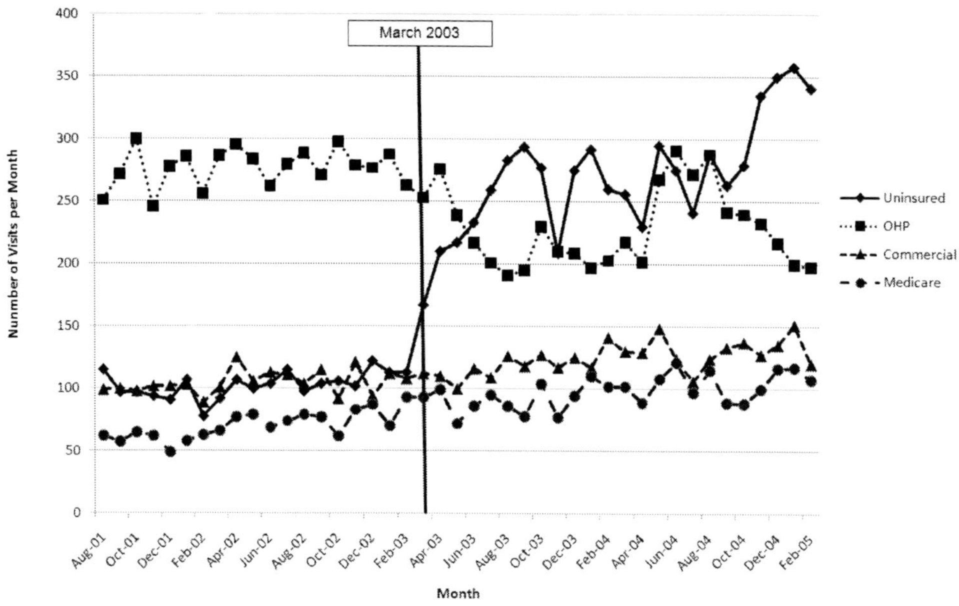

Figure 3. All Drug-related Oregon Emergency Department visits.

Instead, the data suggest that the OHP policy changes were followed almost immediately by an overall rise in drug-related ED visits by the uninsured and under-insured. This finding is consistent with loss of access to outpatient drug treatment programs by the newly-uninsured, and by those chemically-dependent patients remaining in the OHP Standard program for whom such services were no longer covered.

The decline in ED visits among OHP members likely stems from the significant decline in the OHP population. However, even among those who remained enrolled, there is some evidence that the imposition of co-pays between March, 2003 and August, 2004 may have had a suppression effect among those who were still covered by Medicaid. Under the 2003

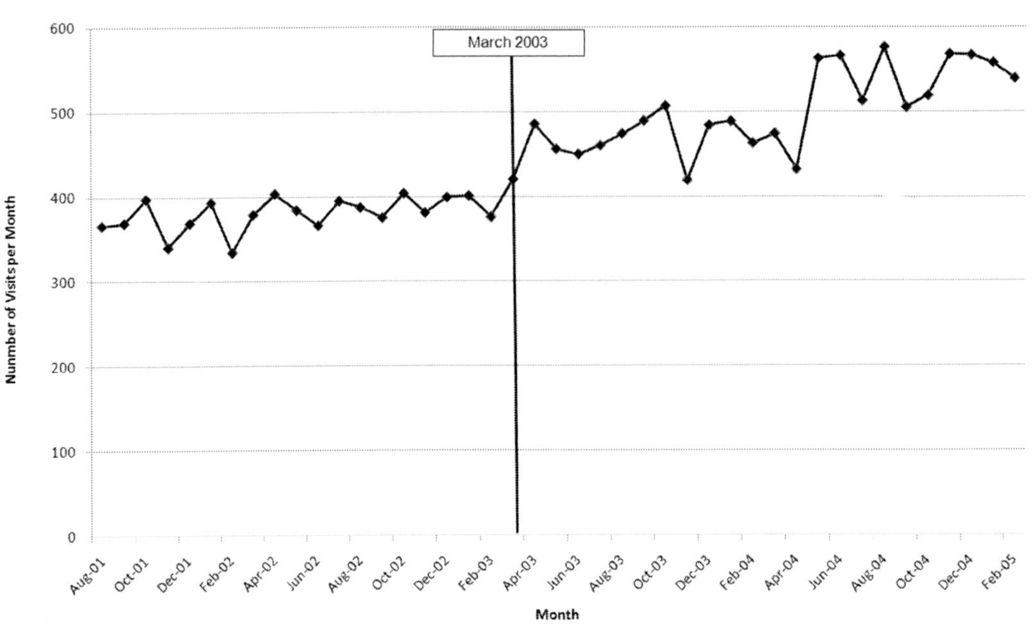

Figure 4. Drug-related Oregon Emergency Department visits by Oregon Health Plan-sponsored and uninsured patients.

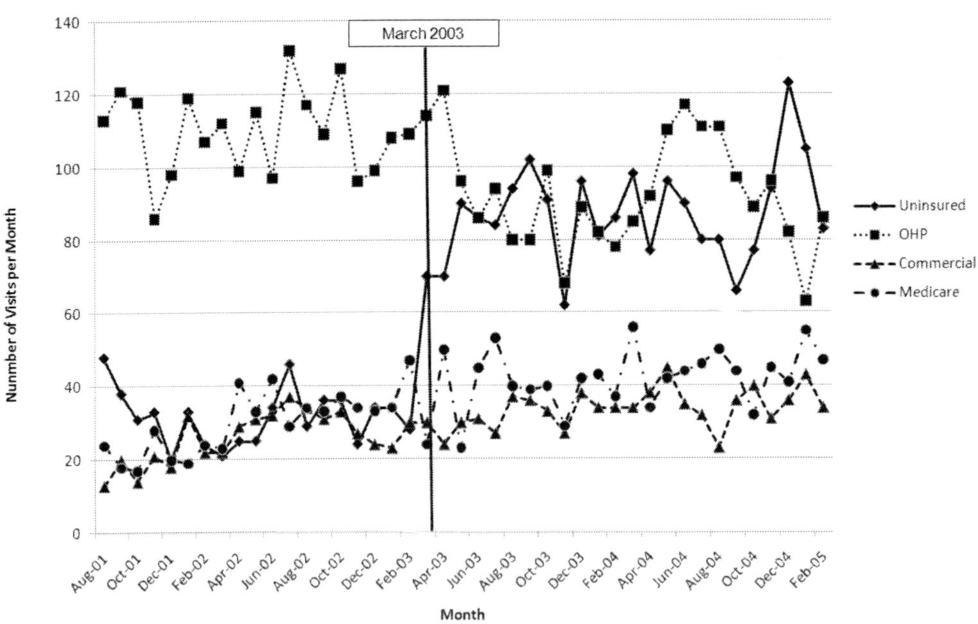

Figure 5. Opioid-Related Emergency Department visits.

program redesign, OHP members who visited the ED incurred a mandatory $50 co-pay, something that had not been present before the redesign. Evidence from the *OHP Panel Study* indicates that the percentage of adults continuously enrolled in OHP Standard who reported visiting the ED at least once declined by nearly 10% in the first 18 months following cutbacks

(Carlson et al., 2006). This finding could suggest that the $50 co-pay did indeed suppress emergency department use among those who remained in OHP after the program redesign.

The pattern of ED utilization for drug-related conditions suggests that the decrease in availability of outpatient chemical dependency services, while triggered by the cuts in OHP Standard, had a spillover effect on a much larger population. Commercially-sponsored and Medicare-sponsored visits increased (Table 1), such that total drug-related visits rose 35%. Thus, these cutbacks not only compromised the clinics' ability to care for uninsured patients but likely affected those who remained able to pay for treatment (Deck, this volume; Oregon OMHAS, 2006).

Other data suggest that the changes in ED use are directly related to the policy changes. Because opioid dependence is particularly amenable to management in drug treatment programs, one would expect reduced access to these programs to have a definite impact on ED use. Figure 5 shows the decrease in OHP-sponsored ED visits and the greater increase in uninsured ED visits for opioid-related diagnoses. As with all drug-related ED visits, there was a "spillover effect," with increased ED use by all payer categories except OHP for opioid-related conditions (Table 2).

Table 2. Opioid-related Oregon Emergency Department visits, 2002 and 2004

Insurance category	2002	2004	% change
Commercial	354	418	+ 18%
Medicare	382	514	+ 34%
Oregon Health Plan (Medicaid)	1,329	1,150	– 13%
Uninsured	367	1,048	+ 185%
Other	130	203	+ 56%
Total	2,562	3,333	+ 30%

CONCLUSION

The OHP policy changes reduced the number of chemically-dependent Oregonians with health insurance coverage and eliminated coverage for outpatient chemical dependency treatment for those remaining in the OHP expansion program. Surveys and administrative data provide consistent evidence that access to substance abuse treatment among both current and former OHP Standard members declined as a result of the policy changes. Furthermore, the reduction in the number of individuals with substance abuse benefits resulted in a substantial decrease of Medicaid revenues on which substance abuse treatment providers across the state depended.

The falling revenues had a devastating effect on treatment providers, reducing treatment capacity statewide for all populations, not just for OHP Standard beneficiaries. The ED utilization data showing increased ED visits among adults covered by commercial insurance and Medicare suggest that the OHP policy changes reduced support for drug treatment programs so severely as to impair their ability to serve patients who would have been able to pay for this care.

Declining access to substance abuse treatment resulted in significant pressure on Oregon's safety net providers. Interviews with Federally Qualified Health Centers conducted six months after the cuts were implemented indicated that lack of mental health and substance abuse treatment benefits created an increased demand for these services that could not be met by the primary care community (Hanes et al., 2003). Moreover, unmet need for treatment combined with increased rates of uninsurance resulted in dramatic increases in rates of uninsured emergency department visits for substance abuse diagnoses.

The purpose of eliminating the substance abuse benefit was to reduce program expenditures in the OHP expansion population. In fact, available evidence suggests that the cuts were only partially successful. A savings of $161 per member per month by eliminating outpatient substance abuse benefits was partially offset by additional costs of $70 to $127 per member per month due to other services required elsewhere (McConnell et al., 2008). These small financial savings were associated with large and devastating impacts to the individuals who relied on treatment, the treatment community itself, and the safety net.

More optimistically, the next chapters address positive innovations in Medicaid including ways to improve organization and financing of this important program.

REFERENCES

Byrne, M., Murphy, A. W., Plunkett, P. K., McGee, H. M., Murray, A., and Bury, G. (2003). Frequent attenders to an emergency department: A study of primary health care use, medical profile, and psychosocial characteristics. *Annals of Emergency Medicine, 41*, 309-318.

Carlson, M. J., DeVoe, J., and Wright, B. J. (2006). Short-term impacts of coverage loss in a Medicaid population: Early results from a prospective cohort study of the Oregon Health Plan. *Annals of Family Medicine, 4*, 391-398.

Carlson, M. J., Wright, B. J., and Mongoue-Tchokote, M. (2006). *The impact of Medicaid program changes on low income adults: Evidence from a three-year panel study of Oregon Health Plan beneficiaries: Final report*. Rockville, MD: Agency for Healthcare Quality and Research.

Carlson, M. J. (2007). *Access to substance abuse treatment services among OHP Standard beneficiaries. Brief.* Portland, OR: Portland State University, Center for Health and Social Inequality Research.

Christakis, D. A., Mell, L., Koepsell, T. D., Zimmerman, F. J., and Connell, F. A. (2001). Association of lower continuity of care with greater risk of emergency department use and hospitalization in children. *Pediatrics, 107*, 524-529.

Cunningham, P. J. (2006). What accounts for differences in the use of hospital emergency departments across U.S. communities? *Health Affairs (Millwood), 25*, w324-36.

Deck, D. D., Wiitala, W. L., and Laws, K. E. (2006). Medicaid coverage and access to publicly funded opiate treatment. *Journal of Behavioral Health Services and Research, 33*(3), 324-334.

D'Onofrio, G., Bernstein, E., Bernstein, J., Woolard, R. H., Brewer, P. A., Craig, S. A., and Zink, B. J. (1998a). Patients with alcohol problems in the emergency department, part 1:

improving detection. SAEM Substance Abuse Task Force. Society for Academic Emergency Medicine. *Academic Emergency Medicine, 5*, 1200-1209.

D'Onofrio, G., Bernstein, E., Bernstein, J., Woolard, R. H., Brewer, P. A., Craig, S. A., and Zink, B. J. (1998b). Patients with alcohol problems in the emergency department, part 2: intervention and referral. SAEM Substance Abuse Task Force. Society for Academic Emergency Medicine. *Academic Emergency Medicine, 5*, 1210-1217.

Fuller, B. E., Rieckmann, T. R., McCarty, D. J., Ringor-Carty, R., and Kennard, S. (2006). Elimination of methadone benefits in the Oregon Health Plan and its effects on patients. *Psychiatric Services, 57*, 686-691.

Gill, J. M., Mainous, A. G., and Nsereko, M. (2000). The effect of continuity of care on emergency department use. *Archives of Family Medicine, 9*(4), 333-338.

Grumbach, K., Keane, D., and Bindman, A. (1993). Primary care and public emergency department overcrowding. *American Journal of Public Health, 83*(3), 372-378.

Halfon, N., Newacheck, P. W., Wood, D. L., and St Peter, R. F. (1996). Routine emergency department use for sick care by children in the United States. *Pediatrics, 98*(1), 28-34.

Hanes, P., Dapcic, B., Hanes, R., and Schau, M. (2003). *Assessing the early impacts of OHP2: FQHC Case Study*. Portland, OR: Oregon Health Policy Institute, Center for Health and Disability Policy. Retrieved from http://www.oregon.gov/OHPPR/OHREC /Docs/Presentations/AssesImpOHP211_01_ppt.pdf

Li, G., Grabowski, J. G., McCarthy, M. L., and Kelen, G. D. (2003). Neighborhood characteristics and emergency department utilization. *Academic Emergency Medicine : Official Journal of the Society for Academic Emergency Medicine, 10*(8), 853-859.

Lombrail, P., Vitoux-Brot, C., Bourrillon, A., Brodin, M., and De Pouvourville, G. (1997). Another look at emergency room overcrowding: Accessibility of the health services and quality of care. *International Journal of Quality in Health Care, 9*, 225-235.

Lowe, R. A., Localio, A. R., Schwarz, D. F., Williams, S., Tuton, L. W., Maroney, S., et al. (2005). Association between primary care practice characteristics and emergency department use in a Medicaid managed care organization. *Medical Care, 43*(8), 792-800.

Lowe, R. A., McConnell, K. J., Vogt, M. E., and Smith, J. A. (2008). Impact of Medicaid cutbacks on emergency department use: The Oregon experience. *Annals of Emergency Medicine, 52*(6), 626-634.

Mandelberg, J. H., Kuhn, R. E., and Kohn, M. A. (2000). Epidemiologic analysis of an urban, public emergency department's frequent users. *Academic Emergency Medicine, 7*, 637-646.

Mann, C. and Artiga, S. (2004). *The impact of recent changes in health care coverage for low-income people: A first look at the research following changes in Oregon's Medicaid program.* Washington, DC: Kaiser Commission on Medicaid and the Uninsured.

Mark, T. L., Coffey, R. M., Vandlvort-Warren, R., Harwood, H. J., and King, E. C. (2005). U.S. spending for mental health and substance abuse treatment, 1991-2001. *Health Affairs (Millwood),* 133-142.

Mark, T. L., Levit, K. R., Buck, J. A., Coffey, R. M., and Vandivort-Warren, R. (2007). Mental health treatment expenditure trends, 1986-2003. *Psychiatric Services, 58*, 1041-1048.

McConnell, K. J., Wallace, N. T., Gallia, C. A., and Smith, J. A. (2008). Effect of eliminating behavioral health benefits for selected Medicaid enrollees. *Health Services Research, 43*, 1348-1365.

Mitchell, T. A., and Remmel, R. J. (1992). Level of uncompensated care delivered by emergency physicians in Florida. *Annals of Emergency Medicine, 21*, 1208-1214.

Mulligan, K. (2004). Fewer of Oregon's poor eligible for MH benefits. *Psychiatric News, July 16*, 10.

Mulligan, K. (2005). Coalition suggests reforms to make Medicaid work. *Psychiatric News, March 18*, 4.

O'Brien, G. M., Stein, M. D., Zierler, S., Shapiro, M., O'Sullivan, P., and Woolard, R. (1997). Use of the ED as a regular source of care: associated factors beyond lack of health insurance. *Annals of Emergency Medicine, 30*, 286-291.

Oregon Division of Medical Assistance Programs. *OHP eligibility reports.*. Salem, OR: Oregon Department of Human Services. Retrieved from http://www.oregon.gov/DHS/healthplan/data_pubs/eligibles/main.shtml

Oregon Office of Mental Health and Addiction Services. (2006). *Overview: The context of substance abuse*. Salem, OR: Oregon Department of Human Services. Retrieved from http://www.theoma.org/Files/OHP%20Committee%20_4_.pdf

Oregon Office of Mental Health and Addiction Services. (2007). *OHP claims data*. Salem, OR: Oregon Department of Human Services.

Rask, K. J., Williams, M. V., Parker, R. M., and McNagny, S. E. (1994). Obstacles predicting lack of a regular provider and delays in seeking care for patients at an urban public hospital. *JAMA : The Journal of the American Medical Association, 271*, 1931-1933.

Richardson, L. D., and Hwang, U. (2001). Access to care: A review of the emergency medicine literature. *Academic Emergency Medicine, 8*, 1030-1036.

Rosenblatt, R. A., Wright, G. E., Baldwin, L. M., Chan, L., Clitherow, P., Chen, F. M., et al. (2000). The effect of the doctor-patient relationship on emergency department use among the elderly. *American Journal of Public Health, 90*, 97-102.

Sarver, J. H., Cydulka, R. K., and Baker, D. W. (2002). Usual source of care and nonurgent emergency department use. *Academic Emergency Medicine : Official Journal of the Society for Academic Emergency Medicine, 9*, 916-923.

Smith, V., Ramesh, R., Gifford, K., Ellis, E., Rudowitz, R., and O'Malley, M. (2004). *The continuing Medicaid budget challenge: State Medicaid spending growth and cost containment in fiscal years 2004 and 2005*. Washington, DC: Kaiser Family Foundation.

Wilson, K. M., and Klein, J. D. (2000). Adolescents who use the emergency department as their usual source of care. *Archives of Pediatrics and Adolescent Medicine, 154*(4), 361-365.

Wright, B. J., and Carlson, M. J. (2005). *Issue Brief: The impact of cost sharing and benefit changes to Oregon Health Plan beneficiaries: Results, two years later*. Salem, OR: The Office for Oregon Health Policy and Research. Retrieved from http://www.oregon.gov/OHPPR/OHREC/Docs/Presentations/OHPCohort_brief_11_05.pdf

Wright, B. J., Carlson, M. J., Smith, J., and Edlund, T. (2005). *Impact of changes to premiums, cost-sharing, and benefits on adult Medicaid beneficiaries: Results from an ongoing study of the Oregon Health Plan, Report No. 848*. New York, NY: The Commonwealth Fund.

Wright, B. J., Carlson, M. J., Edlund, T., DeVoe, J., Gallia, C., and Smith, J. (2005). The impact of increased cost sharing on Medicaid enrollees. *Health Affairs (Millwood), 24*, 1106-1116.

Zuckerman, S., and Shen, Y. C. (2004). Characteristics of occasional and frequent emergency department users: Do insurance coverage and access to care matter? *Medical Care, 42*, 176-182.

In: Medicaid and Treatment for People… ISBN 978-1-61470-742-4
Editor: B.H. McFarland, D.McCarty, et al, pp. 253-269© 2011 Nova Science Publishers, Inc.

Chapter 13

Potential of Enhanced Demographic and Social Data in Prediction of Health Care Costs Related To Substance Abuse In Medicaid And Privately Insured Populations

Frances L. Lynch[1,2], Bentson H. McFarland[1,3], John F. Dickerson[1], Carla A. Green[1,2], Michael R. Polen[1], Donald K. Freeborn[1], and Daniel M. Dickinson[3]

[1] Center for Health Research, Kaiser Permanente Northwest, Portland, OR
[2] Department of Public Health and Preventive Medicine, Oregon Health and Science University, Portland, OR
[3] Departments of Psychiatry and Public Health and Preventive Medicine, Oregon Health and Science University, Portland, OR
[4] Department of Addiction Medicine, Kaiser Permanente, Clackamas, OR, USA

Abstract

States often use capitated payment systems when purchasing health and behavioral health care for Medicaid clients. In capitated (prospective) payment programs, the payer sets payment rates for a future time period. A central problem in the development of Medicaid payment systems is that health plans may attempt to avoid enrolling people who are expected to be costly. In particular, because people with substance abuse may be high utilizers of services, health plans paid through capitation may try to avoid such enrollees — either by not enrolling such persons or by not providing access to high-quality substance abuse care. Risk-adjusted payments may improve this situation by reimbursing health plans based on the expected medical need of actual enrolled populations, rather than on the average community risk. However, risk-adjustment systems that only account for demographics and diagnoses are limited in their ability to reduce health plans' incentives to avoid covering people with substance abuse problems under capitation. Another challenge for risk-adjustment is the transient nature of Medicaid enrollment. Most of the literature on risk adjustment for persons with substance abuse problems includes only people who maintain continuous enrollment over the study period. This chapter reports on several risk-adjustment models focused on Oregon Medicaid clients involved with substance abuse treatment in a large health maintenance organization. Models were designed to predict substance abuse treatment expenditures or total health plan costs. Risk-adjustment models that incorporated new variables such as social, clinical, and Medicaid eligibility indicators predicted substance abuse and total health plan expenditures somewhat better than simpler models typical of current risk-adjustment systems. However, models predicting substance abuse expenditures still performed very poorly and explained no more than 11% of the variation in expenditures. On the other hand, models for total health plan expenditures performed better, explaining as much as 35% of variation in expenditures. Although addition of new variables improved prediction modestly, payments would likely be quite inaccurate in some cases. Risk adjustment for capitated Medicaid substance abuse care remains challenging.

INTRODUCTION

Expenditures on substance abuse and mental health care continue to rise and responsibility for these costs is increasingly borne by the public sector (Levit et al., 2008). Individuals with substance abuse and/or dependence problems have increased overall health care costs (Druss and Rosenheck, 1999; Sturm, 2002) including costs for both specialty substance abuse treatment and for general medical care (Meara and Frank, 2005). State agencies and other public payers are increasingly looking for methods to manage these costs effectively.

Capitated payment systems for Medicaid services are becoming increasingly common (Holahan and Suzuki, 2003; Maglione and Ridgely, 2006). In capitated (prospective) payment programs, the payer sets payment rates for a future time period, typically the following year. Setting the capitated payment rates for each rate cell is a form of risk adjustment. A central problem in the development of payment systems for Medicaid and other groups purchasing insurance (*e.g.*, employers) is that health plans may attempt to avoid enrolling people who are expected to be costly (sometimes called "adverse selection").

In order to manage risk, general medical services adjust payments for the anticipated health status or medical need of health plan enrollees (Ellis et al., 1996; Hornbrook, Goodman, and Bennett, 1991; Hornbrook and Goodman, 1996). Risk-adjusted payments are designed to reimburse health plans based on the expected medical need of actual enrolled populations, rather than on the average community risk. If the payment system makes it costly to identify and avoid potentially high-cost enrollees, risk-adjusted payments can reduce adverse selection significantly. Risk-adjustment systems that include measures of health status or medical need have been shown to improve the predictive power of risk-assessment models compared to models that use only age and gender (Hornbrook, Goodman, and Bennett, 1991; Hornbrook, Goodman, Bennett, and Greenlick, 1991; Newhouse, 1998).

Substance abuse can be particularly costly for health plans. People with substance abuse problems, for example, have significantly higher rates of morbidity and disability, including reduced quality of life (Sturm, 2002), increased work disability (Wickizer, 2001) as well as greater likelihood of involvement with the criminal justice system (Meara and Frank 2005) and increased use of health services (Meara and Frank, 2005; Sturm, 2002). Because substance abuse patients are more likely to be high utilizers of services, health plans paid through capitation may try to avoid attracting "bad" risks—either by not enrolling such persons or by not providing access to high-quality substance abuse care.

Specialty behavioral health carve-out arrangements may help address a health plan's incentives to avoid enrolling persons with substance abuse problems (Frank et al., 1995; Frank et al., 1996). In fact, such arrangements are increasingly used by purchasers to manage the risk of substance abuse services (Arons et al., 1994; Ettner et al., 2000; Frank and McGuire, 1998; Grazier and Eselius, 1999; Grazier et al., 1999). At least 36 state Medicaid programs either have obtained approval for or are currently operating behavioral health carve-out programs. Carve-out vendors also have incentives to limit access in order to control costs because they are typically paid through capitated payments (Ettner et al., 2000).

Savings to health plans can be significant. Research indicates that carve-outs can reduce behavioral health costs by as much as 40% (Bloom et al., 2002; Goldman et al., 1998). However, it is not clear whether these savings are due to improved efficiency or reduced access to services. This research also raises the concern that behavioral health carve-outs may not reduce costs but merely shift them to general medical and pharmaceutical expenses that are not part of their budget (Busch, 1997). Yet even if carve-out regulations limit the ability to shift substance abuse costs, focusing solely on substance abuse costs fails to address potential cost consequences of medical co-morbidities (*e.g.,* alcoholic pancreatitis) caused or exacerbated by individuals' substance abuse conditions. Furthermore, general medical providers can and often do treat substance abuse conditions. Therefore, risk-adjustment systems for persons with substance abuse problems need to address potential impacts on both general medical and specialty substance abuse costs.

Another approach to improving risk adjustment for persons with substance abuse problems is to adapt existing risk-adjustment systems or to develop new systems that more accurately predict expenditures Several studies (see Table 1 for summary) have developed and/or tested risk-adjustment models specifically for people with substance abuse or behavioral health (mental health and substance abuse) problems. These studies have consistently concluded that current models do not adequately or effectively manage risk associated with substance abuse care users. In several studies, Ettner and colleagues (Ettner et al., 2000; Ettner and Notman, 1997; Ettner et al., 1998; Mark et al., 2003; Rosen et al., 2002) found that many widely used general medical risk-adjustment systems did not predict behavioral or substance abuse expenditures very well and would likely not reduce health plans' incentives to avoid persons with substance abuse conditions.

Several of these studies also tested models that used psychiatric diagnostic indicators and indicators of mental health and substance abuse co-morbidity (Ettner et al., 1998, 2000; Ettner et al., 2003; Ettner and Johnson, 2003; Ettner and Notman, 1997). While the psychiatric indicator/co-morbidity models performed somewhat better than the others, substantial incentives to avoid high-utilizing patients would likely remain with each of the systems.

In summary, these studies indicate that current risk-adjustment systems that account for basic demographics (*e.g.,* age, gender) and diagnoses alone are limited in their ability to reduce health plans' incentives to avoid covering people with substance abuse problems under capitation systems that use these types of risk-adjustment models.

Table 1. Selected studies of risk adjustment for behavioral health care

Authors	Data and Population	Models and Methods	Results
Ettner and Notman 1997	30,119 (12,218 adults) continuously enrolled New Hampshire Medicaid Program clients 2956 clients used MH/SA 1992-1994 claims data	Age, gender, diagnoses, ACG NO Split sample Prospective 2 part models separate models for users and non-users of MH/SA	Best model had R^2<0.031 Models underestimated expenditures by 15-49% Mean Absolute prediction errors for total cost of around $18,000 for users of MH/SA; Models estimated MH/SA expenditures better, but still poorly with R^2<0.131 for best model. Mean absolute prediction errors for MH/SA $1500-1800.
Ettner et al. 1998	65,766 (51,621 adults) Claims for service use 1992-1993 data for non-elderly commercial private employers	Age, gender, index of payroll expenditures (to control for geographic region) ACG, Mod ADG, HCC, new psych co-morbidity NO Split sample Prospective 2 part model includes users and non-users	Modified ADGs and comorbidity Model worked best. No model predicted more than 0.10 of variation. Mean absolute prediction errors of $166-237 for MH/SA expenditures
Ettner et al. 2000	56,174 HMO enrollees and 52,990 MH/SA carve out enrollees – about 12,000 were users of MH/SA 1994-1995 Claims for service use large non-elderly public employer	ACG, ADG, HCC, + psychiatric disability Split sample 70-30 2 part model only continuously enrolled	HCC plus psych disability performed best. Best models R^2 =0.193 for HMO, .141 for Carve out. Underestimated expenditures for Patients with MH disability by 15% or more. Mean absolute prediction errors of $108-256 for all users and non-users
Kapur et al. 2000	1,956 clients with severe mental illness 1991-1994 LA County Mental Health Admin data	Demographics (age, gender, race, marital status, native language), insurance (Medicaid, Medicare, other insurance), homeless, MH diagnoses, GAS, lagged MH cost Prospective 2-part model NO Split Sample	Best models include prior costs R^2 < 0.05 without prior cost variables. With prior cost best model R^2 =0.164. Does not have predictive ability for use in capitation. Predictive error ratios of 0.9-1.3

Authors	Data and Population	Models and Methods	Results
Ettner et al. 2001	70,136 adults 49,136 MH/SA users 1991-1993 Claims for service use Medicaid enrollees in Michigan	Age, gender, ADG, HCC, new MH/SA Split sample 70-30 2 part model only continuously enrolled	No models preformed significantly better Mean absolute prediction errors of $3701-19,067 for adult users of MH/SA No R^2 presented
Ettner et al. 2003	70,952 Maryland Medicaid clients; 4,176 had diagnoses of substance abuse in 1995, 3992 had diagnosis in 1997 1995-1997 Claims for service use Maryland Medicaid	ACG for pts with and without SA No model development – only tests models Looked at gains and losses for concurrent and prospective models	Adjusted Clinical Groups reduced incentives to avoid substance abusers. Found gains and losses of up to 60% for some users of SA depending on rate category assigned by ACG.
Mark et al. 2003	68,904 fee-for-service employed adults 18-65 171,644 mixed fee-for-service, managed care adult employees 1994, 1995 claims data Continuously enrolled (for 2 years) employees in two large firms	Age, gender, area hospital wage rate (to control for geographic region), ACG, ADG, HCC Split sample 60-40 Single model – large sample	Mean prediction ratios of .45-1.67 for people with psychiatric conditions.
Rosen et al. 2002	More than 1,000,000 veterans 1997 administrative data VA patients with SA disorders	Age, gender, DCG/HCC Concurrent models With and without SA markers Dependent variables were utilization	Models with SA markers performed better. $R^2 = 0.32$ for best model

Notes: ACG = Ambulatory Care Groups; ADG = Ambulatory Diagnostic Groups; DLG = Diagnostic Cost Groups; GAS = Global Assessment Scale; HCC = Hierarchical Coexisting Conditions; HMO = Health Maintenance Organization; MH = Mental Health; SA = Substance Abuse; VA = Veterans Affairs.

Another consideration in the development of risk adjustment for persons with Medicaid insurance is the transient nature of Medicaid enrollment. Few Medicaid clients have uninterrupted service eligibility. For many clients, Medicaid eligibility may fluctuate even within a year due to changes in employment, administrative challenges of maintaining enrollment, and instability in lifestyle (such as frequent moves). Consequently, fluctuation may be an important factor in patterns of health care expenditures. However, most of the previous literature on risk adjustment for persons with substance abuse problems includes only people who maintain continuous enrollment over the study period.

Having identified a lack of predictive ability in existing risk-adjustment systems for people with substance abuse problems, we set out to identify additional variables, beyond basic demographic and diagnostic measures, that might help improve current risk-adjustment methods. In doing so, this study attempted to answer the following questions: Can additional demographic and social environment information enhance performance of existing risk-adjustment models? Will addition of these variables reduce problems of under- (or over-) payment for substance abuse and-or general medical care for persons with substance abuse problems? Are these variables more useful for Medicaid populations than for persons with commercial insurance? To address these questions, we examined different combinations of variables based on their probable ability to predict expenditures and their availability to program managers responsible for rate setting, such as state Medicaid administrators.

METHODS

Setting and Data

This chapter's study was conducted at Kaiser Permanente Northwest (KPNW), which is a federally qualified, fully capitated health maintenance organization (HMO) located in Portland, Oregon. At the time of the study, the health plan enrolled over 400,000 members, approximately 5% of whom were Oregon Medicaid clients. The HMO's Committee for the Protection of Human Subjects reviewed and approved all study activities.

Treatment for substance use problems is covered under a separate benefit structure within KPNW. Except for Medicaid members, outpatient substance abuse treatment services require a small co-payment, as do other medical outpatient services, and residential services generally require a 20% co-payment.

The Addiction Medicine Department provides most outpatient and other substance abuse services, with some care provided by contracted treatment agencies outside KPNW. Services include assessment, detoxification (hospital inpatient, residential, or ambulatory as clinically indicated), intensive outpatient, and outpatient treatments. Local methadone providers supply methadone maintenance treatment on a contractual basis. Residential treatment for commercial members is provided through contracts with outside providers. Community-based programs funded by the State of Oregon provide residential treatment for Medicaid clients.

Administrative data systems were used to locate all 1,304 Oregon Medicaid clients, aged 12 to 64, who contacted the Addiction Medicine Department during the "study selection window," between January 1, 1996, and December 31, 1997. The date of this contact is the "index date" for the Medicaid substance abuse subjects. Commercial substance abuse subjects (age and gender probability matched to the Medicaid clients) were health plan members who contacted the Addiction Medicine Department during the study selection window. The comparison subject's first contact with Addiction Medicine during the study selection window generated the person's index date. Table 2 presents descriptive information on the sample.

Table 2. Population characteristics by insurance group (Medicaid vs. Commercial): Adults assessed and recommended for substance abuse treatment (excluding methadone)

Characteristic	Study Group Medicaid (N= 641)	Commercial (N= 474)	p-value
Age Group, %			0.08
19-29	31	27	
30-50	65	67	
51-64	4	6	
Mean (SD)	34.2 (8.3)	35.4 (8.9)	0.02
Percent female, %	52	42	0.01
Race/ethnicity, %			
Caucasian only	75	82	
African-American only	14	7	<0.01
Other/mixed/unknown race	11	11	
Not high school graduate	34	15	<0.01
Married, %	33	52	<0.01
Children in household			
1+ children age 11 and under	31	32	0.67
1+ children age 12 and over	13	15	0.52
Employed or in school, %	34	81	<0.01
Housing, %			<0.01
Own home	50	73	
Other private residence	36	18	
Group home or homeless	14	9	
Referral source, %			<0.01
Legal/work/school	42	27	
Social	3	10	
Medical	15	14	
Other	40	48	
Reason for seeking treatment, %			0.06
Legal/work/school	40	35	
Social	46	53	
Medical	3	4	
Other	11	8	

Table 2. (Continued)

Characteristic	Study Group Medicaid (N= 641)	 Commercial (N= 474)	p-value
Clinical history, %			
Forced sex victim, %	33	21	<0.01
Domestic violence victim, %	54	40	<0.01
Suicide attempt, %	23	14	<0.01
Arrest history, %			
Ever arrested	60	39	<0.01
Ever arrested for drunk driving	23	21	0.50
Prior substance abuse treatment, %	68	53	<0.01
Prior treatment for emotional problems, %	55	52	0.34
Substance use in past year, %			
Alcohol	84	92	<0.01
Amphetamine	39	23	<0.01
Cocaine	34	23	<0.01
Opiate	10	7	0.03
Marijuana	52	43	<0.01
Tobacco	83	68	<0.01
Alcohol/drug diagnoses at intake ssessment, %			<0.01
Alcohol-only	72	62	
Drug-only	15	31	
Alcohol + other drug	12	6	
Treatment modality recommended at intake, %			0.65
Intensive outpatient	14	16	
Outpatient	76	76	
Residential or Detoxification	10	8	
Medical Evaluation	5	5	0.99
Mental health evaluation	< 1	< 1	0.91
Out of KPNW treatment	32	21	<0.01
Treatment initiation – after assessment (%)	80	81	0.79
Completed treatment – per counselor (%)	43	51	0.06
Duration of treatment (weeks)	38	49	0.10
Medicaid eligibility category, %		N/A	
AFDC/TANF	24		
Disabled	6		
Newly eligible – working	26		
Newly eligible – unemployed	38		
Other	6		

Table 2. (Continued)

Characteristic	Study Group Medicaid (N= 641)	Commercial (N= 474)	p-value
Lifetime Enrollment in months, Median (mean)	31 (58)	66 (88)	<0.01
Study Enrollment in months, Median (mean)	11 (15.9)	28 (23.5)	<0.01
Died During Study Period, %	< 1	2	0.27
Specific Health Conditions, %			
Infectious and Parasitic Diseases	6	2	<0.01
Neoplasms	3	< 1	<0.01
Endocrine, Nutritional, Metabolic, Immunity Diseases	4	3	0.30
Mental Disorders	5	7	0.32
Depression	16	13	0.16
Other Mental Health Conditions	3	2	0.28
Specific Health Conditions, % (Continued)			
Nervous System and Sense Organs	7	7	0.82
Circulatory System	8	7	0.63
Respiratory System	35	37	0.35
Digestive System	15	17	0.34
Genitourinary and Reproductive Systems	15	10	0.01
Pregnancy, Childbirth, Puerperium	4	2	0.04
Skin and Subcutaneous Tissue	18	18	0.86
Musculoskeletal/Injury and Poisoning	40	43	0.37

Notes: AFDC / TANF = Aid to Families with Dependent Children / Temporary Assistance for Needy Families.

Individuals typically contact the Addiction Medicine Department by telephone and are usually referred to an orientation meeting. Members wishing to pursue treatment following orientation undergo a comprehensive assessment by a counselor. Patient placement criteria are similar to those suggested by the American Society of Addiction Medicine (2001). The majority of substance abuse subjects underwent assessments that yielded considerable demographic and clinical information.

Administrative encounter and claim data provided information on types of services and health plan expenditures for each subject. Mortality data for all subjects were obtained from the Social Security Death Index. State of Oregon data systems provided information about eligibility and health plan enrollment for Medicaid subjects.

Research Design

We estimated both the concurrent and prospective risk-adjustment models using a split-sample approach. We first estimated each risk-adjustment model on a random 60% sample of subjects and then examined the validity of the model using the remaining 40% sample. Traditionally, risk-adjustment models designed to predict expenditures have been prospective (Ettner et al., 2000)—that is, persons setting rates use historical data to predict costs for some future period, typically one year. However, some researchers have suggested that concurrent models may be useful in some situations, particularly when setting rates for high-cost conditions and when there are substantial shifts in enrollment in a population (Dudley et al., 2003)—both of which are more likely when setting payment rates for persons with substance abuse problems. It was not our goal to test a complete system of risk adjustment exhaustively but rather to identify factors that could enhance model performance.

We selected the covariates for the models using three strategies. First, we reviewed the literature on risk adjustment in substance abuse. Table 1 summarizes the key studies. We included covariates similar to these models in order to compare whether addition of new variables improved on prior models. Previous work has primarily used one or more of three risk-adjustment systems: Ambulatory Care Groups – ACGs; Ambulatory Diagnostic Groups – ADGs; and Hierarchical Coexisting Conditions – HCCs (Ash et al., 1989; Ellis et al., 1996; Weiner et al., 1991). We used the Global Risk Assessment Model (GRAM; Hornbrook, Goodman, and Bennett, 1991; Hornbrook, Goodman, Bennett, and Greenlick, 1991), developed at KPNW, which is similar to these other systems in content and application. We also considered the Andersen behavioral model of health care utilization (Aday and Andersen, 1974; Andersen, 1995) and looked for covariates that fit into the suggested categories of predisposing, need, and enabling characteristics from our available covariates.

Because we were particularly interested in exploring our ability to improve prediction over previous models using new types of variables, we also sought to identify new and useful predictors by conducting four focus group interviews with health care professionals in the substance abuse treatment field. Participants were asked to identify client, system, and other factors affecting treatment-related costs—factors that would affect treatment initiation, use of treatment resources, short- versus long-term costs, or costs related to treatment mandates. Our analyses suggested that the predictive ability of current risk-adjustment models might be enhanced by including data related to individual-level factors, including prior lack of health insurance coverage; treatment mandates; severity of substance abuse problems; client environment, social support, and resources; and need for ancillary services. Details of this qualitative study are presented in another report (Green et al., 2004).

Table 3 lists the covariates tested in each risk-adjustment model. We used several principles to select variables for the models. First, we tried to create models that were somewhat similar to past work to assess whether inclusion of the new variables would aid in prediction using typical risk-adjustment methods. Second, we included variables that we believed would have the greatest ability to predict expenditures. Finally, we included variables that we thought most likely to be available to managers setting rates for Medicaid programs.

Table 3. Covariates for the risk adjustment models

Model Number	Model Name	Variables Included
1	DEM	Sex, age, age-squared, race, marital status, months of eligibility
2	DEM + ALC/DRUG indicators	Sex, age, age-squared, race, marital status, months of eligibility Medicaid Indicator, Diagnosis Alcohol Only, Drug Only, or Alcohol and Drug, Substance use in past year
3	DEM + ALC/DRUG + MH Indicators	Sex, age, age-squared, race, marital status, months of eligibility Medicaid Indicator, Diagnosis Alcohol Only, Drug Only, or Alcohol and Drug, Substance use in past year Prior treatment for MH, MH condition indicators, Suicide
4	DEM + ALC/DRUG + MH + Social/Family Characteristics	Sex, age, age-squared race, marital status, months of eligibility Medicaid Indicator, Diagnosis Alcohol Only, Drug Only, or Alcohol and Drug, Substance use in past year Prior treatment for MH, MH condition indicators, Suicide Housing, Active (employed or in school), Ever Arrested, Referral Source, Forced Sex, Domestic violence victim, Prior SA Treatment
5	DEM + ALC/DRUG + MH + GRAM Conditions	Sex, age, age-squared, race, marital status, months of eligibility, Social/Family + GRAM Conditions Medicaid Indicator, Diagnosis Alcohol Only, Drug Only, or Alcohol and Drug, Substance use in past year Prior treatment for MH, MH condition indicators, Suicide Housing, Active, Ever Arrested, Referral Source, Forced Sex, Domestic violence victim, Prior SA Treatment GRAM codes

Notes: GRAM = Global Risk Assessment Model; MH = Mental Health; SA = Substance Abuse

Statistical Analysis

As expected, our expenditures measures were highly skewed. We therefore estimated expenditures using two-part models (Duan et al., 1983). These models separately estimate the probability of incurring any expenditure in the first part of the model. In the second part, the magnitude of expenditures is estimated separately for persons who had any expenditures. The first part of the model was estimated using logistic regression. The second part of the model was estimated using ordinary least squares estimation with a log-transformed dependent variable. Together, these equations allowed us to calculate expected expenditures for each individual. We used a "smearing" procedure to retransform predictions back to the mean of the original distribution following the methods suggested by Duan (1983). In some of our models, because of the way our sample was defined, all study subjects had non-zero expenditures. In these cases, we fit a single model equivalent to the second part of the models described above.

To examine the proportion of variance explained by each of the risk-adjustment models, we calculated either the standard R^2 (for single-part models) or the "synthetic" R^2 (for the two-part models). The synthetic R^2 is the non-linear counterpart to the R^2 and is defined by (Efron, 1978) as

$$1-[\Sigma(Y_i-\hat{Y}_i)^2/\,\Sigma(Y_i-[1/N]\,\Sigma Y_i)^2],$$

where Y_i is the actual expenditure for the ith *subject,*
$\hat{Y}_i$ is the predicted expenditure for the ith *subject,*
and N is the sample size.

To examine the predictive performance of the models, we computed the predictive ratio, which is calculated by dividing the predicted expenditure value by the actual expenditure value. A predictive ratio of less than 1 indicates that the risk-adjusted payment would not cover the actual expenditures; a predictive ratio greater than 1 indicates the risk-adjusted payment would overpay compared to actual expenditures.

RESULTS

We constructed a series of models to examine whether we could improve upon past risk-adjustment models, which have used only basic demographics and diagnostic information. For each dependent variable (total substance abuse expenditures or total health plan expenditures), we used two approaches to estimation, as follows: 1) include all variables in each model, or 2) use stepwise regression to select models.

Results for the two analysis strategies were markedly similar with no major differences. For brevity we report only the stepwise models. We tested concurrent and prospective models of risk adjustment.

Covariates and dependent variables are observed in the same period for concurrent models. In prospective models, covariates are observed in the first period, and dependent variables are for the following year.

Table 4 presents the adjusted R^2 for the models for substance abuse and total health plan expenditures. The simple demographic model performs the worst, and each addition of new variables improves the model. The models predict substance abuse expenditures poorly with R^2 of .10 for the best performing model. The models predicted total health plan expenditures better, with R^2 ranging from .20-.26.

We also examined the prediction ratio to look at possible gains and losses from each model. Table 5 presents the prediction ratios for the substance abuse and total health plan expenditures. For substance abuse expenditures, the prediction ratios ranged from 1.01 for the demographic-only model to 1.05 for the model including the most predictors. For general medical expenditures, the prediction ratios ranged from 1.09 for the demographic-only model to 1.20 for the model including the most predictors.

Table 4. Comparison of R2 values across risk adjustment models: Split sample estimation (40% validation sample)

		Type of Model and Expenditure			
		Concurrent		Prospective	
Model	Risk Adjustment Model	Substance Abuse	Total HMO	Substance Abuse	Total HMO
1	DEM	0.0800	0.1944	0.0138	0.2948
2	DEM + ALC/DRUG	0.0890	0.2008	0.0238	0.2989
3	DEM + ALC/DRUG + MH	0.0921	0.2198	0.0206	0.3259
4	DEM + ALC/DRUG + MH + Social/Family Characteristics	0.0995	0.2448	0.0292	0.3275
5	DEM + ALC/DRUG + MH + Social/Family + GRAM Conditions	0.1032	0.2614	0.0238	0.3520

Notes:
HMO = Health Maintenance Organization (total health plan expenditures)
For substance abuse in the concurrent model, there is a single model and the R2 is reported.
Other models include non-users so a 2-part model is used and the synthetic R2 is reported.
For prospective models, predictors are observed in year 1 and expenditures in year 2 are predicted.

Table 5. Comparison of prediction ratios for risk adjustment models: Split sample estimation (40% validation sample)

		Type of Model and Expenditure			
		Concurrent		Prospective	
Model	Risk Adjustment Model	Substance Abuse	Total HMO	Substance Abuse	Total HMO
1	DEM	1.01	1.09	1.15	1.01
2	DEM + ALC/DRUG	1.02	1.09	1.17	1.02
3	DEM + ALC/DRUG + MH	1.04	1.18	1.14	1.28
4	DEM + ALC/DRUG + MH + Social/Family Characteristics	1.05	1.19	1.15	1.32
5	DEM + ALC/DRUG + MH + Social/Family + GRAM Conditions	1.05	1.20	1.17	1.30

We also examined the prediction ratios for the Medicaid and commercial groups separately to determine whether potential gains and losses differed for the two groups. We found that for the Medicaid group, prediction ratios for substance abuse services were below 1, indicating potential underpayment.

CONCLUSION

We tested several different types of risk-adjustment models using split sample estimation. Our risk-adjustment models that incorporated new demographic variables (beyond age and gender) and social and clinical indicators predicted substance abuse and total health plan expenditures slightly better than simpler models typical of current risk-adjustment systems (Ettner et al., 1998; Ettner and Notman, 1997). However, our results indicate that our models predicting substance abuse expenditures still performed very poorly. explaining no more than 11% of the variation in expenditures. Our models for total expenditures performed better, explaining as much as 35% of variation in expenditures. Although addition of new variables improved prediction modestly, they did not appear to improve the prediction ratios, indicating that payments would likely be quite inaccurate in some cases.

Although our results are generally in line with previous work on risk adjustment for mental health and substance abuse services, our work is different from previous work in a number of ways. We use a different medical risk adjustment system (GRAM model) than in previous work. We do not restrict our sample to people who are continuously enrolled. We include only people who have been assessed and recommended for substance abuse treatment in our models. These differences may account for some of the differences in results of our models compared to previous work.

Limitations

This work needs to be considered in light of several limitations. This research was conducted in one health plan in one geographic region, and the results may not necessarily be representative of other populations and regions. Nonetheless, this integrated delivery system, which combines physical health care with substance abuse treatment, is very similar to programs elsewhere that are regarded as model arrangements (Weisner et al., 2001).

Compared to previous studies (*e.g.,* Ettner et al., 2000; Ettner and Notman, 1997), our-risk adjustment modeling samples were quite small. However, we note that our results are reasonably similar to previous work on mental health and substance abuse risk adjustment. In addition, rather than testing specific risk-adjustment systems rigorously, the focus of this study was to examine whether enhanced demographic and social data could improve risk-adjustment models. Our diagnostic data did not allow us to use the complete GRAM categorization system as it was developed, so we used a modified and less-refined version of the system. Nonetheless, it is fair to conclude that risk adjustment for capitated Medicaid substance abuse care remains challenging.

These difficulties notwithstanding, the following chapter shows that Medicaid remains a key part of the financing system for substance abuse treatment. Moreover, most states appear to have adopted capitated payment systems to finance chemical dependency services for Medicaid clients (Maglione and Ridgely, 2006). Indeed, as seen in the next chapter, states have been innovative in their use of Medicaid funds to enhance access to substance abuse care.

ACKNOWLEDGMENT

Supported in part by National Institute on Drug Abuse grant number R01 DA 011646

REFERENCES

Aday, L. A., and Andersen, R. (1974). A framework for the study of access to medical care. *Health Services Research, 9*(3), 208-220.

American Society of Addiction Medicine (2001). *ASAM PPC-2R: ASAM patient placement criteria for the treatment of substance abuse-related disorders (2nd edition, rev.)*. Chevy Chase, MD: American Society of Addiction Medicine.

Andersen, R. (1995). Revisiting the Behavioral Model and access to medical care: Does it matter? *Journal of Health and Social Behavior, 36*(1), 1-10.

Arons, B. S., Frank, R. G., Goldman, H. H., McGuire, T. G., and Stephens, S. (1994). Mental health and substance abuse coverage under health reform. *Health Affairs (Project Hope), 13*(1), 192-205.

Ash, A., Porell, F., Gruenberg, L., Sawitz, E., and Beiser, A. (1989). Adjusting Medicare capitation payments using prior hospitalization data. *Health Care Financing Review, 10*(4), 17-29.

Bloom, J., Hu, T., Wallace, N., Cuffel, B., Hausman, J., Sheu, M., et al. (2002). Mental health costs and access under alternative capitation systems in Colorado. *Health Services Research, 37*(2), 315-340.

Busch, S. (1997). Carving-out mental health benefits to Medicaid beneficiaries: a shift toward managed care. *Administration and Policy in Mental Health, 24*(4), 301-321.

Druss, B. G., and Rosenheck, R. A. (1999). Patterns of health care costs associated with depression and substance abuse in a national sample. *Psychiatric Services (Washington, D.C.), 50*(2), 214-218.

Duan, N., Manning, W., Morris, C., and Newhouse, J. (1983). A comparison of alternative models for the demand for medical care. *Journal of Business and Economic Statistics, 1*, 115-126.

Dudley, R., Medlin, C., Hammann, L., Cisternas, M., Brand, R., Rennie, D., et al. (2003). The best of both worlds? Potential of hybrid prospective/concurrent risk adjustment. *Med Care, 41*, 56-69.

Efron, B. (1978). Regression and ANOVA with zero-one data: Measures of residual variation. *Journal of the American Statistical Association, 73*, 113-121.

Ellis, R. P., Pope, G. C., Iezzoni, L., Ayanian, J. Z., Bates, D. W., Burstin, H., et al. (1996). Diagnosis-based risk adjustment for Medicare capitation payments. *Health Care Financing Review, 17*(3), 101-128.

Ettner, S. L., Frank, R. G., McGuire, T. G., and Hermann, R. C. (2001). Risk adjustment alternatives in paying for behavioral health care under Medicaid. *Health Services Research, 36*, 793-811.

Ettner, S. L., Argeriou, M., McCarty, D., Dilonardo, J., and Liu, H. (2003). How did the introduction of managed care for the uninsured in Iowa affect the use of substance abuse services? *Journal of Behavioral Health Services and Research, 30*, 26-40.

Ettner, S. L., Denmead, G., Dilonardo, J., Cao, H., and Belanger, A. J. (2003). The impact of managed care on the substance abuse treatment patterns and outcomes of Medicaid beneficiaries: Maryland's HealthChoice Program. *Journal of Behavioral Health Services and Research, 30*, 41-62.

Ettner, S. L., and Johnson, S. (2003). Do adjusted clinical groups eliminate incentives for HMOs to avoid substance abusers? Evidence from the Maryland Medicaid HealthChoice program. *Journal of Behavioral Health Services and Research, 30,* 63-77.

Ettner, S. L., Frank, R. G., Mark, T., and Smith, M. W. (2000). Risk adjustment of capitation payments to behavioral health care carve-outs: how well do existing methodologies account for psychiatric disabilities. *Health Care Management Science, 3*, 159-169.

Ettner, S. L., Frank, R. G., McGuire, T. G., Newhouse, J. P., and Notman, E. H. (1998). Risk adjustment of mental health and substance abuse payments. *Inquiry: A Journal of Medical Care Organization, Provision and Financing, 35*(2), 223-239.

Ettner, S. L., and Notman, E. H. (1997). How well do ambulatory care groups predict expenditures on mental health and substance abuse patients? *Administration and Policy in Mental Health, 24*(4), 339-357.

Frank, R. G., Huskamp, H. A., McGuire, T. G., and Newhouse, J. P. (1996). Some economics of mental health 'carve-outs'. *Archives of General Psychiatry, 53*(10), 933-937.

Frank, R. G., and McGuire, T. G. (1998). The economics of behavioral health carve-outs. *New Directions for Mental Health Services, (78)*(78), 41-47.

Frank, R. G., McGuire, T. G., and Newhouse, J. P. (1995). Risk contracts in managed mental health care. *Health Affairs (Project Hope), 14*(3), 50-64.

Goldman, W., McCulloch, J., and Sturm, R. (1998). Cost and use of mental health services before and after managed care. *Health Affairs, 17*, 40-52.

Grazier, K. L., and Eselius, L. L. (1999). Mental health carve-outs: effects and implications. *Medical Care Research and Review: MCRR, 56 Suppl 2*, 37-59.

Grazier, K. L., Eselius, L. L., Hu, T. W., Shore, K. K., and G'Sell, W. A. (1999). Effects of a mental health carve-out on use, costs, and payers: a four-year study. *The Journal of Behavioral Health Services and Research, 26*(4), 381-389.

Green, C. A., Lynch, F. L., Polen, M. R., McFarland, B. H., Dickinson, D. M., and Freeborn, D. K. (2004). Talk about costs: Health care professionals' views about expenses related to substance abuse treatment. *Administration and Policy in Mental Health, 31*, 483-494.

Holahan, J., and Suzuki, S. (2003). Medicaid managed care payment methods and capitation rates in 2001. *Health Affairs (Project Hope), 22*(1), 204-218.

Hornbrook, M. C., Goodman, M. J., and Bennett, M. D. (1991). Assessing health plan case mix in employed populations: Ambulatory morbidity and prescribed drug models. In M. C. Hornbrook (Ed.), *Advances in health economics and health services research, vol. 12* (pp. 197-232). Greenwich, CT: JAI Press.

Hornbrook, M. C., Goodman, M. J., Bennett, M. D., and Greenlick, M. R. (1991). Assessing health plan case mix in employed populations: Self reported health status models. In M.

C. Hornbrook (Ed.), *Advances in health economics and health services research, vol. 12* (pp. 233-272). Greenwich, CT: JAI Press.

Hornbrook, M. C., and Goodman, M. J. (1996). Chronic disease, functional health status, and demographics: A multi-dimensional approach to risk adjustment. *Health Services Research, 31*(3), 283-307.

Kapur, K., Young, A. S., and Murata, D. (2000). Risk adjustment for high utilizers of public mental health care. *The Journal of Mental Health Policy and Economics, 3*(3), 129-137.

Levit, K. R., Kassad, C. A., Coffey, R. M., Mark, T. L., Stranges, E. M., Buck, J. A., et al. (2008). Future funding for mental health and substance abuse: Increasing burdens for the public sector. *Health Affairs, 27*, w513-w522.

Maglione, M., and Ridgely, M.S. (2006). Is conventional wisdom wrong? Coverage for substance abuse treatment under Medicaid managed care. *Journal of Substance Abuse Treatment*, 30, 285-290.

Mark, T. L., Ozminkowski, R. J., Kirk, A., Ettner, S. L., and Drabek, J. (2003). Risk adjustment for people with chronic conditions in private sector health plans. *Medical Decision Making: An International Journal of the Society for Medical Decision Making, 23*(5), 397-405.

Meara, E., and Frank, R. G. (2005). Spending on substance abuse treatment: how much is enough? *Addiction (Abingdon, England), 100*(9), 1240-1248.

Newhouse, J. P. (1998). Risk adjustment: Where are we now? *Inquiry, 35*, 121-131.

Rosen, A. K., Loveland, S. A., Anderson, J. J., Hankin, C. S., Breckenridge, J. N., and Berlowitz, D. R. (2002). Diagnostic cost groups (DCGs) and concurrent utilization among patients with substance abuse disorders. Health Services Research, 37(4), 1079-1103.

Sturm, R. (2002). The effects of obesity, smoking, and drinking on medical problems and costs. *Health Affairs (Project Hope), 21*(2), 245-253.

Weiner, J. P., Starfield, B. H., Steinwachs, D. M., and Mumford, L. M. (1991). Development and application of a population-oriented measure of ambulatory care case-mix. *Medical Care, 29*(5), 452-472.

Weisner, C., Mertens, J., Parthasarathy, S., Moore, C., and Lu, Y. (2001). Integrating primary medical care with addiction treatment: a randomized controlled trial. *JAMA: The Journal of the American Medical Association, 286*(14), 1715-1723.

Wickizer, T.M. (2001). The impact of substance abuse treatment on employment outcomes among AFDC clients in Washington state (Technical Assistance Publication Series #25, DHHS Publication #01-3508). Rockville, MD: U.S. Department of Health and Human Services, Public Health Service, Substance Abuse and Mental Health Services Administration, Center for Substance Abuse Treatment.

In: Medicaid and Treatment for People... ISBN 978-1-61470-742-4
Editor: B.H. McFarland, D.McCarty, et al, pp. 271-281 © 2011 Nova Science Publishers, Inc.

Chapter 14

STATE INNOVATIONS FOR ENHANCING ACCESS TO ALCOHOL AND DRUG ABUSE TREATMENT

Dennis McCarty[1], Eldon Edmundson[1], Carla A. Green[2], Bentson H. McFarland[2,3], and Victor Capoccia[4]

[1] Department of Public Health and Preventive Medicine, Oregon Health and Science University, Portland, OR

[2] Kaiser Permanente Center for Health Research, Portland, OR

[3] Departments of Psychiatry and Public Health and Preventive Medicine, Oregon Health and Science University, Portland, OR

[4] Open Society Institute, New York, NY, USA

ABSTRACT

States often use Medicaid as part of innovative strategies to finance publicly funded services for treatment of alcohol and drug dependence. Interviews with officials from eleven states provide case studies and examples of financing innovations. Four management tools (memoranda of understanding, cost-savings analysis, utilization management, and coordinated purchase) and four management strategies (delegated management, dedicated funding, optimization of federal funds, and blended/braided funding) are identified and discussed. Examples from the interviewed states provide concrete illustrations of how these tools and strategies were combined to improve access to alcohol and drug abuse treatment.

INTRODUCTION

States seek innovations in the financing and organization of health care to manage the costs of services for low-income individuals and for the uninsured. The Urban Institute's "Assessing the New Federalism" initiative tracked efforts in 13 states to monitor state health policies. During the 1990s, Medicaid, the State Children's Health Insurance Program (SCHIP), and welfare reform were used creatively to improve access to health care, and to control costs (Holahan et al., 2002). A recessionary environment, however, increased management challenges and demands for cost-control. During the 2003 legislative sessions, 13 states reduced or limited Medicaid eligibility, 23 states reduced or eliminated optional Medicaid benefits, and 31 states froze or reduced provider reimbursements for Medicaid services (Johnson, 2003).

Publicly funded treatments for alcohol and drug disorders are among the services at greatest risk during difficult economic times. Many if not most individuals who seek care are either uninsured or qualify for state Medicaid and general relief programs. Public support is crucial and maintaining such support during times of economic hardship requires significant creativity and innovation. State and federal funds accounted for 78 percent of the estimated $21 billion in 2003 expenditures for substance abuse treatment (state/local funds = 40 percent, Medicaid = 18 percent, other federal = 15 percent, and Medicare = 5 percent) (Mark et al., 2007). The number of individuals who need care for alcohol and drug disorders, moreover, substantially exceeds the resources available – each year, about three million individuals enter treatment and more than 10 million individuals who would benefit from alcohol and drug services are untreated (Substance Abuse and Mental Health Services Administration, 2008).

Changes in public financing, however, are challenging. Medicaid coverage for substance abuse treatment varies substantially among states, per capita spending for substance abuse treatment is uneven, and state financing systems differ.

Innovative examples of state financing and management strategies often include collaboration with Medicaid to expand substance abuse treatment. Telephone interviews in 2002 and 2003 completed with state agency personnel identified the general aspects of benefits and methods for funding substance abuse treatment for individuals eligible and not eligible for Medicaid. The interviews assessed approaches to enhancing access as well as strategies for diverting recipients from the use of more expensive treatments to more efficient levels of care as well as coordination of benefits and integration of funding streams. Finally, substance abuse treatment services for children and adolescents using Early and Periodic Screening, Diagnosis and Treatment (EPSDT) and State Children's Health Insurance Program (SCHIP) were examined and strategies to improve access for individuals who qualify for disability status were assessed. State agency documents posted on the Internet were also reviewed.

Table 1 summarizes key features, innovations and systems for treatment of alcohol and drug disorders found among 11 states: Arizona, Connecticut, Iowa, Maine, Missouri, Nebraska, Ohio, Oregon, Pennsylvania, Washington State, and Wyoming. The states varied in their use of Medicaid for substance abuse treatment services and in the integration of Medicaid and non-Medicaid resources. In most states, collaborations between the state authorities for Medicaid and substance abuse were a key to their accomplishments, regardless of financing and management strategies. These collaborative relationships enabled states to introduce managed care tools, including capitation and utilization management, to integrate and/or braid funding streams, and to dedicate funding for expanded services. They also worked to coordinate services and benefits and increased measurement of performance and outcomes.

Table 1. Study states and innovation strategies

State	Major features	Notable aspects	Strategies
Arizona	Integrated Medicaid and non-Medicaid; regional behavioral health managed care carve-out	Expanded Medicaid eligibility with tobacco settlement funds	Dedicated funding Federal funds optimization Braided/blended funding
Connecticut	Blending substance abuse, mental health, Medicaid and child welfare resources to enhance patient outcomes	Ambitious systems reorganization and interagency coordination	Dedicated funding Federal funds optimization Braided/Blended Funding
Iowa	Integrated Medicaid and non-Medicaid; statewide substance abuse carve-out	Effective use of managed care for Medicaid and non-Medicaid services	Delegated management Braided/blended funding
Maine	Consolidated funding across state agencies	Tobacco settlement funds used to expand services	Delegated funding Braided/blended funding
Missouri	Comprehensive Substance Treatment and Rehabilitation coordinates funding streams and services for eligible patients	History of coordination between Medicaid and substance abuse authorities	Delegated management Braided/blended funding
Nebraska	Early and Periodic Screening, Detection and Treatment used to create full spectrum of behavioral health services including substance abuse treatment for children and adolescents	Redeveloped behavioral health care systems; Medicaid coverage for adult substance abuse treatment had been limited	Delegated management Braided/blended funding
Ohio	Rehabilitation option used to develop 10 ambulatory services for Medicaid recipients	Local Boards coordinate delivery of services and tracking of Medicaid match	Federal funds optimization Dedicated funding
Oregon	Oregon Health Plan (1994 – 2003) expanded eligibility and benefits including coverage for residential substance abuse treatment	Oregon Health Plan II (2003 – present) led to cutbacks in optional benefits (including outpatient substance abuse treatment) for expanded eligibility group	Braided/blended funding
Pennsylvania	Medicaid managed care; county level plans	Disability advocacy program helps individuals complete Supplemental Security Income eligibility determination	Braided/blended funding
Washington State	High level of collaboration between Medicaid and substance abuse authorities	Cost-offset analyses supported expansion of coverage for individuals with disabilities	Delegated management Federal funds optimization
Wyoming	Little use of Medicaid	System reorganization led to stronger linkages with criminal justice services	Dedicated funding

The dominant themes, management strategies, and state innovations for financing treatment of alcohol and drug disorders were abstracted from the interviews and summarized. The report helped stimulate thinking, fostered peer learning and encouraged states to share analytical tools. This chapter summarizes key findings.

Collaborations between the state Medicaid and substance abuse authorities seemed to achieve the most success when policy makers used combinations of four management tools and four management and financing strategies. The tools can be applied to a wide variety of initiatives and multiple tools may be used in one initiative. In general, the management and financing strategies are specific to public financing for substance abuse treatment.

Management Tools

Four sets of tools facilitate collaborative efforts among state agencies: memoranda of understanding, cost savings analyses, utilization management and coordinated purchase.

Memoranda of Understanding

Memoranda are used to facilitate coordination among state agencies and are most common when the state Medicaid authority delegates administrative responsibilities to other state agencies. The roles and functions of each collaborating agency are specified in Memoranda of Understanding that address:

a) the Medicaid administrative activities the substance abuse agency undertakes on behalf of the state Medicaid agency,
b) the use of federal Medicaid administrative funds to support management activities,
c) the source of and accounting for required state Medicaid matching funds, and
d) the coordination of third party benefits.

More comprehensive agreements usually:

a) include collaborative clinical oversight of the program,
b) specify utilization management processes and criteria, and
c) enable the transfer of federal financial participation to the state substance abuse agency for Medicaid treatment services furnished pursuant to the arrangement and for costs necessary for the proper and efficient administration of the Medicaid program (42 Code of Federal Regulations 431.15).

The memorandum of understanding developed for the Connecticut Behavioral Health Partnership (see http://www.ct.gov/ctbhp/LIB/ctbhp/documents/other/303mou.pdf; accessed October 31, 2009) is an excellent example. The document specifies the reasons for the agreement, describes membership and governance of the partnership, lists agency roles and responsibilities, and provides details on contracting and financing issues including items to be negotiated later. The memorandum is a blueprint for the partnership and its activities.

Cost-Savings Analysis

Some states conducted cost-savings analyses to assess the benefits from collaborative initiatives between the Medicaid and substance abuse agencies (*e.g.*, reduction of inpatient admissions and cost savings to the publicly funded health system). These types of studies analyzed Medicaid claims to identify health-related claims for Medicaid recipients who have alcohol and drug disorders. The analyses typically combined queries based on procedure and diagnosis codes, and may have involved sophisticated risk prediction software.

Washington State's cost-analyses, for example, compared recipients on Supplemental Security Income (SSI) who entered treatment for alcohol and drug disorders with SSI recipients who needed but did not enter treatment. Treatment for alcohol and drug disorders was associated with a reduction in medical expenses of more than $300 per month per treated recipient; total annual savings were estimated at $9.6 million if alcohol and drug treatment were provided to all SSI recipients in need of treatment (Estee and Nordlund, 2001, 2003). As a result, the state expanded access to substance abuse treatment for individuals with disabilities.

Utilization Management

Utilization management activities offer state agencies the ability to rely on coordinated efforts to ensure appropriate use of treatment. The American Society of Addiction Medicine's Patient Placement Criteria (American Society of Addiction Medicine, 2001), for example, can be adopted as a common tool across systems for Medicaid and non-Medicaid services. Iowa and Oregon require treatment providers to use level-of-care criteria when treatment placements are made. The standardized criteria help to assure the clinical integrity of the treatment system, and facilitate management of utilization and costs by preventing use of unnecessary high-cost services. State substance abuse authorities have expertise not found in other state agencies, oversee a full continuum of services, and are well positioned to implement utilization management techniques like patient placement criteria.

Coordinated Purchase

States can better coordinate procurement of care if they identify major purchasers of substance abuse treatment services (*e.g.*, corrections, child protection), the sources of their funds (*e.g.*, federal, state and local funds), billing and reimbursement requirements, and needs for specific services. Pooled purchasing enables state agencies to identify the nuances related to each funding stream and to develop and manage resources more effectively.

Using such analyses, states can identify state and local funds being used to purchase services that are, or could be, covered by Medicaid and, therefore, might be used as Medicaid match to permit expansion of services. The additional federal revenue can free up some of the state dedicated funds to increase access for non-Medicaid eligible individuals. By combining this strategy with delegated management and claims and payment information systems, state substance abuse authorities can provide Medicaid matching funds without having to transfer lumped sums to state Medicaid agencies.

Partial or overlapping payment for care can be a problem for both service providers and purchasers. The discrete payment arrangements used by each agency are usually related to the kinds of "strings" attached to the resources, the overall mission of the purchaser, and the politics of their service delivery systems. Sometimes, a review finds that two or more agencies are paying for the same service (*e.g.*, residential services billed to both a substance abuse agency and the state child protection agency). Reviews examine the service, determine the true total cost of that care, and assess what portion of the cost should be paid by which purchaser and with what funds.

Management and Financing Strategies

The four sets of tools support four management and financing strategies. States are aligning purchasing policies for alcohol and drug treatment with clinical practices and investing in information technology to foster improvements in access to substance abuse treatment. Four sets of overlapping strategies can expand publicly funded treatment services for alcohol and drug dependence: 1) delegated management, 2) dedicated funds, 3) federal funds optimization, and 4) blended and braided funding. These strategies have evolved as state substance abuse authorities struggle to meet the demand for treatment services in a funding environment where federal block grant support is not growing rapidly and state funding and local resources are constrained.

Delegated Management

Delegated management strategies reflect collaboration between the state authorities for Medicaid and substance abuse treatment services. The state Medicaid agency delegates responsibility for certain administrative activities to the state alcohol and drug abuse treatment authority. When Medicaid dollars are a major source of funding for the treatment of alcohol and drug dependence, there are advantages and efficiencies if the substance abuse authority directly manages both Medicaid and non-Medicaid financing. Similar regulations and rates can be applied to services provided and there is potential for patients to move seamlessly between Medicaid and non-Medicaid funding. The state substance abuse authority typically provides clinical guidance, manages the publicly funded specialty provider network, and supports utilization management and outreach activities. State funds for substance abuse treatment can be used for the state's Medicaid match and the state substance abuse authority may blend and/or braid multiple funding streams to enhance substance abuse care.

The delegation of authority must ensure that the state Medicaid authority retains the level of program administration and oversight required under federal law (42 Code of Federal Regulations 431.10). States formalize these delegated management arrangements in cooperative agreements or memoranda of understanding as required by federal law (42 Code of Federal Regulations 431.615).

Delegated management and collaboration between Medicaid and substance abuse authorities are key features in Iowa, Missouri, and Washington State. Iowa constructed a behavioral health carve-out that supports relatively distinct systems of care for mental health and addiction services and braids services for Medicaid and uninsured residents, so patients move between funding streams with no disruption of service (Ettner et al., 2003; McCarty and Argeriou, 2003). Missouri aligned regulations so that the Medicaid and substance abuse authorities use similar rules and definitions and conduct joint site visits and integrate funding streams for patients enrolled in the Comprehensive Substance Treatment and Rehabilitation (CSTAR) program. Finally, the state authority for substance abuse treatment in Washington State assumed full responsibility for Medicaid-funded alcohol and drug treatment services and coordinates the state Medicaid match using state and local funds.

Dedicated Funds

Multiple dedicated revenue streams (state general funds, federal block grants, Medicaid and other third party payers, and miscellaneous dedicated funds) are also used to support publicly funded services for treatment of alcohol and drug disorders. States sometimes allocate funding streams specifically for the treatment of alcohol and drug dependence. A portion of the tobacco settlement funds, for example, was allocated in some states for alcohol and drug treatment. Wyoming allocated about $25 million from tobacco settlement funds to support a restructuring of the state's substance abuse treatment services and to increase treatment options for individuals in the custody of corrections and courts. A voter referendum (Proposition 204) in Arizona authorized the use of tobacco settlement funds to increase income eligibility for Medicaid to 100 percent of the federal poverty level. Simultaneously, the state redefined and broadened covered benefits for behavioral health care services, including treatment of alcohol and drug disorders. Other states dedicate funds for specific populations or for specific types of services. Ohio allocated funds from the Temporary Assistance to Needy Families (TANF) block grant for treating TANF participants if alcohol or drug-related disorders inhibited ability to initiate and maintain employment. Ohio also earmarked funds specifically for parents and children involved in child protection services.

Optimization of Federal Funds

States also make us of various federal mechanisms to support substance abuse treatment services. These funds may be in the form of categorical grants with specific requirements for types of services purchased (*e.g.,* Substance Abuse Prevention and Treatment Block Grant or Safe and Drug Free Schools). Other federal funds (*e.g.,* Medicaid) support a broad range of medical services and can include substance abuse treatment. Unlike grants that can be used in their totality to fund substance abuse treatment and prevention services, however, the Medicaid program is a jointly (federal/state) funded health insurance program that requires matching state funds to be used to supplement the federal financial participation.

States participating in the Resources for Recovery program reported a wide range of Medicaid funding for substance abuse treatment services in the public substance abuse system, ranging from none to over one hundred million dollars per year. State substance abuse authorities who understand Medicaid payment policies, eligible matching funds, federal Medicaid regulations, and state Medicaid operational policies, can significantly expand the range of services available and the number of individuals served by a state's substance abuse treatment system. Authorities may also be able to grow the overall capacity of the system to provide services. Several specific federal funds optimization strategies are currently being used by states and include use of three optional Medicaid services: 1) Optional Medicaid Rehabilitative Services (Medicaid Rehabilitation Option), 2) Optional Medicaid Clinic Services (Clinic Option), and 3) Early and Periodic Screening, Diagnosis and Treatment (EPSDT). See the early chapter by Lanhan, Smith, O'Brien and McCarty for details on these strategies.

Medicaid Rehabilitation Option

States seeking to optimize Medicaid reimbursement strive to design their service definitions so that they are, as much as possible, the same for Medicaid and non-Medicaid funding sources (while taking into account Medicaid non-allowable populations and services). Overall, the Medicaid Rehabilitation Option seems underutilized for alcohol and drug treatment services. In our sample, only Connecticut and Ohio used the Medicaid Rehabilitation Option to expand access to care.

Medicaid Clinic Option

The Medicaid Clinic Option supports preventive, diagnostic, therapeutic, rehabilitative, or palliative services provided in outpatient clinics that are not hospital-based. Medicaid Clinic Option services must be rendered on-site "in the clinic" and must be under the direction of a physician (except for homeless individuals). The Medicaid Clinic Option may be difficult to apply to alcohol and drug treatment services because the services are often provided without involvement of a physician and may be provided in the community rather than in a clinic. However, Medicaid Clinic Option services can be used for identification and screening for substance abuse problems, brief interventions and referral to the specialty system, and coordination with physical health programs for treatment of health complications (*e.g.,* uncontrolled diabetes in a person dependent on alcohol).

Early and Periodic Screening, Diagnosis and Treatment (EPSDT)

Early and Periodic Screening, Diagnosis, and Treatment (EPSDT) includes necessary screening, vision, dental, and hearing services for children and adolescents. Nebraska used EPSDT to develop mental health and addiction treatment services for children and adolescents without being required to provide the services for adults. The state plan was then amended and Nebraska covered addiction treatment services for adults and children. States that provide a full-range of services for alcohol and drug problems for children and adults tend not to use EPSDT. The flexible nature of EPSDT is perceived to create administrative and utilization challenges and states fear resulting uncontrolled costs. As a result, few states appear to be exercising EPSDT to improve access to substance abuse treatment for children and adolescents.

Blended and Braided Funding

Blended and braided funding build on delegated management, dedicated funding, and optimization of funds. Strategies to integrate funds include capitation, case rates, and individual budgets funded collaboratively through pooled purchasing. Integration may occur through individualized treatment plans or for specific groups of beneficiaries. This funding approach is an area where states' creativity and innovation are apparent. For example, Arizona has used an 1115 Research and Demonstration Waiver to support a managed behavioral healthcare carve-out (Tompkins and Perloff, 2004). Medicaid recipients and uninsured individuals have been served through the same systems of care with blended funding. Covered services were expanded to include non-traditional services and service providers, with the goal of addressing a full range of patient needs.

The Oregon Health Plan is another example of an 1115 waiver that expanded access to substance abuse treatment services for low-income individuals (Deck et al., 2000). As was described in previous chapters, subsequent legislative action, at least temporarily, eliminated outpatient mental health and substance abuse benefits for many recipients in Oregon's Medicaid health plan. Similarly, Iowa used managed care to expand access to treatment for alcohol and drug dependence, but used a 1915B waiver to support a behavioral health carve-out that combined services for Medicaid and uninsured individuals, and allowed recipients to remain in care even when their eligibility for benefits changed (Ettner et al., 2003; McCarty and Argeriou, 2003). Both Oregon and Ohio have integrated funds from Temporary Assistance to Needy Families (TANF) to provide addiction treatment services if alcohol and drug disorders inhibit employability.

Conclusion

A review of state strategies for integrating Medicaid into the funding for treatment of alcohol and drug disorders found innovative examples of aligning purchasing policy, clinical practices, financing, and administrative infrastructure to expand services but constrain costs. State capacity to address alcohol and drug problems can be enhanced if federal resources are optimized, service recipients are treated in less restrictive settings and funding streams are braided and blended. A key element, in most states, was close collaboration between the state authorities for Medicaid and substance abuse treatment. The review is limited in scope and linked to a moment in time when the study was conducted (2002 – 2003). The state examples, however, remain germane and illustrate creative and innovative management.

In Washington State, the Medicaid and substance abuse authorities conducted cost-savings analysis and used the analyses to guide decisions on resource allocation. The result was an expansion of substance abuse treatment specifically for individuals with Supplemental Security Income or Social Security Disability Insurance. Connecticut blended and braided substance abuse, mental health, child welfare, and Medicaid resources to expand access and improve service delivery coordination. Arizona and Iowa used managed behavioral health care to control costs, assure that services are at an appropriate level of care, and integrate funding for Medicaid and non-Medicaid groups. Iowa expanded access to substance abuse treatment for both Medicaid and non-Medicaid populations without an increase in expenditures. Oregon, conversely, relied on linkages with primary care and experienced substantial increase in individuals admitted to substance abuse treatment services. Links between criminal justice systems and treatment for alcohol and drug disorders were the cornerstone of Wyoming's reorganization of services. Delegated management of Medicaid resources has been central in Missouri, Ohio, and Washington State. Pennsylvania promoted disability determination, while Arizona, Maine and Wyoming allocated tobacco settlement funds toward service expansions. EPSDT was used in Nebraska to foster improved services for children and adolescents.

In brief, a review of state practices found compelling examples of strategies that can expand access to substance abuse treatment. The ultimate challenge for states is to craft a system of services that respond to a diverse and changing population of men, women and adolescents dependent on alcohol and other drugs. It is clearly in the interest of states both to constrain the costs of care and to provide a full continuum of treatment for alcohol and drug disorders. State innovations in financing treatment for alcohol and drug dependence may improve access to a scarce but vital resource – publicly funded treatment for alcohol and drug dependence.

Acknowledgments

An award from the Robert Wood Johnson Foundation (Resources for Recovery: State Practices that Expand Treatment Opportunities) supported the preparation of the manuscript. We thank the state officials who completed the interviews for their time and willingness to participate.

References

American Society of Addiction Medicine (2001). *Patient Placement Criteria for the Treatment of Substance Related Disorders: Second Edition Revised (ASAM PPC-2R).* (Second Edition Revised ed.) Chevy Chase, MD: American Society of Addiction Medicine.

Deck, D., McFarland, B. H., Titus, J. M., Laws, K. E., and Gabriel, R. M. (2000). Access to substance abuse treatment services under the Oregon Health Plan. *Journal of the American Medical Association, 284,* 2093-2099.

Estee, S. and Nordlund, D. J. (2001). *Washington State Supplemental Security Income (SSI) Cost Offset Pilot Projects: 2001 Progress Report* (Rep. No. 11.101). Olympia, WA: Washington State Department of Social and Health Services Research and Data Analysis Division.

Estee, S. and Nordlund, D. J. (2003). *Washington State Supplemental Security Income (SSI) Cost Offset Pilot Project: 2002 Progress Report* (Rep. No. 11.109). Olympia, WA:

Washington State Department of Social and Health Services Research and Data Analysis Division.

Ettner, S. L., Argeriou, M., McCarty, D., Dilonardo, J., and Liu, H. (2003). How did the introduction of managed care for the uninsured in Iowa affect the use of substance abuse services? *Journal of Behavioral Health Services and Research, 30,* 26-40.

Holahan, J., Weiner, J. M., and Lutzky, A. W. (2002). Health policy for low-income people: States' responses to new challenges. *Health Affairs, web exclusive,* W187-W218.

Johnson, P. (2003). *FY 2003-2004 NCSL Medicaid Budget Survey: Executive Summary* Washington, DC: National Conference of State Legislatures.

Mark, T. L., Levit, K. R., Coffey, R. M., McKusick, D., Harwood, H. J., King, E. et al. (2007). *National Expenditures for Mental Health Services and Substance Abuse Treatment: 1993 - 2003.* (SAMHSA Publication No. SMA 07-4227 ed.) Rockville, MD: Aubstance Abuse and Mental Health Services Administration.

McCarty, D. and Argeriou, M. (2003). The Iowa Managed Substance Abuse Care Plan (IMSACP): Access, utilization and expenditures for Medicaid recipients. *Journal of Behavioral Health Services and Research, 30,* 18-25.

Substance Abuse and Mental Health Services Administration (2008). *Results from the 2007 National Survey on Drug Use and Health: National Findings*. (DHHS Publication No SMA 08-4343 ed.) Rockville, MD: Substance Abuse and Mental Health Services Administration.

Tompkins, C. and Perloff, J. (2004). Using information to guide managed behavioral health care. *Journal of Behavioral Health Services and Research, 31, 98-110.*

In: Medicaid and Treatment for People… ISBN 978-1-61470-742-4
Editor: B.H. McFarland, D.McCarty, et al, pp. 283-284

Chapter 15

CONCLUSION: MEDICAID AND SUBSTANCE ABUSE TREATMENT IN THE NEXT HALF-CENTURY

Bentson H. McFarland
Departments of Psychiatry and Public Health and Preventive Medicine, Oregon Health and Science University, Portland, OR

Medicaid has changed continuously since its inception nearly 50 years ago. Major developments of the past two decades include the conversion from Aid to Families with Dependent Children to Temporary Assistance for Needy Families (which affected all states), the switch from fee for service to assorted varieties of Medicaid managed care (which affected most states), expansion and contraction cycles in Medicaid eligibility (which affected many if not most states), and increase in Medicaid as a payer for substance abuse treatment services (which also affected many if not most states). Evaluations of these numerous alterations have, not surprisingly, shown assorted results of interest to people with substance abuse problems, to providers, and to policy makers.

As several chapters in this volume indicate, at least some individuals engaged in specialty sector substance abuse treatment manage to remain in care despite vicissitudes of Medicaid eligibility. But other chapters show that shrinkage of Medicaid eligibility criteria may preclude individuals from entering specialty substance abuse treatment and may adversely affect chemical dependency services delivered in general health care or in mental health care settings. Moreover, sub-groups of Medicaid clients such as persons involved with methadone maintenance treatment may be especially vulnerable to loss of Medicaid coverage.

Recent decades have also seen the rise of evidence-based practices for people with substance abuse problems. Considerable research has shown that chemical dependency services can be helpful for people with addictions and especially so when substance abuse is treated as a chronic condition. As discussed in this volume, methadone maintenance treatment may well be the evidence- based practice with the largest research base showing beneficial impact both for clients and for society. Consequently, it is noteworthy and unfortunate that (as this volume shows) restrictions on Medicaid eligibility often imply decreases in entrance to or continuation of methadone maintenance treatment with resulting adverse outcomes at both individual and community levels.

More optimistic overall are the numerous studies on the conversion from fee for service to Medicaid managed care including those in this volume. While this substantial change has not been entirely free of difficulties, by and large the adverse effects appear to have been minimal even for special populations such as adolescent Medicaid clients entering substance abuse treatment and drug court eligible offenders. As shown in work presented here, there is little or no evidence supporting fears about adverse substance abuse treatment client selection related to Medicaid managed care. Indeed, at least in some states, the switch to Medicaid managed care facilitated expansion of eligibility with subsequent increase in chemical dependency service provision. Of course, numerous challenges remain including (as discussed in this book) suitable rate-setting for capitated Medicaid substance abuse treatment programs.

More worrisome in light of the current financial catastrophe are the numerous studies in this book showing the unfortunate impacts of Medicaid cutbacks. As noted, some clients engaged in substance abuse treatment may be able to continue services even in the absence of insurance coverage. Unfortunately, large numbers of individuals may either be unable to enter chemical dependency care or may not be able to maintain services. In addition, several chapters in this volume make the point that impacts from Medicaid cutbacks can be widespread. Because the addiction treatment system now depends heavily on Medicaid, services are fragile. Substance abuse treatment capacity may evaporate in the face of Medicaid cutbacks. But, of course, people with substance abuse problems do not disappear and, as shown here, may well present themselves to emergency departments in lieu of more appropriate care.

This book, then, presents several lessons regarding treatment for people with substance abuse problems as Medicaid enters its second 50 years. Addiction is common, tragic, but treatable. Medicaid plays several essential roles in providing useful services to clients with chemical dependency. Despite numerous complexities, state workers have developed innovative and productive approaches that take advantage of Medicaid's flexibility to facilitate provision of services. As federal policy makers grapple with implementation of health care reform, it is important to recognize the value of Medicaid in supporting delivery of valuable treatments for people with substance abuse problems.

INDEX

D

H

I

J

S